Nanobiomedicine: Fundamentals and Implementation in Theranostic Applications

Edited by

Soumik Podder
Department of Basic Science & Humanities
Institute of Engineering & Management, New Town
University of Engineering & Management
Kolkata, India

&

Amalesh Samanta
Division of Microbiology & Pharmaceutical Biotechnology
Department of Pharmaceutical Technology
Jadavpur University
Kolkata, India

Nanobiomedicine: Fundamentals and Implementation in Theranostic Applications

Editors: Soumik Podder & Amalesh Samanta

ISBN (Online): 979-8-89881-312-3

ISBN (Print): 979-8-89881-313-0

ISBN (Paperback): 979-8-89881-314-7

First published in 2025.

Bentham Science Publishers Pte. Ltd.
No. 9 Raffles Place
Office No. 26-01
Singapore 048619
Singapore
Email: subscriptions@benthamscience.net

BENTHAM SCIENCE

CONTENTS

FOREWORD

The field of nanobiomedicine stands at the precipice of a transformative era in healthcare. The ability to manipulate matter at the nanoscale has opened unprecedented opportunities for diagnosing, treating, and even preventing diseases. This book, Nanobiomedicine: Fundamentals and Implementation in Theranostic Applications, arrives at a crucial juncture, offering a timely and comprehensive exploration of this dynamic field. From its inception, nanobiomedicine has promised targeted therapies, personalized medicine, and earlier disease detection. This promise is now being realized, thanks in part to the synergistic integration of artificial intelligence. Artificial intelligence has the ability to analyze vast datasets, identify patterns, and optimize processes. These key features have accelerated research and development in nanobiomedicine, leading to breakthroughs that were once considered science fiction.

This book expertly navigates the complex landscape of nanobiomedicine, providing readers with a clear understanding of the fundamental principles, diverse applications, and the exciting potential of AI-driven advancements. It meticulously covers key areas, from the basics of nanomaterials and their interactions with biological systems to cutting-edge applications in theranostics, cancer treatment, and neurodegenerative diseases. The book also thoughtfully addresses the challenges and ethical considerations associated with this rapidly evolving field, including risk management and security in AI-based nanomedicinal applications.

What sets this book apart is its holistic approach. It not only delves into the scientific intricacies of nanobiomedicine but also highlights the crucial role of interdisciplinary collaboration. Researchers, clinicians, engineers, and data scientists must work together to unlock the full potential of this field, and this book serves as a valuable platform for fostering such collaboration. I am particularly impressed by the book's focus on the integration of artificial intelligence. The chapters dedicated to AI in nanomedicine formulation, Alzheimer's disease detection, and spinal surgery offer compelling examples of how AI is revolutionizing healthcare. These applications hold immense promise for improving patient outcomes and transforming the way we deliver care.

Nanobiomedicine and AI: Shaping the Future of Healthcare is a must-read for anyone interested in the future of medicine. It is a valuable resource for researchers, clinicians, students, and policymakers alike. I am confident that this book will inspire further exploration, stimulate innovation, and ultimately contribute to the advancement of nanobiomedicine and the betterment of human health.

Santanu Kumar Sen
Principal
Saheed Anurup Chandra Mahavidyalaya
State-Aided Degree College, Govt. of West Bengal
West Bengal, India

PREFACE

The terminology “Biomedicine,” also referred to as “Professional Medicine,” is predominantly biological medicine. To maintain uniformity in labeling medicine across different cultures, the term Biomedicine was coined by Gaines and Hahn in place of cosmopolitan medicine, western medicine, allopathic medicine, or scientific medicine. This traditional medicine applies physiological and biological principles in clinical practice. This field of medical science is administered by formally trained doctors, nurses, and medical practitioners. The medicinal products are targeted to combat diseases at the macro level and often affect normal cells to a significant extent. Another point of observation in biomedicine is its potential to trigger allergic reactions in patients due to the lack of personalized formulations. There is also no scope for adjusting the shape and size of drugs to achieve highly focused drug delivery.

With the advent of nanotechnology, a branch of physics, a remarkable concept emerged for tuning the shape and size of macro-sized materials in nature. Later, chemical science incorporated synthesis routes to prepare these unique materials. One of the advantages of chemical science is that it offers numerous avenues to control shape and size. These strategies have successfully developed nanomaterials with one-dimensional sizes ranging from 1 to 100 nm. One-dimensional nanotubes, two-dimensional nanosheets, nanoflakes, thin films, three-dimensional hierarchical nanostructures, and zero-dimensional quantum dots have made significant contributions in diverse fields, especially healthcare, due to controlled drug release, targeted drug delivery, and reduced cytotoxicity.

The convergence of nanotechnology and biomedicine, now commonly known as nanobiomedicine, has triggered a revolution in healthcare, offering unprecedented opportunities for diagnostics, therapeutics, and theranostics. For diagnostic purposes, nanomaterials can enter the bloodstream easily due to their extremely small size, enabling effective treatment or faster diagnosis. Various nanomaterials, such as nanoparticles, nanowires, nanoconjugates, and nanorods, have opened new possibilities in medical diagnosis and treatment. These materials not only simplify disease detection by functioning as biomarkers but also highlight medical areas that were previously challenging to diagnose or treat using conventional analytical methods.

Nanomaterials, explicitly referred to as nanomedicine, have transformed therapeutic applications through their remarkable versatility in treating complex diseases. In bacterial inhibition, silver, zinc oxide, and copper nanoparticles demonstrate potent antimicrobial properties by disrupting bacterial cell membranes, generating reactive oxygen species, and interfering with essential cellular processes, offering potential solutions to combat antibiotic resistance. In cancer therapy, engineered nanomaterials, such as liposomes, polymeric nanoparticles, and gold nanostructures, enable targeted drug delivery to tumor sites, minimizing damage to healthy tissues while enhancing therapeutic efficacy. These nanocarriers can be functionalized with targeting ligands that specifically recognize cancer cell receptors, allowing for precise delivery of chemotherapeutic agents, genetic material, or immunomodulatory compounds. Additionally, some nanomaterials exhibit intrinsic therapeutic properties, such as gold nanorods and magnetic nanoparticles, which can convert external energy sources, such as light or magnetic fields, into localized heat for thermal ablation of tumors, creating multifunctional platforms that combine diagnostic and therapeutic capabilities in a single system.

Nanobiomedicine has recently emerged as a revolutionary method for tackling diagnostic and therapeutic challenges. Nanoparticles serve as carriers for drugs and genes in treating various diseases. Their advantageous high surface area-to-volume ratio enables drug- or gene-conjugated nanoparticles to penetrate cell membranes and reach intracellular targets. Through receptor-specific recognition, functionalized nanoparticles can target specific cells, reducing off-target effects. Nanoparticles also protect drugs and genes from the degradation common in conventional delivery methods by encapsulating or shielding these formulations. In addition, nanoparticles offer the benefit of combining therapy and diagnostics into a single theranostic platform, allowing for precise treatment and disease monitoring. These versatile particles can transport both imaging agents and therapeutic molecules (including drugs, DNA, and RNA), enabling simultaneous disease imaging and treatment while eliminating the need for separate procedures. Researchers worldwide are currently investigating nanoparticles' theranostic potential across various applications, from cancer and genetic disorder therapies to vaccine development, demonstrating their remarkable capabilities. This chapter examines various nanoparticles used for drug and gene delivery alongside commonly employed imaging techniques in theranostic approaches.

ABOUT THE BOOK

In the present context, this book, "Nanobiomedicine: Fundamentals and Implementation in Theranostic Applications," focuses on providing an in-depth overview of this rapidly evolving field, exploring its fundamental principles, cutting-edge applications, and the transformative role of artificial intelligence.

Designed with an introductory concept of nanobiomedicine, this book explores its potential applications in healthcare and concludes with AI-assisted patient sentiment analysis. The book deliberately features a diverse examination of nanomedicine's role in healthcare to provide readers with a thorough and progressive understanding of medical advancements.

In this book, an introductory overview of nanobiomedicine with key features, potential applications, future prospects, and challenges such as ethical concerns, toxicity, and regulatory obstacles is presented in a comprehensible manner. Subsequently, implications of nanomaterials in the therapeutic sector, including photodynamic therapy, immunotherapy, and gene therapy, are discussed in detail. Simultaneous performance in diagnosis and therapy is also highlighted, where nanomaterials can act as vectors for drugs and genes in the treatment of various disease conditions. Their high surface area-to-volume ratio is a positive factor, as it allows drug- or gene-conjugated nanoparticles to traverse cell membranes and access intracellular targets. Both imaging agents and therapeutic molecules [drugs, DNA, and RNA] can be carried by nanoparticles, whose multifunctionality enables simultaneous disease imaging and treatment, reducing the need for separate interventions. This book also highlights the diagnostic portfolio of nanomaterials in a profound way so that interested researchers can gain ample guidance from the chapter. In this particular chapter, 2-dimensional nanomaterials, quantum dots, nanocomposites, etc., are explored as disease biomarkers, and nanodispersions are discussed. A special literary discussion focuses on cancer treatment and diagnosis by nanomaterials, where nanomedicine has revolutionized cancer therapy by enabling targeted drug delivery to tumor sites through functionalized nanocarriers, minimizing damage to healthy tissues while maximizing therapeutic efficacy. In cancer diagnosis, nanoparticles serve as contrast agents for enhanced imaging techniques, allowing earlier detection of malignancies at the molecular level before morphological changes become apparent. These nanoscale platforms can also be engineered as theranostic agents that combine both diagnostic and therapeutic functions, permitting real-time monitoring of treatment response while simultaneously delivering anticancer drugs or mediating thermal ablation therapies. Interestingly, the theme of the book has slightly shifted to Artificial Intelligence-based disease detection due to the fact that in the modern healthcare industry 5.0 and 6.0 under smart society 5.0 and 6.0, artificial intelligence is an extensively dominant tool to clinically diagnose, analyze diseases, and assist patients. In this regard, the book includes one chapter on Machine Learning-assisted Alzheimer's disease detection that diligently helps patients achieve better treatment and guides doctors to use suitable artificial intelligence models for improved accuracy in prediction. A spontaneous question arises whether there is any scope for artificial intelligence-mediated nanomedicine formulation to design drugs that are more personalized and effective in combating disease. Of course, the book incorporates one chapter on artificial intelligence-based drug discovery, especially for allergic diseases. A comprehensive and more profound generalized conceptualization of artificial intelligence-based nanomedicine formulation is presented in the succeeding chapter. To account for the challenges of artificial intelligence-based nanomedicine formulation and disease treatment, a risk management and regulatory measurement framework is needed for AI-driven nanomedicine, including preventive security measures and real-time monitoring with a stringent algorithm validation process. Finally, the book encompasses sentiment analysis of patients when they are suffering from neurodiseases or cancer. One chapter is dedicated to these patients, where natural language processing techniques (NLP) are used to analyze their emotions and sentiments for more effective treatment. The selection of this chapter is motivated by the aim of enabling healthcare systems to extract emotional insights from patient feedback, social media posts, and clinical notes. By analyzing patient sentiments, healthcare providers can identify areas of dissatisfaction, monitor mental health trends, and personalize treatment approaches based on emotional responses to care. This technology facilitates a more empathetic healthcare ecosystem by quantifying subjective experiences that traditionally went unmeasured, allowing for continuous improvement of patient experiences while providing early warning signals of potential issues in care delivery. NLP-based sentiment analysis bridges the communication gap between patients and healthcare systems, transforming qualitative expressions into actionable intelligence that drives more responsive and emotionally intelligent healthcare services. This book is truly interdisciplinary in its disposition and emerges as an efficient reference for materials scientists, biotechnologists, AI researchers, and medical practitioners.

ORGANIZATION OF THE BOOK

The journey through this book begins with an introduction to the core concepts of nanobiomedicine, laying the groundwork for understanding the intricate interactions between nanomaterials and biological systems, and the reasoning behind the implications of nanomedicines in the evaluation and diagnostics of cancer and other infectious diseases (Chapter 1). In this chapter, the methodologies of nanomedicine injection for tissue engineering and regenerative medicine are depicted with intense focus. Some recent advancements, including nanorobots for customized medications, are highlighted for readers' interest. Finally, some constraints such as ethical concerns, toxicity, and regulatory obstacles are addressed in this chapter, providing a realistic view of nanomedicines.

The diagnostic prowess of nanomaterials is further explored in Chapter 2, showcasing their utility in early disease detection and personalized medicine. This chapter provides a detailed overview of different nanomedicine structures, including nanoparticles, 2D materials, quantum dots, nanofibers, nanowires, nanorods, nanodispersions, carbon nanotubes, and nanocomposites, and their uses in imaging, biosensing, and diagnostics, aiming to give readers a clear understanding of nanomedicine's applications.

Chapter 3 expands on this, focusing specifically on the exciting realm of theranostics, where diagnosis and therapy are seamlessly integrated at the nanoscale. In this chapter, the implications of different types of nanomaterials, such as micelles, organic nanoparticles, and gold nanoparticles, in drug delivery, imaging, Point of Care (POC) therapy, and gene therapy are explained in a comprehensible fashion with concomitant analysis of strategies for sustained drug release.

The fundamental ideas and key points of nanomedicine-induced theranostic systems are then matured in Chapter 4, where we delve into the diverse applications of nanomaterials in therapeutic interventions, highlighting their potential for targeted drug delivery and enhanced treatment efficacy. The chapter comprehensively discusses major progress in nanomaterials-mediated healthcare, including immunotherapy, gene therapy, tumor treatment, and vaccine development. Additionally, this chapter recommends different clinical translations of nanomedicines and examines associated challenges currently faced by the field.

Chapter 5 examines the use of nanomedicine for combined therapy and diagnosis in cancer treatment. This chapter illustrates how nanomedicine has developed to address limitations in traditional cancer therapies. It pays particular attention to recent progress in using various nanomedicine types, such as upconversion, plasmonic, magnetic, quantum dot, carbon, Prussian blue, mesoporous silica, lipid-based, and polymeric nanoparticles, in clinical cancer treatment. The chapter concludes by discussing the future potential and obstacles of implementing nanomedicine in clinical practice.

Chapter 6 presents a fascinating exploration of machine learning (ML)-based approaches for early detection of Alzheimer's disease, demonstrating the power of AI in neurodegenerative disorders for accurate and early detection of intermediate stages. While the promise of nanobiomedicine is immense, challenges remain.

Chapter 7 delves into AI-mediated drug delivery, including oral, intravenous, intramuscular, subcutaneous, and transdermal routes, especially for allergic patients, by addressing challenges in traditional nanomedicine formulation. This chapter addresses inherent challenges in nanomedicine-mediated traditional theranostic applications, such as pharmacokinetics, bioavailability, and targeted action, acknowledging the complexities and potential limitations. However, these challenges are being actively addressed, particularly with the integration of AI methodologies—including machine learning, deep learning, and natural language processing—into the development of next-generation drug delivery platforms.

Besides experimental synthesis of nanomaterials and their implications in theranostic applications, modern technologies such as Artificial Intelligence (AI) and its associated sister concerns pervade theranostic systems to reduce tedious human efforts and provide a smart, decisive, and justifiable healthcare system. In today's hectic life, hypertension and oxidative stress are natural phenomena for every individual and, in most cases, they are untreated or casually treated, resulting in neurodegeneration in individuals over the age of 65. Alzheimer's and Parkinson's are the two most prevalent diseases frequently developed in adults, especially senior citizens, making early identification and medication of utmost priority.

Keeping this in view, Chapter 8 highlights the crucial role of AI in nanomedicine formulation and applications, showcasing its ability to accelerate research and development. This chapter illustrates revolutionary breakthroughs due to AI regarding existing limitations of nanomedicine, specifically in production scales, regulatory burdens, and nanomaterial toxicity. At the outset, the chapter highlights ethical, regulatory, and data-related issues that arise from the integration of AI with nanomedicine.

This book is intended for a broad audience, including researchers, clinicians, engineers, and students interested in the intersection of nanotechnology, biomedicine, and artificial intelligence. We hope that it serves as a valuable resource, inspiring further exploration and contributing to the advancement of this dynamic field. A tapestry of knowledge, woven with threads of expertise and spun with the dedication of insightful minds, has been presented to us. We stand in gratitude, bathed in the luminescence of our contributory authors' intellectual contributions. These are not merely words on a page, but seeds of wisdom, planted with the intention of nurturing a future harvest. We envision these ideas blossoming, becoming guiding stars for burgeoning researchers and clinicians, illuminating their paths toward a sustainable, intelligent healthcare society. Their work, a beacon in the vast expanse of medical innovation, promises to ignite a chain reaction of discovery, fostering a legacy of healing and progress.

Soumik Podder
Department of Basic Science & Humanities
Institute of Engineering & Management, New Town
University of Engineering & Management
Kolkata, India

&

Amalesh Samanta
Division of Microbiology & Pharmaceutical Biotechnology
Department of Pharmaceutical Technology
Jadavpur University
Kolkata, India

ABOUT THE BOOK

In the present context, this book, " Nanobiomedicine: Fundamentals and Implementation in Theranostic Applications," focuses to provide an in-depth overview of this rapidly evolving field, exploring its fundamental principles, cutting-edge applications, and the transformative role of artificial intelligence.

Designed with an introductory concept of nanobiomedicine, this book explores its potential applications in healthcare while concluding with AI-assisted nanomedicine formulation. The book deliberately features a diverse examination of nanomedicine's role in healthcare to provide readers with a thorough and progressive understanding of medical advancements.

In this book, at first an introductory idea of nanobiomedicine with key features, potential possible applications, future prospects, challenges like ethical concerns, toxicity and regulatory obstacles are presented in a comprehensible manner. Simultaneous performance in diagnosis and therapy is also illuminated in this book where the nanomaterials can act as a vector for drugs and genes in the treatment of various disease conditions. Their high surface area-to-volume ratio is a positive factor as it allows the drug or gene conjugated nanoparticles to traverse cell membranes and access intracellular targets. Both imaging agents and therapeutic molecules [drugs, DNA and RNA] can be made to be carried by nanoparticles, the multi-functionality of which enables simultaneous disease imaging and treatment, reducing the need for separate interventions. Afterwards, implications of nanomaterials in therapeutic sector including photodynamic therapy, immunotherapy, gene therapy is discussed in a detailed fashion. This book also highlights separately diagnostic portfolio of nanomaterials in a profound way so that interested researcher can get ample guidance from the chapter. In this particular chapter, 2-dimensional nanomaterials, quantum dots, nanocomposites etc. are used as disease biomarkers, nanodispersion etc. A special literary discussion was made on cancer treatment and diagnosis by nanomaterials where nanomedicine has revolutionized cancer therapy by enabling targeted drug delivery to tumor sites through functionalized nanocarriers, minimizing damage to healthy tissues while maximizing therapeutic efficacy. In cancer diagnosis, nanoparticles serve as contrast agents for enhanced imaging techniques, allowing earlier detection of malignancies at the molecular level before morphological changes become apparent. These nanoscale platforms can also be engineered as theranostic agents that combine both diagnostic and therapeutic functions, permitting real-time monitoring of treatment response while simultaneously delivering anticancer drugs or mediating thermal ablation therapies. Interestingly the theme of the book has slightly transited to Artificial Intelligence based disease detection because of the fact that, in modern healthcare industry 5.0 and 6.0 under smart society 5.0 and 6.0, artificial intelligence is extensively ruling agent to clinically diagnose, analyze diseases and give assistance to patients. In this regard, the book includes one chapter on Machine learning assisted Alzheimer disease detection that diligently help patients for better treatment and mentoring doctors to use suitable artificial intelligence models for better accuracy in prediction. A spontaneous inquisition arises whether there is any scope of artificial intelligence mediated nanomedicine formulation so as to design the drug more personalized and effective in disease combating. Of course, the book incorporates one chapter on artificial intelligence-based drug discovery specially for allergic diseases. A comprehensive and more profound generalized conceptualization on artificial intelligence-based nanomedicine formulation, has been realized in the succeeding chapter. This book is a truly interdisciplinary in its disposition and startlingly turns out as efficient reference for materials scientist, biotechnologist, AI researchers and medical practitioners.

ORGANIZATION OF THE BOOK

The journey through this book begins with an introduction to the core concepts of nanobiomedicine, laying the groundwork for understanding the intricate interactions between nanomaterials and biological systems (Chapter 1). We then delve into the exciting realm of theranostics, where diagnosis and therapy are seamlessly integrated at the nanoscale. (Chapter 2) Chapter 3 focuses on diverse applications of nanomaterials in therapeutic interventions, highlighting their potential for targeted drug delivery and enhanced treatment efficacy. The diagnostic prowess of nanomaterials is further explored in Chapter 4, showcasing their utility in early disease detection and personalized medicine. A significant portion of the book is dedicated to the application of nanomedicine in combating cancer, a disease that continues to challenge modern medicine. Chapter 5 examines the use of nanomedicine for conjugated therapy and diagnosis in cancer treatment, while Chapter 6 presents a fascinating exploration of machine learning-based approaches for early detection of Alzheimer's disease, demonstrating the power of AI in neurodegenerative disorders. While the promise of nanobiomedicine is immense, challenges remain. Chapter 7 delves into AI-mediated drug delivery, especially for allergic patients, by addressing challenges in traditional nanomedicine formulation. This chapter addresses the inherent challenges in nanomedicine-mediated traditional theranostic applications, acknowledging the complexities and potential limitations. However, these challenges are being actively addressed, particularly with the integration of artificial intelligence. Chapter 8 highlights the crucial role of AI in nanomedicine formulation and applications, showcasing its ability to accelerate research and development.

This book is intended for a broad audience, including researchers, clinicians, engineers, and students interested in the intersection of nanotechnology, biomedicine, and artificial intelligence. We hope that it serves as a valuable resource, inspiring further exploration and contributing to the advancement of this dynamic field. We are indebted to the contributing authors for their expertise and dedication, and we hope that it serves as a valuable resource, inspiring further exploration and contributing to the advancement of this dynamic field. A tapestry of knowledge, woven with threads of expertise and spun with the dedication of insightful minds, has been gifted to us. We stand in gratitude, bathed in the luminescence of our contributory authors' intellectual contributions. These are not merely words on a page, but seeds of wisdom, planted with the intention of nurturing a future harvest. We envision these ideas blossoming, becoming guiding stars for burgeoning researchers and clinicians, illuminating their paths towards a sustainable, intelligent healthcare society. Their work, a beacon in the vast expanse of medical innovation, promises to ignite a chain reaction of discovery, fostering a legacy of healing and progress.

List of Contributors

Abhishek Mohanta	Division of Microbiology & Pharmaceutical Biotechnology, Department of Pharmaceutical Technology, Jadavpur University, Kolkata, India
Aniket Hazra	Department of Biotechnology, Institute of Engineering & Management, New Town, University of Engineering & Management, Kolkata, India
Aritra Nandi	Department of Biotechnology, Institute of Engineering & Management, New Town, University of Engineering & Management, Kolkata, India
Amalesh Samanta	Division of Microbiology & Pharmaceutical Biotechnology, Department of Pharmaceutical Technology, Jadavpur University, Kolkata, India
Arnab De	Department of Pharmaceutics, Bharat Technology, Uluberia, Howrah, West Bengal, India
Abhishek Mukherjee	Agricultural and Ecological Research Unit, Biological Science Division, Indian Statistical Institute, Giridih, Jharkhand, India
Chandan Kumar Ghosh	School of Materials Science and Nanotechnology, Jadavpur University, Kolkata, India
Debaprasad Das	Department of Electronics and Communication Engineering, Assam University, Silchar, Assam, India
Mousumi Das	Division of Microbiology & Pharmaceutical Biotechnology, Department of Pharmaceutical Technology, Jadavpur University, Kolkata, India
Mousumi Tudu	Division of Microbiology & Pharmaceutical Biotechnology, Department of Pharmaceutical Technology, Jadavpur University, Kolkata, India
Mrinmoy Dasgupta	Department of Biotechnology, Institute of Engineering & Management, New Town, University of Engineering & Management, Kolkata, India
Milan Karmakar	Department of Biotechnology, Institute of Engineering & Management, New Town, University of Engineering & Management, Kolkata, India
Mandira Das	School of Materials Science and Nanotechnology, Jadavpur University, Kolkata, India
Moloy Dhar	Guru Nanak Institute of Technology, Panihati, West Bengal, India
Pratik Talukder	Department of Biotechnology, Institute of Engineering & Management, New Town, University of Engineering & Management, Kolkata, India
Pranab Naskar	Division of Microbiology & Pharmaceutical Biotechnology, Department of Pharmaceutical Technology, Jadavpur University, Kolkata, India
Panchanan Sahoo	Division of Biochemistry, ICMR-National Institute for Research in Bacterial Infections, Kolkata, West Bengal, India School of Materials Science and Nanotechnology, Jadavpur University, Kolkata, India
Swastika Mohanta	Department of Biotechnology, Institute of Engineering & Management, New Town, University of Engineering & Management, Kolkata, India
Suparna Garai	Division of Microbiology & Pharmaceutical Biotechnology, Department of Pharmaceutical Technology, Jadavpur University, Kolkata, India
Suparna Karmakar	Guru Nanak Institute of Technology, Panihati, West Bengal, India

Snehika Sengupta	Department of Biotechnology, Institute of Engineering & Management, New Town, University of Engineering & Management, Kolkata, India
Sayani Konar	Guru Nanak Institute of Technology, Panihati, West Bengal, India
Sayantan Biawas	Department of Biotechnology, Institute of Engineering & Management, New Town, University of Engineering & Management, Kolkata, India
Shouvik Sarkar	Department of Computer Science and Engineering-AI, Brainware University, Barasat, Kolkata, West Bengal, India Department of Electronics and Communication Engineering, Assam University, Silchar, Assam, India
Shreeja Sinha	Guru Nanak Institute of Technology, Panihati, West Bengal, India
Sohini Chatterjee	Division of Microbiology & Pharmaceutical Biotechnology, Department of Pharmaceutical Technology, Jadavpur University, Kolkata, India
Soumik Podder	Department of Basic Science & Humanities, Institute of Engineering & Management, New Town, University of Engineering & Management, Kolkata, India
Souvick Das	Department of Biotechnology, Institute of Engineering & Management, New Town, University of Engineering & Management, Kolkata, India
Shaheen Sultana	Department of Biotechnology, Institute of Engineering & Management, New Town, University of Engineering & Management, Kolkata, India
Subham Adhikari	School of Materials Science and Nanotechnology, Jadavpur University, Kolkata, India
Suparna Biswas	Guru Nanak Institute of Technology, Panihati, West Bengal, India
Sucharita Bhattacharyya	Guru Nanak Institute of Technology, Panihati, West Bengal, India
Sreejita Das	Department of Botany, University of Calcutta, Kolkata, West Bengal, India
Sayantika Hore	Department of Biotechnology, Institute of Engineering and Management, New Town, University of Engineering & Management, Kolkata, India

CHAPTER 1

Fundamentals of Nanomedicine

Amalesh Samanta[1,*], Suparna Garai[1], Pranab Naskar[1], Sohini Chatterjee[1], Mousumi Das[1], Abhishek Mohanta[1] and **Mousumi Tudu[1]**

[1] *Division of Microbiology & Pharmaceutical Biotechnology, Department of Pharmaceutical Technology, Jadavpur University, Kolkata, India*

Abstract: Nanomedicine is a multidisciplinary field merging nanotechnology with medicine to address complicated health challenges at the cellular and molecular levels. The fundamental theory involves operating with materials at the nanoscale (1-100 nanometers), where distinctive physical, chemical, and biological characteristics become apparent. These nanoscale substances can interact with cellular systems in novel ways, allowing precise diagnostics, selective drug delivery, and novel therapeutic methods. Key developments include the progress of nanoparticle-derived delivery systems that enhance the bioavailability and singularity of treatments, decreasing side effects. Nanobiomedicine also plays a crucial role in evaluation and diagnostics, where nanosensors and imaging agents enable the early detection of diseases, including cancer and other infectious diseases. Additionally, nanotechnology has potential in regenerative medicine and tissue engineering, where nanomaterials help in tissue repair and cell growth. Recent advancements, for instance, the incorporation of nanorobots for minimum invasive processes and the utilization of biocompatible nanostructures for customized medications, highlight the revolutionary potential of nanobiomedicine. Although challenges like ethical concerns, toxicity, and regulatory obstacles must be recognised for widespread clinical application, with continuous research, nanobiomedicine promises to transform healthcare, providing more potent, personalized, and reduced invasive medical solutions.

Keywords: Cancer therapy, Diagnostic imaging , Nanomedicine , Nanoparticles, Regenerative medicines, Targeted drug delivery.

INTRODUCTION

Definition and Scope: Nanomedicine is a multidisciplinary field of science that includes physics, chemistry, engineering, biology, medicine, and allied sciences for the detection and treatment of diseases with the help of nanotechnology. The

* **Corresponding author Amalesh Samanta:** Division of Microbiology & Pharmaceutical Biotechnology, Department of Pharmaceutical Technology, Jadavpur University, Kolkata, India;
E-mail: amalesh.samanta@jadavpuruniverity.in

Soumik Podder & Amalesh Samanta (Eds.)

ultimate goal of nanomedicine is to target the human body at the atomic and molecular levels, repairing it in a manner similar to how we maintain conventional machines today [1]. The spectrum of nanobiomedicine is vast, encompassing areas such as advanced diagnostic imaging methods, targeted drug delivery, tissue engineering, and regenerative medicines. By utilizing the noble and unique aspects of nanomaterials such as high surface-area volume ratio, quantum effects, nanobiomedicine can achieve much higher accuracy in targeting tissues (more specific), thereby increasing the therapeutic efficacy and decreasing the adverse effects.

Historical Background: It is recognized that the original foundation of nanotechnology dates back to Richard Feynman's 1959 lecture, "There's Plenty of Room at the Bottom," in which he proposed the concept of nanotechnology. Feynman is known for his work in the theory of quantum electrodynamics. In that seminar, he proposed the idea of directly manipulating atoms and molecules [2]. Although the term "nanotechnology" was introduced by Norio Taniguchi, a professor at the Tokyo University of Science, to describe processes such as semiconductor-like thin film deposition and ion beam machining that demonstrate precise control at the nanometer scale, in 1974 [3]. A significant milestone was marked with the introduction of Scanning Tunneling Microscopy (STM) by Gerd Binning and Heinrich Rohrer in the 1980s [4]. The unification of nanotechnology and biomedical sciences, which began in the late 1990s and 2000s, is driven by the advancements in nanofabrication techniques and nanomaterials. Developments in nano-materials-based delivery of drugs and nanoscale imaging methods highlight the prospect of this multidisciplinary field in revolutionizing the healthcare system [5, 6].

Interdisciplinary Nature: The fundamentals of nanomedicine are inherently interdepartmental, leveraging wisdom and methodologies from several fields, which include physics, chemistry, biology, engineering, and medicine. This intersection is crucial for addressing the complex design and implementation of nanoscale tools and materials for biomedical applications. For example, the formation of nanoparticles for drug delivery requires expertise in chemistry and material science to ensure functionality and biocompatibility [7].

Medicine and cell biology also play an important role in understanding the relationship and interaction between nanoparticles and biological systems. It is crucial to focus on collaborative efforts from diverse disciplines in order to translate the findings in the laboratory into clinical applications, thereby nurturing innovation and accelerating the evolution of novel nanobiomedical technologies (Fig. **1**).

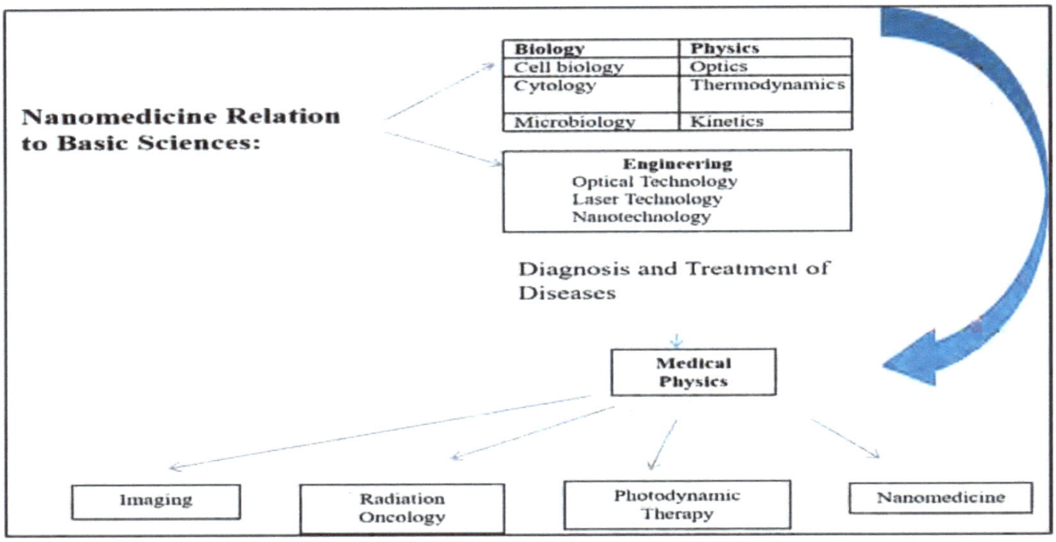

Fig. (1). Relation between nanomedicine and basic sciences.

Basic Concepts of Nanotechnology

Nanomaterials and Nanostructures

Materials with structural characteristics smaller than 100 nanometers in one or more dimensions are known as nanomaterials. They can be zero-dimensional, known as nano-particles, one-dimensional, called nanotubes and nano-wires, two-dimensional, known as nanofilms and nanosheets, or can be three-dimensional, which are called nanocomposites. Nanostructures are attributed to the specific configuration of atoms or molecules at the nanoscale, which often provide materials with unique physical and chemical properties compared to their bulk counterparts [8].

Properties: Due to increased surface area and quantum effects, materials at the nanoscale exhibit distinct properties. These characteristics include electrical conductivity, enhanced mechanical strength, chemical reactivity, and optical behaviour. For example, gold particles in their nano form can be used in imaging and therapeutic applications, as they exhibit optical properties that are size-dependent [9]. Carbon Nanotubes are used in biosensor applications and tissue engineering because of their exceptional mechanical strength [10].

Fabrication and Characterization Techniques

Nanobiomedicine uses nanotechnology to address challenges in healthcare, such as targeted drug delivery, diagnostics, and imaging. This field relies on robust fabrication techniques to generate precise nanostructures, as well as advanced characterization methods to ensure their suitability for biomedical applications.

Fabrication Techniques

Top-Down Approaches

Top-down techniques reduce macroscopic materials into nano-structures through physical, chemical or mechanical techniques.

- Lithography: Various techniques such as electron-beam lithography (EBL) and photolithography are utilized to generate patterns on substrates, which are essential for nanoscale structures like nanowires or nanopillars [11].
- Etching: Wet Chemical Etching or Reactive Ion Etching (RIE) is utilized to sculpt materials, delivering fine accuracy for biomedical devices such as biosensors [12].

Bottom-Up Approaches

These approaches put together nanoparticles molecule-by-molecule or atom-b--atom.

- Self-Assembly: Substances such as lipid and protein structure themselves organize into specified structures like micelles or liposomes, which are widely utilized for the delivery of drugs [13].
- Sol-Gel Method: This chemical reaction uses metal alkoxides to generate nanostructured ceramics, generally implemented in generating drug-loaded nanocarriers [14].

Green Synthesis

Green synthesis utilizes biological agents such as microorganisms or plant extracts for the production of eco-friendly nanoparticles. For example, silver nanoparticles fabricated using plant extracts illustrate excellent biocompatibility and antimicrobial properties [15].

Fabrication of Drug Delivery Systems

- Electrospinning: This procedure is employed to generate nanofibers for purposes like wound repair or controlled medication release [16].
- Nanoprecipitation: This is a bottom-up method for fabricating polymeric nanoparticles that encase drugs, increasing their solubility and bioavailability [17].

Techniques of Characterization

Structural and Morphological Analysis

- Scanning Electron Microscopy (SEM) and Transmission Electron Microscopy (TEM): These tools with high-resolution imaging capacity provide insights into shape, nanoparticle size, and surface morphology [18].
- Atomic Force Microscopy (AFM): It analyses the surface features as well as the mechanical characteristics of the nanomaterials at an extremely small scale [19].

Spectroscopic Techniques

- Fourier-Transform Infrared Spectroscopy (FTIR): It identifies the functional groups as well as the chemical bonding present in the nanoparticles [20].
- UV-Visible Spectroscopy: It delivers information on nanoparticle size distribution and optical properties depending on the absorption of light [21].

Surface Characterization

- X-ray Photoelectron Spectroscopy (XPS): It offers details regarding chemical states and surface composition, which is important for biocompatibility studies [22].
- Zeta Potential Measurement: It helps to measure surface charge, which is crucial for ascertaining the colloidal stability of nanoparticles present in biological systems [23].

Crystallinity and Phase Identification

- X-ray Diffraction (XRD): It is used to understand the crystalline structure and the degree to which nanoparticles consist of a single, uniform crystalline phase without contamination or secondary phases [24].

Biological Interaction Studies

- Dynamic Light Scattering (DLS): It measures the polydispersity and the hydrodynamic size, which are the key parameters for a nanoparticle's behaviour in biological fluids [25].
- Cellular Imaging: Confocal microscopy and fluorescence facilitate monitoring the movement and localization of nanoparticles inside cells, providing insight into the intracellular interactions and biodistribution [26].

The advancement of nanobiomedicine relies on the precise fabrication and thorough analysis of nanomaterials. Fabrication techniques enable the creation and design of nanoparticles with specific properties and functions, tailored for targeted applications, while sophisticated characterization verifies their effectiveness and biocompatibility. Through sustained advancements, these techniques will enhance the prospects of nanotechnology in medicine.

Nanomedicine in Disease Treatment

Nanomedicine represents a transformative strategy for medical therapies, utilizing the unique features of nanomaterials to achieve improved and targeted approaches. Fundamental to nanomedicine's role in the treatment of diseases is its ability to design nanoparticles capable of transporting medications, genes, and therapeutic agents right away to disease sites, like infected tissues or tumors, diminishing harm to adjacent healthy cells.

Among the most promising applications of nanomedicine are in cancer therapy. Nanoparticles can be designed to administer anticancer drugs specifically to cancer cells, using their increased permeability and retention impact. This allows for elevated levels of medications at tumor sites while minimizing systemic side effects connected with traditional chemotherapy. Nanoparticles like liposomes, gold nanoparticles and dendrimers have revealed significant promise in improving drug delivery and increasing the bioavailability for drugs with low solubility, making treatments more efficient and less toxic [27, 28].

Along with cancer, nanomedicine has achieved significant improvements in treating infectious diseases. For instance, nanoparticles have been employed to enhance the delivery of antibiotics to bacterial infection sites, thereby circumventing the bacterial cell membrane and facilitating more effective treatment of antibiotic-resistant infections. Particularly, silver nanoparticles have proven antimicrobial effects, assisting in wound healing as well as preventing infection in chronic and persistent wounds [29]. Additionally, nanomaterials, such as magnetic nanoparticles, have been studied for potential use in gene delivery systems, which facilitate targeted treatment for genetic disorders by transporting corrective genes directly to the affected cells [30].

Nanomedicine plays a significant role in treating neurodegenerative diseases. In neurodegenerative diseases, the blood-brain barrier frequently reduces the effectiveness of conventional delivery of drugs. Nanoparticles, like polymeric nanoparticles, have been engineered to surmount this barrier and thus deliver the drugs directly into the brain. This offers a new potential opportunity for treating neurodegenerative conditions like Parkinson's disease and Alzheimer's disease. The capability to develop nanoparticles that can navigate inside the brain's complex environment paves the way for innovative possibilities in treating these hard-to-manage diseases [31].

Moreover, the combination of immunotherapy with nanomedicine has shown significant potential in increasing immune responses to diseases such as cancer. Nanoparticles can also be utilized to deliver vaccines, immune-stimulating agents or antigens, directly to the immune cells, thus improving vaccine efficiency and stimulating more robust immune responses [32].

In summary, nanomedicine can be mentioned as a revolutionary way of treating diseases by enabling precise, targeted, and controlled therapy. Its utilization in cancer, neurodegenerative conditions, infectious diseases, and immunotherapy is growing continuously, offering hope for effective as well as personalized treatments.

Principles of Operation

Nanomedicine is an advanced domain of medical science, harnesses nanotechnology for diagnostic and advanced therapeutic purposes. Various approaches, including photothermal therapy, targeted drug delivery, and cancer therapy are being scrutinized for their ability to increase treatment outcomes, improve patient care and reduce side effects.

Targeted Drug Delivery: The fundamental principle of targeted drug delivery includes the use of nanomaterials, such as nanoparticles, dendrimers, or liposomes, to selectively transfer therapeutic agents to specific sites in the body, commonly affected tissues and organs. This strategy aims to enhance drug concentration at the designated site while minimizing exposure to healthy tissues and reducing side effects [33].

Mechanism

Surface Modification: Ligands are used to functionalize the nanoparticles (*e.g.*, antibodies, small molecules or peptides) that associate specifically with receptors, which are overexpressed on diseased cells, like the cancer cells [34] (Fig. **2**).

Passive Targeting: This happens *via* the improved permeability and retention mechanism effect, where nanoparticles aggregate in tumor tissues because of their poor lymphatic drainage and leaky vasculature (Fig. **2**).

Active Targeting: Nanoparticles are precisely engineered to bind specifically to receptors present on the surface of target cells, ensuring the precise delivery of the drug [35] (Fig. **2**).

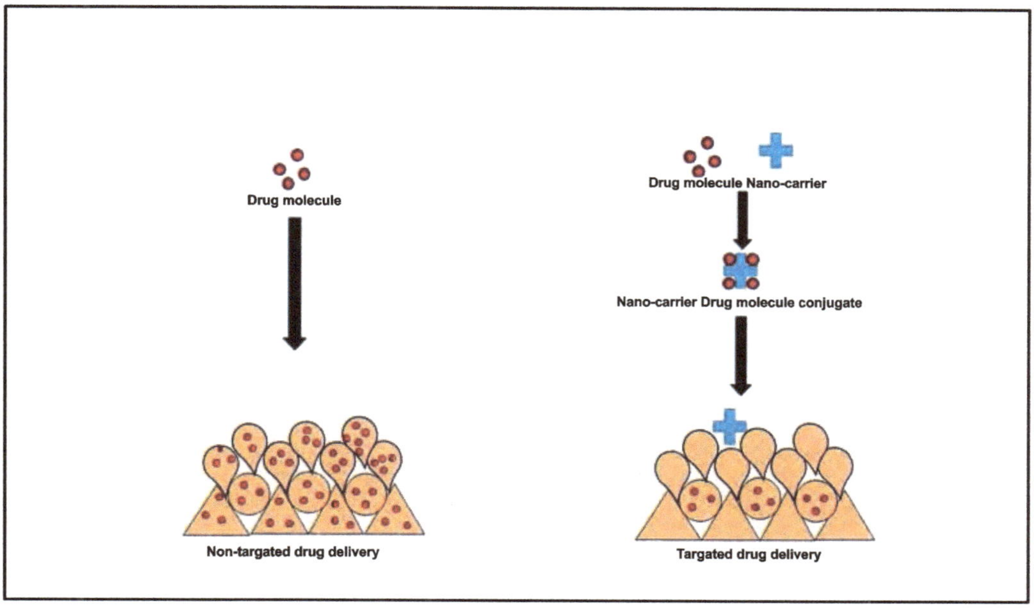

Fig. (2). The diagram shows the nanoparticle, which is loaded with the drug and circulates in the bloodstream, then directs it towards a tumour cell. Another diagram shows a drug attached through the receptor-ligand interactions. Here, the drug is directly released within the tumour tissue, thus avoiding systemic circulation.

Photothermal Therapy (PTT): This therapy utilizes nanoparticles that absorb light and then convert it into heat. It can selectively target and demolish specific cells, such as cancer cells, without damaging the surrounding healthy tissues. The method is non-invasive and relies on the localized thermal properties of nanoparticles when exposed to specific light wavelengths [35].

Mechanism: Nanoparticles' Selection: Substances such as gold nanoparticles (AuNPs) and carbon-based nanomaterials (like graphene oxide) are selected for their capability to absorb near-infrared light and transmute it into heat [35].

Laser Irradiation: Either through active or passive targeting, the nanoparticles are directed towards the tumor site. Then they are irradiated with the help of near-infrared light. The energy absorbed is then transformed into heat, which leads to the thermal annihilation of tumor cells [36] (Fig. **3**).

Localized Treatment: This localized thermal effect minimizes damage to surrounding healthy tissues. It is effective in the treatment of superficial lesions or tumours [37].

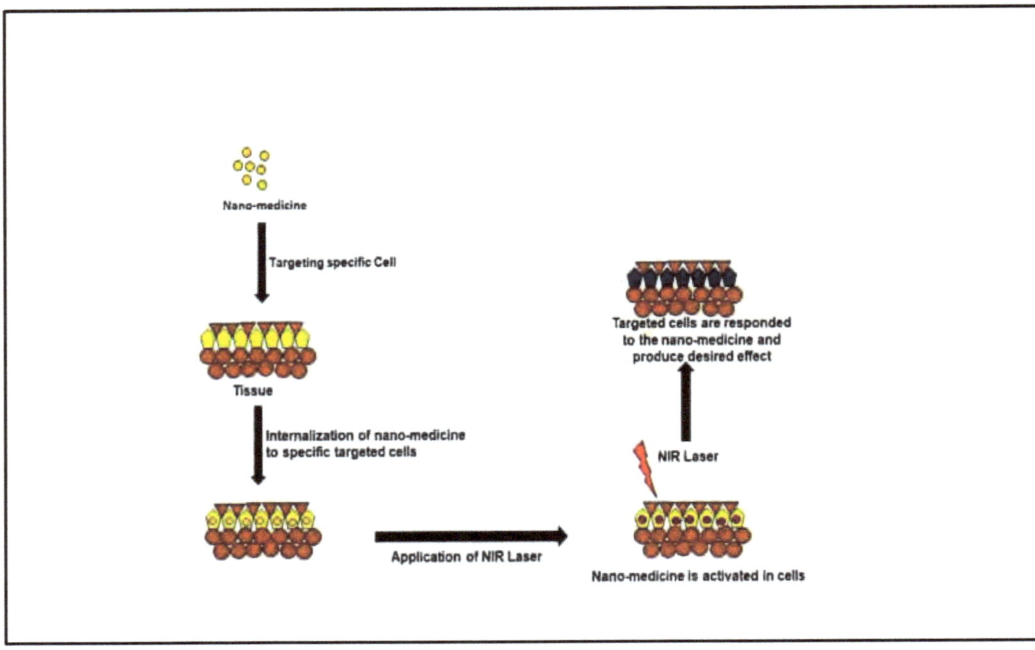

Fig. (3). Schematic diagram showing the eradication of tumour cells by Laser Irradiation.

Cancer Therapy Using Nanomedicine: This therapy includes both photothermal therapy and drug delivery, besides emerging methodologies such as, immunotherapy and gene therapy, all focused on optimizing the treatment of cancer [37].

Mechanism: Delivery of drugs for the treatment of cancer: Chemotherapeutic agents are encapsulated by nanoparticles and protect them from degradation as well as ensure controlled release specifically at the site of the tumor [37]. This methodology can be unified with targeting mechanisms to enhance precision and diminish effects that are off-target.

Gene Therapy for Cancer: Therapeutic genes, like RNA-based drugs or tumor-suppressor genes, are delivered directly to cancer cells by the nanoparticles. This modulates the gene expression and inhibits the growth of the tumor [38].

Immunotherapy: The immune-stimulating agents and checkpoint inhibitors are also delivered with the help of nanonanoparticles, thus enhancing the body's immune response against cancer [38].

The principles underlying nanomedicine therapies, such as targeted drug delivery, cancer treatment, and photothermal therapy, rely on the capability to specifically engineer nanoparticles for designated applications. These strategies have proven to increase the therapeutic efficacy and reduce side effects, thus offering an encouraging future for personalized medication [38].

Current Applications and Relevant Research

Nanomedicine, which applies nanotechnology to medication, has revolutionized the diagnosis of diseases, their treatment, as well as prevention. The aim of nanomedicine is to increase the bioavailability, efficacy and specificity of the therapeutic agents using nanoparticles (NPs), simultaneously minimizing side effects. Mentioned below are some notable examples concerning nanomedicine and relevant research associated with these substances:

Drug Delivery Systems: Nanoparticles are of great potential in delivering drugs to the targeted site of the body, thus improving the precision as well as the effectiveness of the treatments for conditions such as cancer, infections, and cardiovascular diseases. A study performed by Panyam *et al.* displayed the use of nanoparticles in delivering chemotherapeutic drugs to cancer cells, thus increasing tumour-targeting capability and alleviating systemic toxicity. The nanoparticles can also be engineered to respond to specific cellular conditions, like enzyme activity or pH, thus improving the release profile of the drugs at the site of the disease and reducing their impact on healthy cells [39].

Further study by Moghimi *et al.* (2013) investigated the use of polymeric nanoparticles and liposomes for the controlled release of oncologic drugs. The drug delivery systems demonstrated improved pharmacokinetics and enhanced drug concentrations near the tumor sites, exhibiting their therapeutic potential in clinical oncology [40].

Gene Therapy: Nanomedicine has also advanced in gene delivery, providing newer methodologies for genetic disorders. Gene Therapy, which involves the presentation of corrective genes to affected cells, has been increased by nanoparticles such as dendrimers, viral vectors, and liposomes. Wang *et al.* examined the progress of gene delivery systems based on nanoparticles that can efficiently transport genetic material to target cells. These systems improve the stability genes delivered as well as ensure their specific release inside the cell, enhancing treatment outcomes for genetic disorders like muscular dystrophy and cystic fibrosis [41].

Antibiotic Resistance: Nanoparticles also play a crucial role in combating antibiotic-resistant infections, a growing global issue. Wang *et al.* showcased that silver nanoparticles have strong antibacterial properties, which help to combat infections that are caused by resistant bacteria, such as MRSA (Methicillinresistant *Staphylococcus aureus*) [42]. In the same way, research by

Niżnik *et al.* emphasized the use of nanoparticles made of gold to enhance the antimicrobial efficacy of certain antibiotics, potentially minimising the need for high doses of drugs as well as side effects [43].

Diagnostic Imaging: Nanomedicine, applied to medical imaging, allows better visualization as well as early diagnosis of diseases. Sun *et al.* created magnetic nanoparticles for MRI (magnetic resonance imaging), which enhanced image resolution and allowed for the detection of lesions smaller in size, such as those present in cancer patients. They can also serve as transporters for imaging agents, transporting them specifically to the targeted tissue, thus improving the precision of diagnostic techniques [44].

Regenerative Medicine: Nanoparticles are being more widely utilised in regenerative medicine, specifically in wound healing and tissue engineering. Research by Wang *et al.* explored the usage of nanomaterials like hydrogels and nanofibers for healing wounds and regeneration of tissue. These nanostructures have the ability to mimic the extracellular matrix, promoting cell adhesion and providing structural support. They also promote migration and differentiation, essential for tissue repair [45].

Nanomedicine has created opportunities for novel paths for treating diseases that are complex in nature, by enhancing the drug efficacy, and offering therapies that are targeted with low side effects. Studies in this field keep advancing, with nanoparticles leading the way in revolutionizing medicinal treatments. The usage of nanomaterials in gene therapy, drug delivery, infection control, regenerative medicine, and diagnostics showcases their wide-ranging potential in the transformation of healthcare [46].

Ethical and Regulatory Considerations in Translating Nanotechnologies to Clinical Practice

The advancement and implementation of nanotechnologies in healthcare, specifically nanomedicine, have an immense possibility for improving diagnosis, patient outcomes, and treatment. Translating this advancement in clinical practice shows significant ethical, regulatory, and safety challenges.

Regulatory Challenges

Nanotechnologies often resist easy categorization into prevailing regulatory frameworks due to their unique properties, such as shape, size, and surface chemistry. These characteristics impact the behavior of the nanoparticles present in biological systems, further complicating their categorization and assessment under device regulatory and traditional drug pathways.

Classification Issues: Nanomedicine exhibits both device-like and drug-like properties, which raise questions about how they should be regulated [46]. A few examples are regulatory bodies like the EMA and FDA, which must decide whether the nanoparticle-based therapy can be classified as a drug, medical device or biologic. The hybrid nature of such systems necessitates all regulatory decisions, which leads to inconsistency and delays in the approval processes [47].

Standardization: The scarcity of standardized protocols for the testing of nanoparticles is a critical barrier in regulation. Instituting guidelines for characterizing the physicochemical properties of nanoparticles, as well as their interaction with biological systems and bio-distribution, is essential for ensuring safety and consistency in clinical applications [48]. Efforts, such as the ISO/TC 229 technical committee, as well as the FDA's Nanotechnology Regulatory Science and Research Plan, represent various attempts to address the gap; however, global harmonization remains limited [49].

Safety and Toxicology Concerns: The small size and high reactivity of nanoparticles can lead to unintended interactions with biological systems, raising concerns about safety and toxicity [50].

Toxicity Mechanisms: Reactive oxygen species (ROS) are generated by Nanoparticles, leading to inflammation, oxidative stress, and cytotoxicity. Moreover, their capability to cross the biological barriers (*e.g.*, the blood-brain barrier) increases the potential for accumulation of unintended organ [49]. Their clearance mechanisms, especially in immunocompromised individuals, need further investigation [51].

Long-term Effects: The biocompatibility and clearance of the nanoparticles from the body remain ambiguous. -degradable nanoparticles can accumulate in organs such as the liver and spleen, thus posing potential health risks [52].

Case Study: Further Research on carbon nanotubes has shown that inflammatory responses can be induced, similar to those caused by asbestos when inhaled, underscoring the need for comprehensive toxicological evaluations [53].

Ethical Concerns: Nanomedicine brings up ethical concerns about access, safety, and equitable distribution.

Informed Consent: The sophistication of nanotechnologies challenges patients' understanding of associated potential risks and advantages, further complicating the process of acquiring informed consent. This is actually problematic in the early phase of clinical trials and in populations with constricted scientific literacy [54].

Equity and Accessibility: Significant development expenses may limit the availability of nanomedicine therapies, specifically in low and middle-income countries, aggravating healthcare inequalities. Targeted policies as well as pricing strategies are essential for preventing inequality in access to the advanced therapies [55].

Dual-Use Concerns: Nanotechnologies designed for healthcare purposes could be potentially misused, such as in non-therapeutic contexts or for enhancement issues, expressing worries about ethical boundaries. The dual-use dilemma calls for a robust governance frameworks that consider medical benefit as well as misuse potential [53].

Present Regulatory Frameworks and Progress: Approaches of FDA and EMA: The Food and Drug Administration U.S. FDA and the European Medicines Agency (EMA established task groups to confront specific challenges related to nanomedicine. These efforts encompass the creation of classification systems for nanomaterials and the development of risk assessment tools customized to nanotechnology [56].

ISO Standards: The ISO or International Organization for Standardization, issued standards for the nanomaterial characterization to support regulatory bodies as well as developers [55].

CONCLUSION

Nanotechnology in healthcare offers transformative possibilities but requires consideration of regulatory, ethical, and safety aspects to assure its equitable and safe translation into clinical practice. Collaborative initiatives among scientists, ethicists, and regulators are important to address these obstacles and realise the potential of nanomedicine.

REFERENCES

[1] Adabi M, Naghibzadeh M, Adabi M, *et al.* Biocompatibility and nanostructured materials: applications in nanomedicine. Artif Cells Nanomed Biotechnol 2017; 45(4): 833-42. [http://dx.doi.org/10.1080/21691401.2016.1178134] [PMID: 27247194]

[2] Feynman RP. There's plenty of room at the bottom 1960. https://resolver.caltech.edu/CaltechES:23.5.1960Bottom

[3] Taniguchi N. On the basic concept of 'nano-technology' 1974.https://www.scribd.com/document/372768443/On-the-Basic-Concept-of-Nano-technology

[4] Binnig G, Rohrer H. Scanning tunneling microscopy. Helv Phys Acta 1982; 55(6): 726-35. [http://dx.doi.org/10.5169/seals-115309]

[5] Blanco E, Shen H, Ferrari M. Principles of nanoparticle design for overcoming biological barriers to drug delivery. Nat Biotechnol 2015; 33(9): 941-51. [http://dx.doi.org/10.1038/nbt.3330] [PMID: 26348965]

[6] Bayda S, Adeel M, Tuccinardi T, Cordani M, Rizzolio F. The History of Nanoscience and Nanotechnology: From Chemical–Physical Applications to Nanomedicine. Molecules 2019; 25(1): 112.
[http://dx.doi.org/10.3390/molecules25010112] [PMID: 31892180]

[7] Jain KK. Nanomedicine: application of nanobiotechnology in medical practice. Med Princ Pract 2008; 17(2): 89-101.
[http://dx.doi.org/10.1159/000112961] [PMID: 18287791]

[8] Cao G, Wang Y. Nanostructures and nanomaterials: synthesis, properties, and applications. World Scientific 2005.
[http://dx.doi.org/10.1142/p305]

[9] Daniel MC, Astruc D. Gold nanoparticles: assembly, supramolecular chemistry, quantum-size-related properties, and applications toward biology, catalysis, and nanotechnology. Chem Rev 2004; 104(1): 293-346.
[http://dx.doi.org/10.1021/cr030698+] [PMID: 14719978]

[10] Iijima S. Helical microtubules of graphitic carbon. Nature 1991; 354(6348): 56-8.
[http://dx.doi.org/10.1038/354056a0]

[11] Bhushan B. Springer Handbook of Nanotechnology. 3rd ed., Berlin: Springer 2010.
[http://dx.doi.org/10.1007/978-3-642-02525-9]

[12] Wang J, Zhang B, Sun J, Hu W, Wang H. Recent advances in porous nanostructures for cancer theranostics. Nano Today 2021; 38: 101146.
[http://dx.doi.org/10.1016/j.nantod.2021.101146] [PMID: 33897805]

[13] Zhang L, Gu FX, Chan JM, Wang AZ, Langer RS, Farokhzad OC. Nanoparticles in medicine: therapeutic applications and developments. Clin Pharmacol Ther 2008; 83(5): 761-9.
[http://dx.doi.org/10.1038/sj.clpt.6100400] [PMID: 17957183]

[14] Nasirizadeh N, Asadi P, Karami A, *et al.* Green synthesis of nanoparticles and their biomedical applications. Environ Chem Lett 2020; 18: 703-27.
[http://dx.doi.org/10.1007/s10311-020-00984-0] [PMID: 32206050]

[15] Ahmed S, Saifullah , Ahmad M, Swami BL, Ikram S. Green synthesis of silver nanoparticles using Azadirachta indica aqueous leaf extract. Journal of Radiation Research and Applied Sciences 2016; 9(1): 1-7.
[http://dx.doi.org/10.1016/j.jrras.2015.06.006]

[16] Li D, Xia Y. Electrospinning of nanofibers: Reinventing the wheel? Adv Mater 2004; 16(14): 1151-70.
[http://dx.doi.org/10.1002/adma.200400719]

[17] Fessi H, Puisieux F, Devissaguet JP, Ammoury N, Benita S. Nanocapsule formation by interfacial polymer deposition following solvent displacement. Int J Pharm 1989; 55(1): R1-4.
[http://dx.doi.org/10.1016/0378-5173(89)90281-0]

[18] Reimer L. Transmission Electron Microscopy: Physics of Image Formation and Microanalysis. 5th ed., Berlin: Springer 2012.

[19] Binnig G, Quate CF, Gerber C. Atomic force microscope. Phys Rev Lett 1986; 56(9): 930-3.
[http://dx.doi.org/10.1103/PhysRevLett.56.930] [PMID: 10033323]

[20] Stuart B. Infrared Spectroscopy: Fundamentals and Applications. 1st ed., Hoboken: Wiley 2004.
[http://dx.doi.org/10.1002/0470011149]

[21] Jain PK, Huang X, El-Sayed IH, El-Sayed MA. Noble metals on the nanoscale: optical and photothermal properties and some applications in imaging, sensing, biology, and medicine. Acc Chem Res 2008; 41(12): 1578-86.
[http://dx.doi.org/10.1021/ar7002804] [PMID: 18447366]

[22] Briggs D, Seah MP. Practical Surface Analysis by Auger and X-ray Photoelectron Spectroscopy. Chichester: Wiley 1990.

[23] Hunter RJ. Zeta Potential in Colloid Science: Principles and Applications. London: Academic Press 1981.

[24] Cullity BD, Stock SR. Elements of X-Ray Diffraction. 3rd ed., Boston: Addison-Wesley 2001.

[25] Zetasizer Nano Series User Manual. Worcestershire, UK: Malvern Instruments 2013.

[26] Lakowicz JR. Principles of Fluorescence Spectroscopy. 3rd ed., New York: Springer 2006. [http://dx.doi.org/10.1007/978-0-387-46312-4]

[27] Aslan B, Ozpolat B, Sood AK, Lopez-Berestein G. Nanotechnology in cancer therapy. J Drug Target 2013; 21(10): 904-13. [http://dx.doi.org/10.3109/1061186X.2013.837469] [PMID: 24079419]

[28] Yechezkel B, Liposome application: problems and prospects,Current Opinion in Colloid & Interface Science,2021;6((1):66-77.

[29] Prabhu S, Poulose EK. Silver nanoparticles: mechanism of antimicrobial action, synthesis, medical applications, and toxicity effects. Int Nano Lett 2012; 2(1): 32. [http://dx.doi.org/10.1186/2228-5326-2-32]

[30] Rai M, Yadav A, Gade A. Silver nanoparticles as a new generation of antimicrobials. Biotechnol Adv 2009; 27(1): 76-83. [http://dx.doi.org/10.1016/j.biotechadv.2008.09.002] [PMID: 18854209]

[31] Bondarenko O, Mortimer M, Kahru A, *et al.* Nanotoxicology and nanomedicine: The Yin and Yang of nano-bio interactions for the new decade. Nano Today 2021; 39: 101184. [http://dx.doi.org/10.1016/j.nantod.2021.101184] [PMID: 36937379]

[32] Hu J, Arvejeh PM, Bone S, Hett E, Marincola FM, Roh KH. Nanocarriers for cutting-edge cancer immunotherapies. J Transl Med 2025; 23(1): 447. [http://dx.doi.org/10.1186/s12967-025-06435-0] [PMID: 40234928]

[33] Choi YS, Lee MY, David AE, Park YS. Nanoparticles for gene delivery: therapeutic and toxic effects. Mol Cell Toxicol 2014; 10(1): 1-8. [http://dx.doi.org/10.1007/s13273-014-0001-3]

[34] Liu Q, Zou J, Chen Z, He W, Wu W. Current research trends of nanomedicines. Acta Pharm Sin B 2023; 13(11): 4391-416. [http://dx.doi.org/10.1016/j.apsb.2023.05.018] [PMID: 37969727]

[35] Huang X, Jain PK, El-Sayed IH, El-Sayed MA. Plasmonic photothermal therapy (PPTT) using gold nanoparticles. Lasers Med Sci 2008; 23(3): 217-28. [http://dx.doi.org/10.1007/s10103-007-0470-x] [PMID: 17674122]

[36] Han X, Feng G, Li X, *et al.* Functional nanomaterials for enhanced tumor photothermal therapy - the mechanisms and applications. Front Pharmacol 2025; 16: 1604965. [http://dx.doi.org/10.3389/fphar.2025.1604965] [PMID: 40727107]

[37] Ali MS, Gupta G, Alsayari A, Wahab S, Kesharwani P. Biotinylated nanoparticles: A new frontier in nanomedicine and targeted cancer therapy. Biomaterials Advances 2025; 176: 214366. [http://dx.doi.org/10.1016/j.bioadv.2025.214366] [PMID: 40479769]

[38] Markman JL, Rekechenetskiy A, Holler E, Ljubimova JY. Nanomedicine therapeutic approaches to overcome cancer drug resistance. Adv Drug Deliv Rev 2013; 65(13-14): 1866-79. [http://dx.doi.org/10.1016/j.addr.2013.09.019] [PMID: 24120656]

[39] Panyam J, Labhasetwar V. Biodegradable nanoparticles for drug and gene delivery to cells and tissue. Adv Drug Deliv Rev 2003; 55(3): 329-47. [http://dx.doi.org/10.1016/S0169-409X(02)00228-4] [PMID: 12628320]

[40] Moghimi SM, Hunter AC, Murray JC. Nanomedicine: Current status and future prospects. FASEB J 2013; 27(3): 1007-19.
[PMID: 15746175]

[41] Wang F, Liang L, Wang C, *et al.* Non-Viral Gene Delivery Systems: Current Advances and Therapeutic Applications. Chem Asian J 2025; 20(20): e00684.
[http://dx.doi.org/10.1002/asia.202500684] [PMID: 40874945]

[42] Wang L, Hu C, Shao L. The antimicrobial activity of nanoparticles: present situation and prospects for the future. Int J Nanomedicine 2017; 12: 1227-49.
[http://dx.doi.org/10.2147/IJN.S121956] [PMID: 28243086]

[43] Niżnik Ł, Noga M, Kobylarz D, *et al.* Gold Nanoparticles (AuNPs)—Toxicity, Safety and Green Synthesis: A Critical Review. Int J Mol Sci 2024; 25(7): 4057.
[http://dx.doi.org/10.3390/ijms25074057] [PMID: 38612865]

[44] Sun C, Lee JSH, Zhang M. Magnetic nanoparticles in MR imaging and drug delivery. Adv Drug Del Rev 2008; 60(11): 1252-65.
[http://dx.doi.org/10.1016/j.addr.2008.03.018]

[45] Wang Q, Wang X, Feng Y. Chitosan Hydrogel as Tissue Engineering Scaffolds for Vascular Regeneration Applications. Gels 2023; 9(5): 373.
[http://dx.doi.org/10.3390/gels9050373] [PMID: 37232967]

[46] Etheridge ML, Campbell SA, Erdman AG, Haynes CL, Wolf SM, McCullough J. The big picture on nanomedicine: the state of investigational and approved nanomedicine products. Nanomedicine 2013; 9(1): 1-14.
[http://dx.doi.org/10.1016/j.nano.2012.05.013] [PMID: 22684017]

[47] Halamoda-Kenzaoui B, Holzwarth U, Roebben G, Bogni A, Bremer-Hoffmann S. Mapping of the available standards against the regulatory needs for nanomedicines. Wiley Interdiscip Rev Nanomed Nanobiotechnol 2019; 11(1): e1531.
[http://dx.doi.org/10.1002/wnan.1531] [PMID: 29923692]

[48] Fadeel B, Farcal L, Hardy B, *et al.* Advanced tools for the safety assessment of nanomaterials. Nat Nanotechnol 2018; 13(7): 537-43.
[http://dx.doi.org/10.1038/s41565-018-0185-0] [PMID: 29980781]

[49] Hurst SJ. Biomedical Nanotechnology. Methods Mol Biol 2011; 726: 1-13.
[http://dx.doi.org/10.1007/978-1-61779-052-2_1] [PMID: 21424439]

[50] Oberdörster G, Oberdörster E, Oberdörster J. Nanotoxicology: an emerging discipline evolving from studies of ultrafine particles. Environ Health Perspect 2005; 113(7): 823-39.
[http://dx.doi.org/10.1289/ehp.7339] [PMID: 16002369]

[51] de Jong WH, Borm PJ. Drug delivery and nanoparticles: Applications and hazards. Int J Nanomedicine 2008; 3(2): 133-49.
[http://dx.doi.org/10.2147/IJN.S596] [PMID: 18686775]

[52] Donaldson K, Poland CA, Schins RPF. Possible genotoxic mechanisms of nanoparticles: Criteria for improved test strategies. Nanotoxicology 2010; 4(4): 414-20.
[http://dx.doi.org/10.3109/17435390.2010.482751] [PMID: 20925449]

[53] Allhoff F, Lin P, Moor JH, Weckert J. 2007. Nanoethics: The ethical and social implications of nanotechnology. John Wiley & Sons; 2007 Aug 10.

[54] Shepherd CCJ, Li J, Cooper MN, Hopkins KD, Farrant BM. The impact of racial discrimination on the health of Australian Indigenous children aged 5–10 years: analysis of national longitudinal data. Int J Equity Health 2017; 16(1): 116.
[http://dx.doi.org/10.1186/s12939-017-0612-0] [PMID: 28673295]

[55] Matteucci F, Giannantonio R, Calabi F, Agostiano A, Gigli G, Rossi M. Deployment and exploitation

of nanotechnology nanomaterials and nanomedicine. AIP Conf Proc 2018; 020001. [http://dx.doi.org/10.1063/1.5047755]

[56] Guidance D. Guidance for industry considering whether an FDA-regulated product involves the application of nanotechnology. Biotechnol Law Rep 2011; 30(5): 613-6. [http://dx.doi.org/10.1089/blr.2011.9814]

CHAPTER 2

Nanobiomedicine: Fundamentals and Implementation in Theranostic Applications

Pratik Talukder[1,*], Sreejita Das[2], Mrinmoy Dasgupta[1], Aniket Hazra[1], Sayantan Biawas[1], Swastika Mohanta[1], Sayantika Hore[1] and **Milan Karmakar[1]**

[1] *Department of Biotechnology, Institute of Engineering and Management, New Town, University of Engineering & Management, Kolkata, India*

[2] *Department of Botany, University of Calcutta, Kolkata, West Bengal, India*

Abstract: In recent years, nanobiomedicine has emerged as a transformative approach to addressing challenges in diagnosis and therapy. Nanoparticles can act as a vector for drugs and genes in the treatment of various diseases. Their high surface area-to-volume ratio is a positive factor, as it allows the drug- or gene-conjugated nanoparticles to traverse cell membranes and access intracellular targets. Functionalized nanoparticles can target specific cells using receptor-specific recognition, thereby minimizing off-target effects. Degradation of drugs is common in conventional delivery methods, but nanoparticles help prevent this by encapsulating or shielding the drug formulations. In addition to the aforementioned benefits, nanoparticles can be used to integrate therapy and diagnostics into a single platform, known as theranostics, enabling precise treatment and monitoring of diseases. Both imaging agents and therapeutic molecules (drugs, DNA, and RNA) can be carried by nanoparticles, whose multifunctionality enables simultaneous disease imaging and treatment, reducing the need for separate interventions. Currently, studies are being conducted worldwide on the theranostic potential of nanoparticles under various conditions, ranging from cancer therapy and treatment of genetic disorders to vaccine development, which speaks volumes about their capabilities. In this chapter, we review various nanoparticles used for drug and gene delivery alongside commonly utilized imaging techniques for theranostic applications.

Keywords: Biosensors, DNA, Gene therapy, Nanobiomedicine, Nanomaterials, Point-of-care devices, RNA detection, Targeted drug delivery.

* **Corresponding author Pratik Talukder:** Department of Biotechnology, Institute of Engineering and Management, New Town, University of Engineering & Management, Kolkata, India; E-mail: pratik.talukder@uem.edu.in

Soumik Podder & Amalesh Samanta (Eds.)

INTRODUCTION

A fundamental benefit of nanotechnology in medicine is the nanoscale size of the particles, which generally range from 1 to 100 nm. This small size allows nanoparticles to easily penetrate human cells, making them especially efficient in targeted drug delivery as well as disease detection. Moreover, nanoparticles function as a protective armor around therapeutic agents, preventing their degradation in the blood by the time they reach the target site. Nanoparticles, designed with antibodies or other biomolecules, help in the precise targeting of diseased cells while sparing healthy tissues, thereby reducing systemic side effects [1]. There are many types of nanoparticles, like liposomes, polymeric nanoparticles, dendrimers, gold nanoparticles, and quantum dots, which are now widely used for diagnostic purposes [2].

Modern drug delivery systems based on nanotechnology address many limitations of traditional therapies by enhancing efficacy and reducing side effects. For example, ions have great potential in targeted drug delivery with applications in cancer treatment. Such nanoparticles can exhibit high binding efficiency and be magnetically guided to specific locations in the body. Functionalization of ions with antimicrobial peptides, such as lasioglossin III from bee venom, exhibits enhanced antimicrobial activity, and the cationic nature of these peptides improves the potential for binding. Studies have shown that drug-loaded nanoparticles exhibit enhanced antimicrobial activity and reduced cytotoxicity compared to free drugs, making them promising candidates for controlled and precise drug delivery [3]. The nano-bio interface has also transformed personalized medicine, enabling highly precise therapeutic interventions. The leading players in this transformation are multifunctional nanoparticles, capable of simultaneously delivering and imaging drugs. These so-called "theranostic" nanoparticles enable real-time monitoring of treatment responses, thereby enhancing the efficacy of therapies while simultaneously reducing systemic toxicity. The same principles that underlie the development of nanoparticle-based platforms for vaccines emphasize the enhancement of antigen delivery and immune stimulation. Such approaches have proven to be particularly effective in generating robust and durable immune responses against infectious diseases and cancers. Additionally, antimicrobial nanomaterials primarily aid in infection control, while nanovaccines and prophylactic drug delivery systems help mitigate the spread of infectious agents, underscoring the versatility of nanotechnology in addressing global health challenges [4].

Although the toxicity of nanomaterials remains a significant consideration in their biomedical applications, the cytotoxicity of nanoparticles proves invaluable for targeting cancer cells, whereas uncontrolled exposure can affect healthy tissues.

Thus, it has become very important to understand nanotoxicity in designing safer nanomaterials. Recent advances in nanotoxicity research have led to the development of this aspect of nanomaterials, where surface modifications, biodegradable materials, and functional coatings are being used to minimize adverse effects. These strategies ensure selective toxicity to diseased cells while maintaining biocompatibility. Such advances are pivotal in developing safe and effective nanobiomedicine solutions for treating complex diseases, such as cancer [5]. Nanocarrier technologies have proven vital in overcoming many limitations associated with conventional drug delivery. Among these nanocarriers, those with unique physicochemical properties are used to treat a wide range of conditions, from microbial infections to genetic disorders and cancers. Despite this tremendous potential, challenges are still related to the limited drug capacity of these nanocarriers, poor solubility, and suboptimal targeting. Innovations in nanocarrier systems, such as micelles, hydrogels, nanocomposites, and microneedles, could address such issues. Advanced features that allow sustained drug release, increased solubility, and responsive releasing mechanisms have made these systems indispensable in modern medicine. An example is the combination of multiple material properties that gives nanocomposites superior functionality, while hydrogels represent a versatile platform for encapsulating and releasing drugs. Microneedles are an innovative method for delivering drugs and vaccines in a minimally invasive way while maintaining efficacy and patient compliance [6].

Another very intriguing innovation in this field of nanotechnology and biomedical science is autonomous nanobiomedicine. Currently, it is becoming possible to eliminate external intervention by launching nanoparticles that can autonomously navigate the body and release therapeutic agents with precision and control. Such interfacial engineering between nanoscale tools and disease detection and treatment processes of autonomous nanobiomedicine promotes the possibility of rapid, personalized assessment and intervention. However, before successful translation to the clinic, there are concerns regarding reproducibility and safety, as well as regulatory hurdles. Prerequisites for understanding the behaviour of autonomous systems include appropriate preclinical studies for the safe application of them in patients. One factor that would determine the success of such a promising field is finding the right balance between innovation and patient safety [7]. The advanced properties, such as high surface-to-volume ratios and a balance of strength and flexibility, of nanomaterials have been exceedingly useful in medicine. These nanomaterials are utilized in disease diagnosis kits in an easy and non-invasive manner, serve as bioimaging agents in biological imaging, and are incorporated into formulations for therapeutic purposes. Liposomal nanocarriers, for example, encapsulate drugs for targeted delivery, while nano-based scaffolds are engineered to enhance bone tissue regeneration. Improvements in biocompatibility and stability make it possible to obtain better treatment outcomes and expand the scope of medical applications [8]. AI-powered nanomedicine accelerates personalized drug delivery, diagnostics, and theranostics by enabling the logical design of smart nanoparticles—optimizing size, surface chemistry, targeting efficiency, and toxicity through machine learning. AI enhances the synthesis of nanoparticles, forecasts nanobio interactions, and directs self-governing nanorobots for the management of infectious diseases and precision oncology.

Therapeutic Nanobiomedicine: Targeted Drug Delivery

Therapeutic nanobiomedicine opens the way for a whole novel approach to the challenge in drug delivery and cancer treatment, especially aggressive cancer subtypes like HER2-positive [HER2+] tumors. Such tumors are therapy-resistant, exhibit a high rate of recurrence, and correspond to a poor prognosis in comparison with conventional treatments. Enhanced drug targeting, modulated TME, and diagnostic-therapeutic functionality combined with nanotechnology have prompted further development of advanced nanobiomedicine platforms. This chapter discusses the applications of biomimetic nanoplatforms, modulation of the tumor microenvironment, theranostic systems, and photothermal innovation in treating HER2+ tumors and other solid malignancies, addressing the challenges and opportunities this approach poses for clinical translation. A promising area of therapeutic nanobiomedicine is the integration of biomimetic drug delivery. By mimicking elements of biological systems using synthetic components, these drug delivery systems promise to target the location of interest with greater precision and amplify drug efficacy. A prime example is a nanoplatform consisting of PLGA nanoparticles encapsulating chemotherapeutic agents, such as doxorubicin [DOX] or near-infrared dyes. These nanoparticles are coated with engineered macrophage membranes that have been modified to express anti-HER2 affibodies, which specifically target HER2+ tumor cells. Compared to traditional macrophage-coated nanoparticles, these advanced platforms demonstrate superior pharmacokinetics and higher tumor accumulation, as confirmed through *in vivo* imaging studies [9]. Mechanistically, these nanoparticles result in the inhibition of tumor growth *via* the induction of apoptosis and inhibition of the PI3K/AKT pathway. These provide promising prospects for targeted, synergistic treatment of cancer. Biomimetic systems have been created as templates for multifunctional nanoplatforms that potentially overcome the deficits associated with traditional treatments. Another emerging area in nanobiomedicine relates to the modulation of the TME. The TME is a complex network of cancer cells, immune cells, stromal cells, and extracellular matrix that significantly plays a role in tumor progression, invasion, and resistance to therapy. One of the integral components of the TME, TAMs, could thus be therapeutically reprogrammed to exhibit tumor-suppressing properties. Nanoparticle-based strategies for modulating TAMs include reprogramming macrophages from the pro-tumorigenic M2 phenotype to the anti-tumorigenic M1 phenotype, depletion of TAMs, inhibition of the recruitment of monocytic myeloid-derived suppressor cells, and delivery of immune checkpoint inhibitors. All these may potentially result in the transformation of an immunosuppressive environment into an immunostimulatory one, leading to improved therapeutic agents for cancer immunotherapy [10, 11]. Microvesicles released from macrophages have also been explored as drug delivery vehicles to take advantage of their intrinsic ability to target inflammatory sites and improve the localization and release of drugs within tumors. These advances highlight the potential of nanobiomedicine in redirecting TME for improved therapeutic benefits [12]. Theranostics, the integration of therapy and diagnostics, represents a groundbreaking innovation in nanobiomedicine. For instance, biomimetic decomposable nanotheranostics, such as MMV-Au-C-s-DOX, which utilize macrophage-derived microvesicles, are employed for tumor-specific drug delivery. They utilize TME-specific stimuli, such as high glutathione [GSH] levels, to trigger nanoparticles to disintegrate into functional parts. This targeted approach helps realize multimodal therapies, such as chemotherapy and chemodynamic therapy, while monitoring chemotherapy resistance in parallel through fluorescence-based GSH detection. By combining therapeutic and diagnostic capabilities, theranostic platforms effectively overcome challenges, such as low targeting, early clearance, and multidrug resistance, thereby advancing precision oncology [13, 14]. Photothermal therapy [PTT] is one of the alternative treatments that accompany traditional cancer therapies, particularly for deep-seated tumors. By using the second near-infrared [NIR-II] bio window, PTT provides deep biological penetration and minimal off-target effects. Recently, substantial progress has been made in the MXene-based photothermal agents, which exhibit tunable light absorption and excellent photon-to-thermal conversion efficiency. Specifically, anionic regulation within the MXene framework maximizes light-harvesting capabilities, thus optimizing the efficacy of tumor eradication at low nano-drug dosages [15]. In fact, by encapsulating photothermal agents within an imaging modality, such as photoacoustic [PA] imaging, real-time monitoring and targeted therapy of tumors are feasible. These innovations demonstrate that PTT can be utilized to improve the treatment outcome while minimizing the adverse long-term effects associated with high doses of medication. Although such a significant success has been achieved, the medical translation of nanobiomedicine remains challenging. Barriers include challenges in designing nanoparticles, scaling up their production, and potential systemic toxicity. Ensuring biocompatibility and stability of nanoparticles within the human body is essential for their use in clinical applications. The need for personalized nanobiomedicine strategies for different types of cancer, the heterogeneous nature of the TME, and variability among patients requires the development and synthesis of completely novel nanoparticles. However, optimizing nanoparticle design and function will be necessary to solve these challenges in an interdisciplinary manner, incorporating cutting-edge technologies, such as AI and gene editing [9].

Nanoparticles in Gene Therapy

Gene therapy, on the other hand, is a technique where vectors or systems carrying engineered genetic constructs are employed to repair or modify genes in genetic and acquired disorders. The majority of gene delivery therapeutics utilize viral vectors due to their high efficiency. Despite the high efficiency of viral vectors, there is also a high probability of them inducing immunogenicity or causing insertional mutagenesis. For this reason, non-viral vectors like lipid nanoparticles [LNPs] offer more safety and biocompatibility. LNPs have played a pivotal role in gene delivery since their introduction by Felgner *et al.* in 1987 [16]. These lipids are designed to form complexes with negatively charged nucleic acids, such as DNA or RNA [17]. Solid Lipid Nanoparticles [SLNs] offer advantages over liposomes and nanoemulsions, including protection of active ingredients, modulated release profiles, long-term stability, and compatibility with sterilization and lyophilization techniques. They are typically under 500 nm and possess a solid lipid core and a surfactant layer, which are usually cationic for nucleic acid binding. Nucleic acids get electrostatically condensed by them, providing protection from degradation [18]. A study conducted by Truong *et al.* [19] demonstrated the usage of LNPs to encapsulate Arginase (ARG1) mRNA for systemic administration in a murine model of ARG1 deficiency. LNPs were administered every three days, leading to remarkable outcomes. Treated mice showed 100% survival beyond 11 weeks, compared to controls, whereas control mice died by day 22. Plasma ammonia, arginine, and glutamine levels were effectively normalized, with no accumulation of neurotoxic guanidino compounds. Liver arginase activity reached 54% of wild-type levels, restoring near-normal urea cycle function and enabling successful metabolism of toxic ammonium challenges. Importantly, the nanoparticle delivery system demonstrated excellent safety, with no evidence of hepatotoxicity or adverse effects, emphasizing the massive potential of LNPs in human gene and mRNA therapy.

As depicted in Fig. (**1**), there are various kinds of nanoparticles that are routinely used in gene therapy and drug delivery studies. Polymers are another widely used category of nanocarriers for drug and gene delivery due to their versatility, biodegradability, and ease of synthesis. Naturally occurring polymers like cellulose and lignin, along with synthetic polymers, such as PLA, PLGA, and

PCA, offer tailored structures for efficient gene delivery while minimizing toxicity. Biodegradable polymers like PLGA degrade into natural metabolites, ensuring safe elimination, and have been used in clinical trials for brain tumor therapies. Polymers like PEG enable facile functionalization and stability, supporting advancements in green nanotechnology. The scalable production of polymer nanoparticles (PNPs) has advanced with the integration of automation and optimized techniques, such as emulsification and nanoprecipitation, thereby improving consistency and reducing costs. These innovations have expanded the applications of PNP in gene therapy, bioimaging, and the treatment of complex diseases. Other commonly used nanoparticles in gene therapy include peptide-based NPs and inorganic NPs.

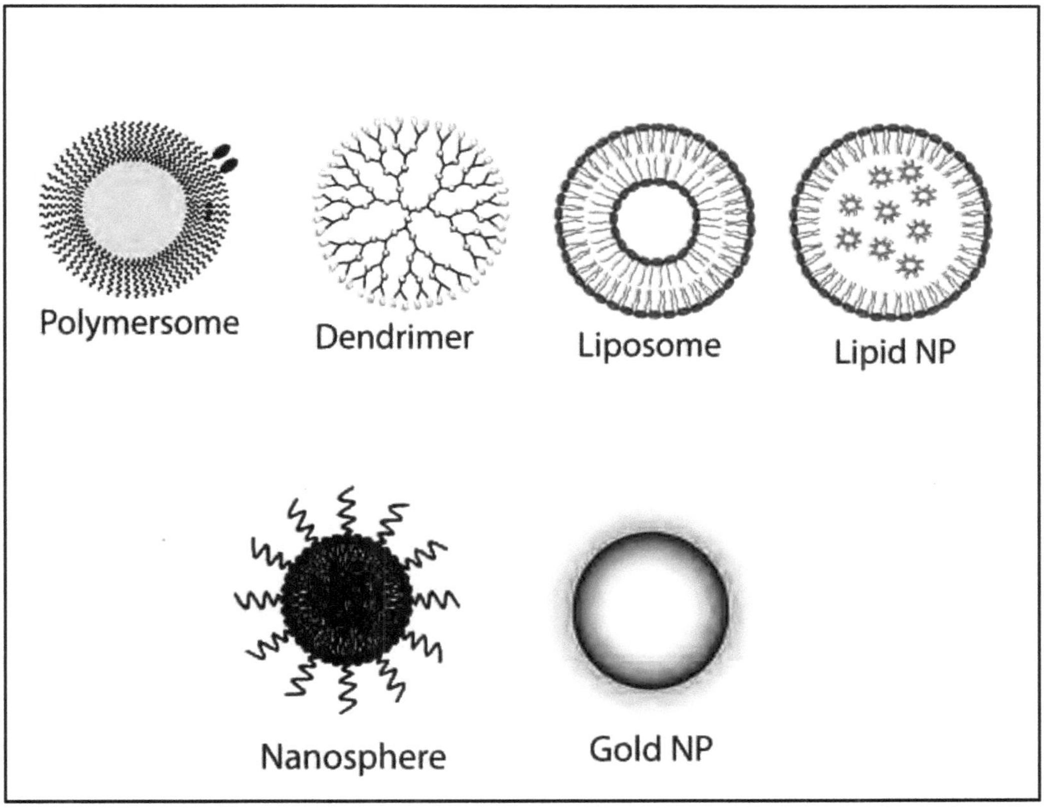

Fig. (1). The figure illustrates the structural diversity of nanocarriers, including polymersomes, dendrimers, liposomes, lipid nanoparticles (NPs), nanospheres, and gold nanoparticles. These systems are widely employed for improving the precision, stability, and efficiency of therapeutic and gene delivery applications [2].

Gold NPs are among the most popular inorganic nanocarriers as they are non-toxic, biocompatible, and detectable by various spectroscopic methods, including

Rayleigh spectroscopy [20]. One significant study reported the delivery of 2-kDa polyethyleneimine in the cornea of rabbits (*in vivo*) and human corneas (*in vitro*) using gold nanoparticles [21]. The successful uptake of gold NPs was identified using Transmission Electron Microscopy (TEM). Transgene delivery at high concentrations resulted in several negative effects, including moderate keratocyte apoptosis and reduced cellular density. The findings demonstrated that gold nanoparticles are bioinert, safe, and effective for corneal gene delivery.

While nanoparticle-mediated gene therapy is an experimental field, numerous pre-clinical and clinical studies have reported the potential of NPs in successfully delivering genes and mRNAs. Further research is required until nanoparticles can be established as a common vector in large-scale therapies.

Nanotechnology in Disease Diagnosis

Early and accurate disease diagnosis is a crucial step in protecting public health and achieving optimal clinical outcomes; it is, therefore, an essential component in ensuring that proper medical treatment is provided. The process involves establishing the nature or cause of a disease, analyzing the patient's medical history, and interpreting all relevant lab findings [22]. Diagnosis must be rapid, accurate, and specific to minimize the possibility of false positives and false negatives. The high sensitivity and specificity of diagnostic tools enable the earlier identification of diseases, thereby maximizing the success of treatment and improving patients' prognosis. Rapid and precise identification of illnesses, infections, and organ dysfunction is made possible by AI-driven diagnostics, which utilize machine learning and deep learning to evaluate clinical records, omics data, and medical images. By reducing diagnostic errors and shortening the time to treatment, these tools enhance risk prediction, facilitate early detection, and enable individualized care. The advances in diagnostic technology have an immediate impact on the general health of populations, so innovation in this domain is an important goal of modern applied science. Researchers in the field of biotechnology are working on the development of fast, accurate, portable, and inexpensive diagnostic devices to enable patients to monitor their own health [23].

A wide range of assays and techniques have been commonly used for disease diagnosis, such as immunoassays, genetic testing, medical imaging, and biosensing methods. Commonly employed diagnostic bioassays include polymerase chain reaction (PCR) for genetic analysis, enzyme-linked immunosorbent assay (ELISA) for detecting specific proteins, and staining techniques like Gram and Giemsa staining for identifying bacterial and viral infections [24]. Traditional detection techniques have several disadvantages, including low sensitivity, low specificity, and limited addressing capability.

Nanotechnology addresses these limitations through the unique properties of nanoparticles, such as an extremely high surface area-to-volume ratio, tunable surface chemistry, and the ability to interact specifically with biological molecules. These features have led to revolutionary improvements in diagnostic tools, offering enhanced sensitivity, specificity, and functionality. Nanostructured materials, therefore, hold great promise for the future of diagnostics [25]. The convergence of nanotechnology with fields, such as genomics, proteomics, and molecular machinery, makes it efficient and reliable to have on-site diagnostic tools. Nanotechnology is transforming these fields by providing avenues for the development of new materials used in medical diagnostic devices [26].

Techniques that facilitate health, science, and diagnosis with nanotechnology encompass nanobiosensors, imaging techniques, point-of-care devices, and DNA-RNA detections. These techniques have potentially paved a better and more advanced path for the medical world [27].

Biosensors

They comprise bio-receptors that identify the target molecules, transducers that convert biological interactions into observable signals, and a signal-reading device that analyzes the data for interpretation. Analytical devices, such as biosensors, have become a cutting-edge tool with remarkable precision in sensitivity for the detection of disease biomarkers. The biological sensing elements, coupled with nanoscale materials, are used to identify specific molecules, such as proteins, metabolites, and nucleic acids, that are related to different devices. This tool has been applied in various fields, including cancer diagnostics for the identification of circulating tumor cells, DNA mutations, and proteins. Attached with antibodies, gold nanoparticles can identify the tumor-specific antigens with high accuracy. Graphene-based sensors can also detect cancer biomarkers like HER2 present in breast cancer patients, which facilitates early diagnosis and aids in treatment [28]. Detection of infectious diseases using plasmonic biosensors that can detect viral RNA to diagnose COVID-19, and magnetic nanoparticle-based systems that can be used to isolate and identify bacteria in blood samples, can also be used to expedite the diagnosis of sepsis or tuberculosis. Neurological diseases, such as Alzheimer's or Parkinson's, are often identified by the detection of particular proteins in blood or cerebrospinal fluid. Nanobiosensors further enhance this capability with high sensitivity in detecting biomarkers, such as beta-amyloid peptides and tau proteins [29]. Nanobiosensors facilitate the early diagnosis of heart conditions by detecting biomarkers, including troponin, a specific protein released during heart attacks. With the use of nanotechnology in point-of-care devices, results may be available in a matter of minutes, saving valuable emergency time. Glucose monitoring systems incorporating nanobiosensors are more efficient than conventional methods. For instance, graphene-based sensors offer non-invasive monitoring by detecting glucose levels in sweat or saliva.

Imaging Techniques

Conventional imaging technologies, X-rays, MRI, and CT, often fail to detect diseases at earlier stages and also do not deliver detailed molecular-level information. The presence of such specific properties in nanomaterials has improved contrast and enabled targeted imaging, as well as the opportunity to facilitate *in situ* and real-time monitoring of disease progression by overcoming these limitations. Supermagnetic iron oxide nanoparticles serve as contrast agents in MRI. They enhance resolutions and detect lesions or tiny tumors of such an early stage that may not be visible otherwise. These SPIONs can be functionalized with antibodies or peptides to specifically target tissues, such as cancer cells or inflamed areas. The potential of CT imaging by gold nanoparticles is based on their absorption properties towards X-rays. Quantum dots exhibit intense and stable fluorescence, which facilitates the visualization of biological processes at the cellular or subcellular level, thereby improving optical imaging. Radiolabeled nanoparticles enhance the sensitivity of PET imaging by enabling the precise detection of molecular targets. Nanoparticles carrying radioisotopes can locate and image tumors, thus offering critical information about their metabolic activity and spread. Nanotechnology-enhanced ultrasound contrast is achieved using microbubbles or gas-loaded nanoparticles [30]. These agents enhance the signal, leading to improved visualization of blood flow, vascular structures, and tissue abnormalities. Functionalized nanoparticles with ligands, antibodies, or nucleic acids enable imaging of molecular-level changes associated with diseases. This is essential for understanding disease mechanisms and responses to therapy [31].

Point-of-Care Devices

Nanotechnology has also led to the development of portable diagnostic devices that yield results promptly. In lateral flow assays, which resemble home pregnancy tests, nanoparticles are now utilized to enhance their sensitivity. These devices are crucial for rapid tests used to diagnose HIV, tuberculosis, COVID-19, malaria, and many other diseases, which are critical in controlling outbreaks. Portable nucleic acid-based tests allow pathogens to be quickly detected in resource-limited settings. Devices, such as glucose meters for diabetes, INR meters for blood clotting, and cholesterol monitors, make it possible to manage the disease continuously. Biomarkers that can be measured with POC devices include troponin for the detection of heart attacks or monitoring of blood pressure and heart rate. Tests for human chorionic gonadotropin levels detect pregnancy, while ovulation kits assist with fertility tracking. Liquid biopsy-based POC devices detect circulating tumor DNA (ctDNA) or cancer biomarkers for the early detection of cancer. Electrolyte and lactate rapid tests, as well as infection tests, offer critical information in emergency rooms and intensive care units [32].

DNA and RNA Detection

Another area where nanotechnology excels is in the detection of genetic material specific to pathogens or disease-associated mutations. Nanoparticles can be functionalized with strands of complementary DNA or RNA for capturing target sequences. Techniques such as nano-plasmonic arrays and nanopore sequencing enable precise and rapid genetic analysis, which can lead to the early detection of diseases like COVID-19 and hereditary disorders.

CHALLENGES AND FUTURE TRENDS IN NANOBIOMEDICINE

Nanobiomedicine has the potential to enhance/change healthcare, but it is encumbered by pressing issues. The large extent of the problem lies in the complexity of NPs' behavior in biological systems and their potential for unwanted toxicity or interaction with the immune system. Safety improvements focus on biodegradable materials, green synthesis approaches, and knowledge of nanoparticle pharmacodynamics and pharmacokinetics. Nevertheless, these attempts are limited by the need for detailed, patient-specific experimental data, especially for delivery mechanisms, such as the EPR effect, which has been found to be variable in clinical settings [33]. Regulatory and manufacturing barriers further hinder progress. Additionally, current frameworks often lack clarity on evaluating the safety and efficacy of nanobiomedicine, while scaling up production to ensure uniformity and cost-effectiveness remains a significant challenge. Intellectual property concerns and high development costs also slow down commercialization.

Future developments in nanobiomedicine focus on incorporating new technologies and advancements. Artificial intelligence (AI) and machine learning (ML) are increasingly crucial in enhancing nanoparticle design, forecasting toxicity, and customizing therapies. Utilizing advancements in gene editing, such as CRISPR-Cas9, may lead to more targeted and accurate treatment options [34]. Furthermore, theranostic platforms that combine diagnostics and therapeutics are becoming increasingly popular for the real-time monitoring and effective treatment of diseases, such as cancer.

Advancements in active targeting systems, utilizing ligands, such as antibodies and peptides, for precise nanoparticle delivery, offer improved effectiveness. Innovative methods in photothermal therapy, which utilize substances, such as iron oxide nanoparticles and MXenes, offer non-invasive treatment options that minimize systemic side effects. Collaboration across disciplines is essential for addressing these challenges, maintaining a balance between innovation and patient safety, and successfully transitioning nanobiomedicine from research to widespread clinical application.

Regulatory translation of nanobiomedicine remains a significant challenge. Organizations, such as the U.S. Food and Drug Administration (FDA) and the European Medicines Agency (EMA), require a thorough assessment of nanomaterials for toxicity, biodistribution, pharmacokinetics, and long-term safety to ensure approval. Yet, there are no generally accepted standards for characterizing nanocarriers, particularly multifunctional platforms, such as theranostics, which are capable of functioning as both drug and diagnostic agents [35]. This absence of definitive classification makes regulatory approval more challenging, as these systems often fall between the definitions of drug, device, or combination products in regulatory regulations [36]. In addition, interspecies variation in EPR effect and immune reactions between animal and human models makes it challenging to translate successful preclinical experience to clinical outcomes [37]. For example, a study indicated that as little as 0.7% of the injected nanoparticles penetrate solid tumors in humans, which is much lower than preclinical expectations [38].

CONCLUSION

Nanobiomedicine stands at the forefront of a new era in precision healthcare, offering multidimensional solutions for both therapeutic and diagnostic challenges. For a holistic understanding of this chapter, theranostic systems transform disease monitoring into real-time capabilities, gene therapy, and targeted drug delivery using engineered nanoparticles. Nanobiomedicine enables improved outcomes in treatment and minimizes off-target effects by integrating biomimetic platforms, modulating the tumor microenvironment (TME), and utilizing advanced imaging techniques, offering a level of control and specificity previously unattainable in conventional medicine.

Furthermore, in gene therapy, the application of non-viral nanocarriers, such as lipid nanoparticles (LNPs), polymeric nanoparticles, and gold nanostructures, suggests that they offer a safer, more efficient alternative to conventional viral vectors. They minimize immunogenic responses while providing strong protection to nucleic acids, thus leading to some promising results within preclinical disease models. In diagnostics, nanotechnology has enabled the creation of both biosensors and imaging agents with unmatched sensitivity and specificity, allowing for early disease detection, real-time monitoring, and treatment regimens customized based on individual patient profiles. The rise of personalized medicine benefits greatly from this advancement.

Nanotechnology is integrating with artificial intelligence (AI), machine learning (ML), gene editing tools (*e.g.*, CRISPR-Cas9), and point-of-care (POC) technologies. This convergence marks a shift in the medical science model. These integrations enable researchers to refine nanoparticle design and achieve therapeutic precision, also allowing them to model predictively, provide real-time feedback, and strategize therapeutically and adaptively.

Even with progress like this, the clinic still faces challenges in translating nanobiomedicine due to key barriers. These include nanoparticle toxicity concerns, unpredictable interactions with the immune system, patient response heterogeneity, and large-scale manufacturing challenges, as well as the absence of a standardized regulatory framework for approval. We must also consider ethics in conjunction with cost-effectiveness and accessibility in low-resource settings. This ensures adoption is equitable for all.

When researchers, clinicians, industry leaders, and regulatory bodies work together closely across disciplines, they will overcome these challenges. Thorough preclinical and clinical evaluations are necessary for safely transitioning nanobiomedicine from the bench to the bedside. Adaptive policy-making is also effective for sustainable manufacturing practices.

Nanobiomedicine has the potential to transform healthcare. This pathway holds great promise for future developments, driven by its ability to harmonize innovation with safety. Targeted, personalized, and intelligent therapies—once considered mere possibilities—are now becoming a reality for patients worldwide.

LIST OF ABBREVIATIONS

APCs	Antigen-Presenting Cells
HER2+	Human Epidermal Growth Factor Receptor 2 Positive
DNA	Deoxyribonucleic Acid
RNA	Ribonucleic Acid
PLGA	Poly(lactic-co-glycolic acid)
DOX	Doxorubicin
TME	Tumor Microenvironment
TAMs	Tumor-Associated Macrophages
GSH	Glutathione
PTT	Photothermal Therapy

NIR-II	Second Near-Infrared Window
MXene	Transition Metal Carbide/Nitride-Based Nanomaterial
SPIONs	Superparamagnetic Iron Oxide Nanoparticles
PET	Positron Emission Tomography
POC	Point-of-Care
ELISA	Enzyme-Linked Immunosorbent Assay
PCR	Polymerase Chain Reaction
SLNs	Solid Lipid Nanoparticles
ARG1	Arginase 1
mRNA	Messenger Ribonucleic Acid
LNPs	Lipid Nanoparticles
PEG	Polyethylene Glycol
PNPs	Polymer Nanoparticles
TEM	Transmission Electron Microscopy
CT	Computed Tomography
MRI	Magnetic Resonance Imaging
PA	Photoacoustic
AI	Artificial Intelligence
ML	Machine Learning
CRISPR-Cas9	Clustered Regularly Interspaced Short Palindromic Repeats - CRISPR-associated Protein 9
INR	International Normalized Ratio
ctDNA	Circulating Tumor DNA
PLA	Polylactic Acid
PCA	Polycyanoacrylate

REFERENCES

[1] Haseeb Q, Hamdani SDA, Akram A, Khan DA, Rajput TA, Babar MM. Nanobiotechnology: Paving the way to personalized medicine. In: Saxena S, Khurana S, Eds. NanoBioMedicine. Singapore: Springer 2020; pp. 17-32.
[http://dx.doi.org/10.1007/978-981-32-9898-9_2]

[2] Karnwal A, Sharma V, Kumar G, Jassim AY, Dohroo A, Sivanesan I. Transforming Medicine with Nanobiotechnology: Nanocarriers and Their Biomedical Applications. Pharmaceutics 2024; 16(9): 1114.
[http://dx.doi.org/10.3390/pharmaceutics16091114] [PMID: 39339152]

[3] Turrina C, Berensmeier S, Schwaminger SP. Bare iron oxide nanoparticles as drug delivery carrier for the short cationic peptide lasioglossin. Pharmaceuticals (Basel) 2021; 14(5): 405.
[http://dx.doi.org/10.3390/ph14050405] [PMID: 33923229]

[4] Singh D. Nano-Bio Interfaces: Pioneering Targeted Approaches for Disease Treatment and Prevention. J Macromol Sci Part B Phys 2024; 1-18.

[http://dx.doi.org/10.1080/00222348.2024.2395693]

[5] Wang Y, Santos A, Evdokiou A, Losic D. An overview of nanotoxicity and nanomedicine research: principles, progress and implications for cancer therapy. J Mater Chem B Mater Biol Med 2015; 3(36): 7153-72.
[http://dx.doi.org/10.1039/C5TB00956A] [PMID: 32262822]

[6] Patra JK, Das G, Fraceto LF, *et al.* Nano based drug delivery systems: recent developments and future prospects. J Nanobiotechnology 2018; 16(1): 71.
[http://dx.doi.org/10.1186/s12951-018-0392-8] [PMID: 30231877]

[7] Chohan DP, Dey B, Tarkunde A, Vyas V, De Sarkar S, Sundara BK. Advancing Autonomous Nanomedicine: Bridging the Gap from Concept to Potential Clinical Studies. J Cluster Sci 2024; 35(8): 2607-35.
[http://dx.doi.org/10.1007/s10876-024-02691-0]

[8] Saxena SK, Nyodu R, Kumar S, Maurya VK. Current advances in nanotechnology and medicine. In: Saxena S, Khurana S, Eds. NanoBioMedicine. Singapore: Springer 2020; pp. 3-16.
[http://dx.doi.org/10.1007/978-981-32-9898-9_1]

[9] Hua S, de Matos MBC, Metselaar JM, Storm G. Current trends and challenges in the clinical translation of nanoparticulate nanomedicines: pathways for translational development and commercialization. Front Pharmacol 2018; 9: 790.
[http://dx.doi.org/10.3389/fphar.2018.00790] [PMID: 30065653]

[10] Ning P, Yao H, Du F, *et al.* Gene reprogramming armed macrophage membrane-camouflaged nanoplatform enhances bionic targeted drug delivery to solid tumor for synergistic therapy. Mol Pharm 2023; 20(5): 2362-75.
[http://dx.doi.org/10.1021/acs.molpharmaceut.2c00929] [PMID: 36989419]

[11] Wang F, Yu Q, Li J, Jiang J, Deng T, Yu C. Biomimetic macrophage membrane-coated gold-quantum dots with tumor microenvironment stimuli-responsive capability for tumor theranostic. Mater Today Bio 2022; 16: 100359.
[http://dx.doi.org/10.1016/j.mtbio.2022.100359] [PMID: 35937575]

[12] Khan MM, Li Y, Zhou Z, *et al.* Macrophage-modulating nanomedicine for cancer immunotherapy. Nanoscale 2024; 16(15): 7378-86.
[http://dx.doi.org/10.1039/D3NR06333J] [PMID: 38511468]

[13] Maeda H. Toward a full understanding of the EPR effect in primary and metastatic tumors as well as issues related to its heterogeneity. Adv Drug Deliv Rev 2015; 91: 3-6.
[http://dx.doi.org/10.1016/j.addr.2015.01.002] [PMID: 25579058]

[14] Suhag D, Kaushik S, Taxak VB. Nanomaterials in biomedicine. InHandbook of biomaterials for medical applications, Volume 1: fundamentals 2024 Jul 24 (pp. 91-120). Singapore: Springer Nature Singapore.
[http://dx.doi.org/10.1007/978-981-97-4818-1_4]

[15] Wang S, Zhou L, Tian H, *et al.* Site-specific nanomodulator capable of modulation apoptosis for enhanced colorectal cancer chemo-photothermal therapy. J Nanobiotechnology 2023; 21(1): 24.
[http://dx.doi.org/10.1186/s12951-023-01779-5] [PMID: 36670444]

[16] Hua S, De Matos MB, Metselaar JM, Storm G. Current trends and challenges in the clinical translation of nanoparticulate nanomedicines: pathways for translational development and commercialization. Frontiers in pharmacology. 2018 Jul 17;9:790.Felgner PL, Gadek TR, Holm M, Roman R, Chan HW, Wenz M, Northrop JP, Ringold GM, Danielsen M. Lipofection: a highly efficient, lipid-mediated DNA-transfection procedure. Proc Natl Acad Sci USA 1987; 84(21): 7413-7.
[PMID: 2823261]

[17] Liu C, Zhang N. Nanoparticles in gene therapy principles, prospects, and challenges. Prog Mol Biol Transl Sci 2011; 104: 509-62.
[http://dx.doi.org/10.1016/B978-0-12-416020-0.00013-9] [PMID: 22093228]

[18] del Pozo-Rodríguez A, Solinís MÁ, Rodríguez-Gascón A. Applications of lipid nanoparticles in gene therapy. Eur J Pharm Biopharm 2016; 109: 184-93.
[http://dx.doi.org/10.1016/j.ejpb.2016.10.016] [PMID: 27789356]

[19] Truong B, Allegri G, Liu XB, *et al.* Lipid nanoparticle-targeted mRNA therapy as a treatment for the inherited metabolic liver disorder arginase deficiency. Proc Natl Acad Sci USA 2019; 116(42): 21150-9.
[http://dx.doi.org/10.1073/pnas.1906182116] [PMID: 31501335]

[20] Louit G, Asahi T, Tanaka G, Uwada T, Masuhara H. Spectral and 3-dimensional tracking of single gold nanoparticles in living cells studied by Rayleigh light scattering microscopy. J Phys Chem C 2009; 113(27): 11766-72.
[http://dx.doi.org/10.1021/jp9018124]

[21] Sharma A, Tandon A, Tovey JCK, *et al.* Polyethylenimine-conjugated gold nanoparticles: Gene transfer potential and low toxicity in the cornea. Nanomedicine 2011; 7(4): 505-13.
[http://dx.doi.org/10.1016/j.nano.2011.01.006] [PMID: 21272669]

[22] Holmboe ES, Durning SJ. Assessing clinical reasoning: moving from *in vitro* to in vivo. Diagnosis (Berl) 2014; 1(1): 111-7.
[http://dx.doi.org/10.1515/dx-2013-0029] [PMID: 29539977]

[23] Weatherall D, Greenwood B, Chee HL, *et al.* Science and technology for disease control: past, present, and future. In: Disease Control Priorities in Developing Countries. 2nd edition. Washington (DC): The International Bank for Reconstruction and Development / The World Bank; 2006.

[24] Laoboonchai A, Kawamoto F, Thanoosingha N, *et al.* PCR□based ELISA technique for malaria diagnosis of specimens from Thailand. Trop Med Int Health 2001; 6(6): 458-62.
[http://dx.doi.org/10.1046/j.1365-3156.2001.00736.x] [PMID: 11422960]

[25] Retèl VP, Hummel MJM, van Harten WH. Review on early technology assessments of nanotechnologies in oncology. Mol Oncol 2009; 3(5-6): 394-401.
[http://dx.doi.org/10.1016/j.molonc.2009.05.001] [PMID: 19540817]

[26] Safari J, Zarnegar Z. Advanced drug delivery systems: Nanotechnology of health design A review. J Saudi Chem Soc 2014; 18(2): 85-99.
[http://dx.doi.org/10.1016/j.jscs.2012.12.009]

[27] Scida K, Stege PW, Haby G, Messina GA, García CD. Recent applications of carbon-based nanomaterials in analytical chemistry: Critical review. Anal Chim Acta 2011; 691(1-2): 6-17.
[http://dx.doi.org/10.1016/j.aca.2011.02.025] [PMID: 21458626]

[28] Thévenot DR, Toth K, Durst RA, Wilson GS. Electrochemical biosensors: recommended definitions and classification. Biosens Bioelectron 2001; 16(1-2): 121-31.
[PMID: 11261847]

[29] Patel PD. (Bio)sensors for measurement of analytes implicated in food safety: a review. Trends Analyt Chem 2002; 21(2): 96-115.
[http://dx.doi.org/10.1016/S0165-9936(01)00136-4]

[30] Demetzos C. Pharmaceutical nanotechnology. Fundamentals and practical applications. 2016.

[31] Cormode DP, Skajaa T, Fayad ZA, Mulder WJM. Nanotechnology in medical imaging: probe design and applications. Arterioscler Thromb Vasc Biol 2009; 29(7): 992-1000.
[http://dx.doi.org/10.1161/ATVBAHA.108.165506] [PMID: 19057023]

[32] Thwala LN, Ndlovu SC, Mpofu KT, Lugongolo MY, Mthunzi-Kufa P. Nanotechnology-based diagnostics for diseases prevalent in developing countries: current advances in point-of-care tests. Nanomaterials (Basel) 2023; 13(7): 1247.
[http://dx.doi.org/10.3390/nano13071247] [PMID: 37049340]

[33] Tang X, Zhu Y, Duan D, *et al.* Anionic Solid Solution MXene for Low□Dosage NIR□II Tumor

Photothermal Therapy. Adv Funct Mater 2023; 33(42): 2305965.
[http://dx.doi.org/10.1002/adfm.202305965]

[34] Song X, Qian R, Li T, *et al.* Imaging-guided biomimetic M1 macrophage membrane-camouflaged magnetic nanorobots for photothermal immunotargeting cancer therapy. ACS Appl Mater Interfaces 2022; 14(51): 56548-59.
[http://dx.doi.org/10.1021/acsami.2c16457] [PMID: 36521052]

[35] Park K. The beginning of the end of the nanomedicine hype. Journal of controlled release: official journal of the Controlled Release Society. 2019 Jun 4;305:221-2.
[http://dx.doi.org/10.1016/j.jconrel.2019.05.044]

[36] Ventola CL. Progress in nanomedicine: approved and investigational nanodrugs. P&T 2017; 42(12): 742-55.
[PMID: 29234213]

[37] Anselmo AC, Mitragotri S. Nanoparticles in the clinic: An update. Bioeng Transl Med 2019; 4(3): e10143.
[http://dx.doi.org/10.1002/btm2.10143] [PMID: 31572799]

[38] Wilhelm S, Tavares AJ, Dai Q, *et al.* Analysis of nanoparticle delivery to tumours. Nat Rev Mater 2016; 1(5): 16014.
[http://dx.doi.org/10.1038/natrevmats.2016.14]

CHAPTER 3

Nanomaterials in Therapeutic Application

Pratik Talukder[1,*], **Aritra Nandi**[1], **Souvick Das**[1], **Shaheen Sultana**[1] and **Snehika Sengupta**[1]

[1] *Department of Biotechnology, Institute of Engineering and Management, New Town, University of Engineering & Management, Kolkata, India*

Abstract: Using the special phenomenon known as the increased permeability and retention (EPR) effect, the idea of nanomedicine has seen tremendous development in recent decades. Integration of principles based on nanotechnology into diagnostics and medicines has led to major progress in imagining, precision medicine, and targeted delivery of drugs. With a special focus on cancer therapy, countless nanomedicines have been invented and used for the treatment of a variety of diseases. Nanomedicine has recently been applied in a number of cutting-edge sectors, such as tissue engineering, immunotherapy, vaccines, gene transfer, and diagnostics. Concurrent drug administration, therapeutic monitoring, and imaging are made possible by multifunctional nanomedicines, enabling prompt reactions and individualized treatment regimens. This chapter mainly highlights the major progress made in nanomaterials and their probable beneficial uses in the fields of biology and medicine. In addition to this, this chapter also refers to the different clinical translations of nanomedicines and the significant problems that are currently being faced by nanomedicine to overcome the clinical translation barrier.

Keywords: Nanomedicine, Photodynamic Therapy, Tissue Engineering , Targeted drug delivery.

INTRODUCTION

The knowledge of nanotechnology was primarily introduced by Richard Feynman, a Physicist, in the year 1959 during a conversation on developing objects at the molecular and atomic levels. These days, most scientists have faith that nanotechnology is the most capable technology development in the 21st century. They have premeditated that nanotechnology was the new method that has the capability for studying medical conditions. In the last 10 years, the funding for the development and research of nanotechnology has increased, which signifies that nanotechnology will lead the new generation towards productivity

* **Corresponding author Pratik Talukder:** Department of Biotechnology, Institute of Engineering and Management, New Town, University of Engineering & Management, Kolkata, India; E-mail: pratik.talukder@uem.edu.in

Soumik Podder & Amalesh Samanta (Eds.)

and success [1]. Additionally, the usage of nanomedicine has widened new possibilities, predominantly in the treatment of cancer because it has accuracy, pointing, high effectiveness, and lower antagonistic effects [2]

Abundant NPs, such as inorganic NPs, polymeric NPs, are providing advantages in the therapy field, which include both *in vivo* and *in vitro* drug stability, smooth surface modification, and easy therapeutic efficacy [3]. It has been recently discovered that NPs can now couple with bispecific molecules by the action of physical or chemical techniques, and NPs can also attach to certain biological events like interaction between receptor-ligand, antigen-antibody collaboration, and DNA-DNA hybridization [4]. The engineered NPs are planned to regulate the release of drugs and partially interact with specific cells that safeguard the targeted medication transfer while preventing enzymatic degradation [3]. During the nanoparticles design, there are a few things that are kept in mind while using them, such as particle shape, surface charge, size, and hydrophobicity. All of these factors are sensitive reasons for the nanoparticles to reach the targets. The nanoparticles that are smaller than <5 nm may be washed out from the blood vessels during movement, whereas the larger nanoparticles that are larger than >100 nm are retained in the ECM, and the medium-sized nanoparticles of size between 5 nm to 100 nm stay inside the bloodstream and are smoothly conveyance to the targeted sites. The size as well as the shape are the substantial important factor that impacts the clearance of nanoparticles from the lymph nodes. Most of the nanoparticles are spherical, but due to the advancement of nanoparticle engineering, different diversity forms have been developed, such as prisms, stars, rods, and discs. In addition to shape and size, the surface charge carrier plays a significant function in immune response activation and cellular internalization, also it influences how cells efficiently engulf the nanoparticles. Comparing the positively and negatively charged, it shows that positively charged nanoparticles have a sturdier immunological response, but they show decreases in the tissue permeability because they often get trapped in the ECM of negatively charged [5]. That's why engineered nanoparticles are more beneficial than conventional therapeutics, which include preventing biological depletion, and targeting tumor cells *via* active targeting while reducing the toxicity of cells and enhancing bioavailability and *in vivo* stability. Nanoparticles are designed in such a manner that they release the payload at a particular targeted site [6]. However, the precise application is identified by the surface of physics, chemistry, thermodynamics, and toxicological impacts [4].

The application of nanomedicine serves as a key approach in cancer treatment, leveraging the enhanced permeability and retention effect [7]. In different book chapters and articles, the mechanism, history, and future perspective of EPR have been well documented [2]. Therefore, it acts as a dynamic role in the accumulation of nanomedicine for the tumor tissue, as it boosts the effectiveness, along with decreasing side effects and systemic exposure. The impact of EPR signifies the process of accumulation of selective macromolecule particles in the tumor tissue, and is eased by the exceptional pathophysiological and anatomical features of tumor blood vessels. The legitimacy of EPR effects has been recognized not only in animal models, but also in humans, which include situations like renal, metastatic, and liver breast cancer [8 - 10]. In a study, it has been discovered that human metastatic breast cancer and renal tumors have shown a substantial impact on the development of the anti-cancer nanomedicines [8, 9]. According to the effects of EPR, it has been demonstrated that nanomedicine is beneficial for the treatment of cancer, in contrast to earlier traditional smaller molecular anti-cancer drugs that have a tendency to accumulate extensively in ordinary organs, tissues, which leads to adverse systemic impacts [11 - 13]. Hence, nanomedicine offers an improved and promising treatment option. In the last two decades, there has been significant advancement and growth in the arena of anti-cancer nanomedicine.

In recent years, various nanomedicines have been developed and designed for cancer therapy, which are less invasive, such as photodynamic therapy, which is a nanoprobe-based approach, and magnetic hyperthermia therapy using magnetite, as well as BNCT; all of these have therapeutic potential [2]. Moreover, the use of nanomedicine in advanced biomedical fields like gene therapy, immunotherapy, and deterrent medicine has gained substantial consideration. A prominent illustration is the accomplishment of the COVID-19 mRNA vaccine that uses nanoparticles composed of lipids for the drug delivery process [14]. In this framework, this article examines the potential uses of nanomedicines in the development of cancer therapy and various biological fields.

The Applications of Nanomedicine in Photodynamic Therapy

Nano-Engineered Photosensitizers Propose a Promising Strategy for Cancer Treatment

In spite of the constant development of various methods of tumor treatment, substantial challenges continue, which include resistance to drugs, non-specificity, lower response rates, and various side effects related to toxicity [15]. PDT is a targeted alternate and is non-intrusive, whereas activated-light PS produces ROS, which acts as a cell death of tumor cells. Therefore, PDT provides an effective and prominent approach for addressing the upcoming strategies for the treatment of tumor cells [16]. Though the process of PDT clinical trial is resisted by the restrictions of old-style photosensitizers, mainly for the absence of tumor selectivity, consequential in its relatively lesser number of applications in recent clinical practice [17]. Therefore, the development of the NanoPS acts as an overwhelming challenge by permitting the advantages of the improved retention and permeation impact to be tumor specific, and providing a substantial potential to enhance the PDT effectiveness and its specificity [18]. Since most of the PSe shows fluorescence in nature, it is possible to distinguish between normal tissue and tumor using the help of fluorescent imaging, which is known as PDD.

Uses for Nanops for the Targeting of Tumor Tissue

On comparing NanoPSs and PS, NanoPSs show better tumor-targeting capabilities because of their surface alterations and their nanoscale size [19]. Moreover, NanoPSs can be further functionalized for targeting specific antibodies or ligands on their surface that act as particular binding and recognition to tumor cells that enhance the efficacy of therapy and reduce the injury to normal tissues [26]. By various approaches like active targeting and EPR-effect-mediated passive accumulation with the help of antibodies and ligands, NanoPSs can be confined exactly inside tumors, reduce the effects of off-targets, and enhance the therapeutic results [20]. However, the NanoPSs optical properties can be altered by adjusting the size, structure, and morphology that allow maximum absorption of photosensitizers at a particular wavelength, which helps to improve the efficiency of PDT and improve the more precise treatment of tumors [21].

The Potential Uses of Nanoparticles and the Clinical Applications of PDT

In the earlier few eras, clinical studies about PDT have gained speedy expansion, where many PS have already been approved for clinical treatment. For example, 5-ALA and MAL have been accepted by the FDA for basal cell carcinoma treatment, actinic keratosis, and squamous and basal cell carcinoma. Radachlorin has also gained rights from the MHRF for the treatment of skin cancer [2]. Temoporfin also obtained approval from the EMA for the action of palliative treatment of neck and head squamous cell carcinoma [22]. PDT was a comparatively modern advanced application for the cutaneous malignancies, treatment specifically for skin cancer, like basal and squamous cell carcinoma [33]. It is a localized treatment method as it not only provides high efficacy cosmetic outputs, but also reduces the effect on the appearance of the patient, showing well lower recurrence rates and anti-tumor effects [23]. PDT is one of the vital therapeutic sensory systems that has been accepted and used commonly, specifically for the small non-cancer cells in the early stage [35]. In various other fields like urogenital malignancies, intracranial malignancies, gastrointestinal malignancies, and neck and head malignancies, PDT has exhibited extensive potential impact.

Furthermore, there is an abundance of clinical studies being done on PDT for a variety of cancers, which include ovarian, endometrial, cervical, osteosarcoma, and hematologic malignancies. PDT has promising in an increasing array of cancer treatments as research advances [24, 25]. To sum up, PDT, as a targeted treatment approach, along with advancements in new photosensitizers and nanotechnology, has an enormous amount of opportunity for offering more individualized and reliable cancer treatments, which could ultimately enhance patient outcomes, rates of survival, as well as quality of life.

Versatile Therapeutic Approaches for Utilizing Nanoparticles

The constant development and upgradation of NanoPSs were capable of certain types that not only exhibited photosensitivity but also possessed the properties of photothermal and sonosensitivity. These typical features allow PDT to unite with photothermal therapy or sonodynamic therapy, which provides efficient resilience to participate with various additional treatment modalities for achieving synergistic impacts [2]. For example, the study done by Liao *et al.* has discovered that Chlorin e6 shows effective sonosensitivity and photosensitivity that play an important part in sonodynamic therapy combined with PDT [26]. Moreover, using NanoPSs for the transfer of immune modulators, drugs responsible for chemotherapy, or gene therapy agents provides an understanding of strategies for the treatment of cancer [27]. Additionally, integrating NanoPSs into imagining probes permits real-time monitoring for the treatment response, which facilitates specific treatment approaches [28].

Challenges and the Upcoming Progress of Photodynamic Therapy

The widespread applications and usages of NanoPSs in the treatment of cancer have played a crucial role, while showing an excellent result not only in the research field but also in medical studies. The therapeutic usefulness for the treatment of cancer is closely connected with different aspects, like NanoPSs' own characterization, their process of transportation in the organism, and the target of cellular damage. All of these reasons, along with functional and loading alteration of smaller size drug molecules, the tumor accumulation and *in vitro* transportation of nanomedicines, the microenvironmental regulator release and intratumoral diffusion, and particular injury to the tumor cells and biosafety of healthier cells [29]. But, in spite of potential progress, the extensive application of NanoPSs intermediated PDT still faces various challenges and obstructions. These challenges such as concerns about the use in the long-term, approval from the regulatory process, biocompatibility, and the normalization of synthesis approaches. Upcoming research direction may rely on the upgradation of the multifunctional NanoPS platform, which refines various targeting strategies and optimizes the treatment routines, examining the transportation mechanism of drug delivery and the impact on multiple phases in the process of *in vivo* treatment, to maximize the effectiveness of the therapeutic effect and minimize the adverse reactions [2].

Currently, a smaller number of NanoPSs have been approved for clinical use, mostly in the phase of an undeveloped study or clinical trials. As the study goes on, a growing number of clinical trials have been started. A rapid growth in basic studies and research on NanoPSs in photodynamic therapy (PDT) for anti-tumor treatment can be expected, increasing the likelihood of clinical trials in the near future and promoting the broader application of NanoPSs in clinical practice (**Fig. 1**).

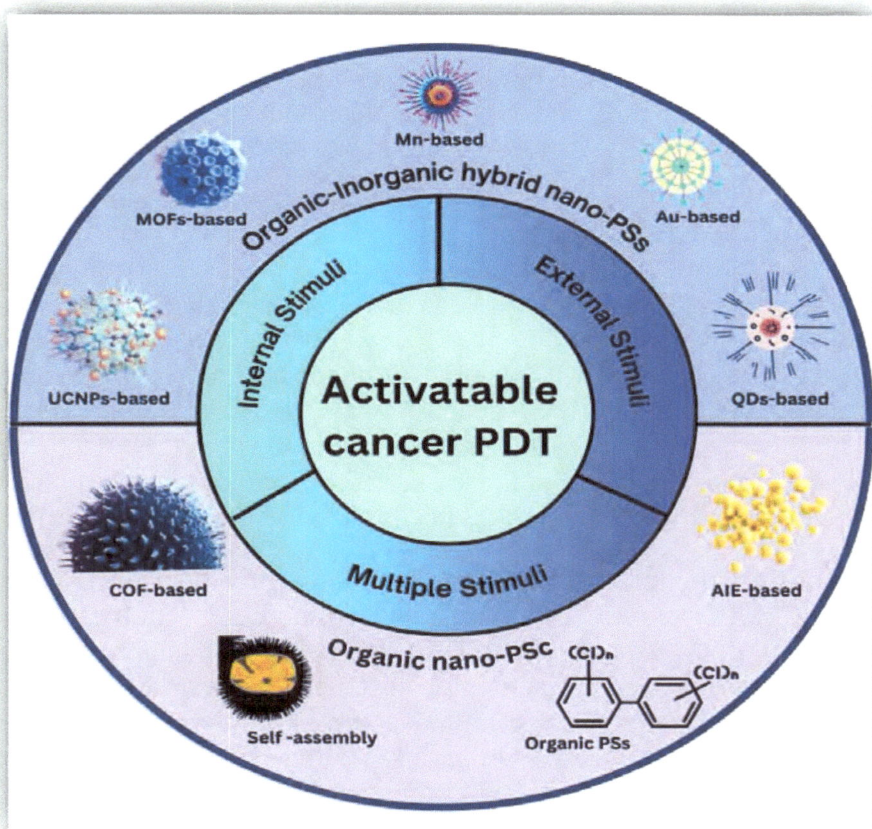

Fig. (1). Diagrammatic representation of the role PDT plays in therapeutic applications.

Nanomedicine: Applications in Immunotherapy [2]

The convergence of nanotechnology and medical science, called Nanomedicine, has heralded a new dimension in immunotherapy by overcoming the intricacy of the TME. Examples of immune cells that could be targeted by NanoPs are regulatory T cells, myeloid-derived suppressor cells, and tumor-associated macrophages to free the TME of immunosuppression and restore anti-tumor immune reprogramming. These are polypeptide-modified multifunctional nanocarriers, which encapsulate and deliver compounds that induce an immunomodulatory response, such as those that include cytokines, siRNA, and checkpoint inhibitors, with the aim of enhancing activation and function of immune cells. With improved NP designs, which involve surface functionalization and controlled release, targeted therapy and longer therapeutic effects with minimal or fewer side effects are possible. Besides, NPs can reprogram immune cells, such as polarizing tumor-associated macrophages or suppressing Tregs, for restoring the immune balance in TME [30]. With advancements in the field come innovations and inventions aimed at improving tumor penetration, reducing systemic toxicities, and combination therapies in nanomedicine to eventually lead to safer, more efficacious, and personalized approaches to immunotherapy.

Targeting Tumor Immune Microenvironment

The TIME is an interactive terrain of cells and molecules that inhibit or enhance cancer propagation. Nanotechnology has recently emerged as a powerful tool for modulating TIME and allows the use of nanocarriers to evade obligatory immunosuppression. Tregs, MDSCs, and TAMs contribute significantly to the immunosuppression within the TIME. Nanoparticles may restore effector immune cell anti-cancer functions, such as those exerted by cytotoxic T lymphocytes, by selectively inhibiting the activity of these cells.

Therapeutically active nano-carriers present a long-term advantage by delivering agents, such as cytokines, siRNAs, monoclonal antibodies, or immune checkpoint inhibitors, directly into the tumor site. They will help enhance immune responses locally with low off-target effects. For instance, nanoparticles loaded with siRNAs may silence yet-stormy immune-suppression-related specific genes in immune cells, while NPs loaded with cytokines may boost immune activation. Nanoparticles provide a favorable environment for cancer immunotherapy by reprogramming macrophage polarization from immunosuppressive to pro-inflammatory. In addition, the hypoxic and nutrient-deprived conditions of LOTIE may inhibit immune cell activity [31]. In particular, NPs aimed at modulating the oxygen concentration or at delivering agents that normalize tumor vasculature can relieve these barriers. For example, oxygen technologies or those that manipulate vascular permeability improve immune cell access to the tumor. Various types of advances that can co-deliver various agents make the area of nanomedicine a powerful strategy to target the TIME.

Although advances have been made in this regard, there are still many challenges for effective optimization of nanocarriers, including those related to tumor penetration, rapid clearance after systemic administration, and sustained effect.

Targeting and Reprogramming T-Cells

T cells are central to the immune system's ability to recognize and eradicate cancer cells and hence are a key target in cancer immunotherapy. Nanotechnology offers a new avenue for the targeting and reprogramming of T cells to enhance their therapeutic potential. NPs deliver therapeutics by modulating T-cell activity with high precision and less on-target effects. One promising approach is the use of NPs to provide siRNA to silence inhibitory signals in T cells. Examples include using siRNA to target genes responsible for immune checkpoints, such as PD-1 or CTLA-4, and to relieve T cell functional suppression to enhance their cytotoxic functions. NPs can also deliver genetic material, mRNA, or DNA to reprogram T cells, allowing them to express CARs or other specific receptors on their surface to enhance recognition and killing of cancer cells. Compared with traditional CAR-T cell therapy, NP-mediated reprogramming is less invasive and believed to be more accessible [32].

Nanotechnology works to instill these two modes of action in the suppression of Tregs in the tumor microenvironment on one hand, while at the same time, improving effector T-cell function on the other hand. Tregs inhibit effector T cells and contribute to immune evasion by tumors. NPs may be engineered to selectively target and suppress Tregs and help restore a balanced immune response with anti-tumor immunity. These two-wave operations of both enhancing effector T cells while obstructing Tregs will amplify the overall effectiveness of cancer immunotherapy.

On top of that, NPs could prove to be better carriers with respect to the co-delivery of multiple agents - for example, cytokines or co-stimulatory molecules - to T cells and would specifically be directed toward improving activation and proliferation of T cells. All these assure prolonged T-cell role against tumors while reducing the chances of immune exhaustion [33].

Activation of NK Cells and their Enhancement

NK cells are a type of innate immune cell that is inherently responsible for directly identifying and killing tumor cells and cells infected by viruses, without prior sensitization. There are major hurdles posed by the limited proliferation, short lifespan, and decreased activity of NK cells in the immunosuppressive tumor microenvironment, preventing therapeutic application of NK cells. Herein, nanotechnology may provide a convenient solution to bend these inconsistencies in favor of NK cells by providing NK cell modulation, such as NK activation, proliferation, and cytotoxic activity.

Nanoparticles can be engineered to directly target and activate NK cells through the targeted delivery of stimulatory agents. In this case, the NPs might be loaded with NKG2D receptor agonists, which bind the activating receptor on NK cells, thereby indirectly augmenting their cytotoxic activity. NKG2D receptors actively recognize stress-induced ligands in human tumors, allowing NK cells to selectively engage and destroy them [34]. By enhancing NKG2D signaling, the NPs amplify NK cell-mediated immune responses. NPs can also be designed to serve a dual purpose in various situations. They can carry cytokines like IL-15 or IL-12 to proliferate NK cells and maintain their activity. These cytokines are important for NK cell maturation and expansion, which secures a better and prolonged immune response for tumor eradication.

Additionally, NPs may relapse the co-delivery of multiple such drugs, such as stimulatory cytokines and chemokines to the tumor site in conjunction with improving the NK cells' function. Nanoparticles also alleviate the immunosuppressive effects of the tumor microenvironment that usually antagonizes NK cell activity. For example, NPs can deliver siRNA that silences genes involved in immune evasion mechanisms or neutralizes suppressive factors like TGF-β. The NPs indeed give this gift to reprogram the tumor microenvironment in favor of the NK cells to mount an enhanced anti-tumor response [35]. Further advancements in NP inventions and their designs, such as biodegradable and targeted delivery systems, will perhaps drive prospects for further enhancement of NK-based immunotherapies. Scientists are using nanotechnology to design more effective, durable, and accessible NK therapies to treat cancer and infectious diseases.

Expressed from the Activation of NKG2D Receptors

The NKG2D receptor plays an important role in the immune system on how it will mold the recognition and elimination of cancer and virus-infected cells. This activating receptor has its expression in NK cells and certain T cells, and it responds through activating ligands, often overexpressed on the tumors or infected cells, which engages the mechanistic response to cell death of the targeted cells involved. However, tumor microenvironments and tumors downregulating NKG2D ligands limit the effectiveness of NKG2D-mediated immunity, which helps in immune evasion from these cells.

On the other hand, functionalized NPs are popular candidates for enhancing immunity triggered against the NKG2D receptor. NPs, functionalized with NKG2D ligands, could also develop tumor targeting specificity and provide greater recognition of tumor cells by NK cells. The NKG2D receptors on NK cells and the tumor cell ligands are bridged by these bivalent molecules, resulting in enhanced NB cell activation and cytotoxicity. Because of this, off-target effects are reduced, and the therapeutic efficacy is improved. One of the major advantages of nanoparticles functionalized with NKG2D ligands is re-sensitization of tumor cells to immune detection. Tumors often downregulate NKG2D ligands to escape immune responses, but the addition of exogenous ligands *via* nanoparticles will restore these targets and make tumor cells more susceptible to destruction mediated by NK cells [36]. This approach will be particularly advantageous for tumors that have evolved mechanisms to evade immune attacks.

In addition, NPs can be engineered to deliver multiple agents at the same time, such as cytokines or immune modulators, enhancing NK cell activity. For example, nanoparticles can supply IL-15.

Nanoparticles in Targeting Antigen-Presenting Cells

Nanoparticles have now emerged as potent agents in immunology, targeting and delivering antigens to antigen-presenting cells such as dendritic cells, macrophages, or B cells, whose role is critical in the initiation of an immune response. Antigen targeting through conventional means does not allow much cellular uptake and has a fast clearance; however, by mimicking natural pathogens, NPs would solve these challenges, enabling much-efficient antigen presentation.

NPs can shape themselves as pathogens so as to give a clear signal for the immune system to recognize. Targeting NP surfaces through antibody or peptide-conjugation to the NP surface allows selective binding with APC on an enhanced basis for antigen presentation, much like bodily processes of infection, thus eliciting stronger responses from the immune system. Antigens include proteins, peptides, nucleic acids, or tiny molecules that may be encapsulated into small volumes, such as NPs. NPs do allow for the controlled release of antigens and therefore for prolonged recruitment of immune cells, similar to what happens following natural infection, but also support long-term memory. Polymeric NPs are made of biodegradable materials, such as polylactic acid and poly(lactic-c--glycolic acid), and have been used in vaccine formulations. Different NPs can control the release profile of encapsulated antigens and enhance immune activation. PEGylation refers to the attachment of PEG to NP surfaces, which prolongs their circulation time and reduces their clearance by the immune system. Thus, bioavailability and APC targeting of NPs further improve [37].

NPs have shown promise in both cancer and viral vaccines to augment the effect of cell-mediated and humoral immune responses. Antigens delivered by NPs to APCs enhance CD4+ and CD8+ T cell response through MHC class I and II pathways due to cross-presentation, which results in better T cell memory and enhanced antibody production to give optimum protection against infections and decrease cancer recurrence. NPs can help in cancer immunotherapy by enabling direct targeting of the tumor-attached antigens or by being an enabler for immune-modifying agents like cytokines or checkpoint inhibitors into APCs or the tumor microenvironment to boost the anti-tumor immune responses. NP also allows selective modulation of immune responses, such as promoting a Th1 response for viral infections or a Th2 response for allergies. Such control can be applied for vaccines, autoimmune diseases, or allergies, opening up novel possibilities for their intervention [38]. Cumulatively, NPs have become a milestone development in immunology, where optimized antigen delivery to APCs is likely to improve vaccine and immunotherapy efficiency and how cancer and other immune-related diseases will be treated.

Advancing Immune Checkpoint Inhibitors through Targeted Carriers

Among the most cutting-edge and sophisticated cancer therapies for today are immune checkpoint inhibitors, specifically anti-PD-1 and anti-CTLA-4 monoclonal antibodies. While mainly treatment options, the use of these inhibitors as monotherapy has a limited effect on certain patients due to inadequate tumor penetration, the off-target effects, immune-related adverse events, and resistance to ICIs. Thus, nanoparticle-mediated delivery of ICIs will take care of these concerns through better targeting, increased tumor penetration, and decreased systemic toxicity. Nanoparticles can be surface-modified to recruit specific targeting ligands. This allows the ICIs to direct their action toward the tumor sites, thus blocking inhibitory signals and restoring the immune function. They will also improve the pharmacokinetics by increasing circulation time, avoiding rapid immune clearance, and protecting ICIs from degradation by enzymes. Small-sized nanoparticles increase tumor penetration, thanks to the physical barriers posed by dense extracellular matrices and the irregular vasculature of tumors. Besides, nanoparticles can liberate their pincers, aimed towards specific tumor microenvironment characteristics, such as acidic pH [39].

Nanoparticles allow for the co-delivery of multiple agents, thus improving the extent of anticancer effects. This could include immunomodulators such as cytokines, adjuvants, or small molecule inhibitors that activate immune cells (*e.g.*, T cells and NK cells) in the tumor microenvironment. This would enable prolonged required exposure to therapy for the efficacy of ICIs, especially in therapies requiring long or repeated dosing. Moreover, nanoparticles can carry other agents, such as chemotherapeutics, and then work synergistically with the ICIs to cause greater tumor cell killing and reduce the resistance mechanisms. A lot of evidence from preclinical and clinical studies indicates that delivery systems based on nanoparticles are more effective in the delivery of immune-checkpoint inhibitors while also minimizing adverse effects to the patient. For example, anti-PD-1 antibody-loaded nanoparticles exhibited greater tumor growth suppression in conjunction with immunotherapy or chemotherapy in animal models but reduced systemic side effects. However, considerable challenges still exist, such as precisely controlling the size and surface characteristics of nanoparticles; mass production of nanoparticles for clinical application; and the complicated nature of the tumor microenvironment, which may still thwart ICI activity [40]. Notwithstanding, there is a ray of hope for better clinical efficacy given the speedy evolution in nano drug delivery research.

Clinical Development of Nano Immunotherapy

Nano-immunotherapy combines nanotechnology with immunotherapy to enhance immunogenicity and reduce side effects, thus promising to become revolutionary in cancer treatment. It commonly employs nanoparticles (NPs) to deliver an immunomodulatory agent to immune cells in the tumor microenvironment. These therapeutic agents enhance immune targeting, stability, and delivery. It can induce a strong immune response against the tumor-associated antigens delivered effectively *via* APCs. To this end, mRNA-based vaccines allow cells to produce tumor-specific antigens, targeted immunity, and very few off-target effects. Nanogels sustainably release agents like cytokines and antibodies, enhancing their therapeutic effects while partly mitigating systemic toxicity against certain immune cells, such as NK and T cells. Nanoparticle delivery of receptor agonists or immune checkpoint inhibitors can modulate NK and T cell activity and boost anti-tumor immunity. Challenges in the development of the new way include the optimization of nanoparticle design so that there is sufficient biodistribution and systemic uptake and the avoidance of immune clearance and immunogenicity [41]. Nanoparticle transport through tumor tissue can be hindered by the physical dimensions of nanoparticles, leaky blood vessels, dense ECM, and hypoxic conditions. Stimuli-responsive designs may help overcome these hurdles.

Thus, limiting off-target effects is vital for providing acceptable safety, and the use of targeting ligands to guide nanoparticles to the tumor or immune cells can be of real help in this regard. Imaging and biodistribution studies will then allow optimization of the therapeutic indices. Preclinical research and ongoing clinical trials demonstrate encouraging results on regression of tumors, the design of immune responses, and diminished side effects across a panel of cancers, including melanoma, lung, and breast cancers.

Challenges and Perspective

Nano Immunotherapy is hopeful in its efficacy, but several challenges still need addressing for it to achieve clinical significance. The first, in order of priority, will be the design of the nanoparticles to improve drug-specific functions while reducing off-target effects. The size, charge, and composition of such nanoparticles need to be finely tuned to deliver the therapeutic cargo to the tumor site effectively, better target the immune cells, and avoid being taken up by liver and spleen macrophages. Penetration into the tumor has other significant problems arising from the heterogeneous and complex nature of the tumor microenvironment, including a very dense extracellular matrix and an irregularity in the arrangement of the blood vessels. These barriers indeed obstruct the effective distribution of nanoparticles within solid tumors. In addition, off-target effects, or in other words, nanoparticles accumulating in healthy tissues, pose safety concerns and also impair therapeutic efficacy. The solution to these challenges has to lie in interdisciplinary research incorporating nanotechnology, immunology, and cancer biology. Rapid advances in the innovation of nanotechnology provide an avenue for the inventiveness of new therapies, which may revolutionize cancer management at a much lower toxic level and with better therapeutic dispositions.

Nanomedicine in Gene Delivery

Diagnostics have come up with various techniques to edit/modify specific regions of the human genome since DNA is the primary component of hereditary [42]. By inserting, deleting, or replacing genetic material, gene therapy can correct specific alterations or mutations [43]. On September 14, 1990, a 4-year-old child with SCID had the first authorized gene therapy surgery. This was performed by W. French Anderson of NIH along with his colleagues [44].

Viruses are the most commonly used vectors because they can transfer their own genetic material into host cells. Yet, at the same time, viruses cannot be used for gene therapy as they have many potential adverse effects. For instance, the startling demise of a University of Pennsylvania student who took part in a gene therapy experiment in 1999 [45]. For this particular reason, researchers are working hard to synthesize carriers that are synthetic and from non-viral sources. Furthermore, non-viral vectors have shown enhanced potential for targeted delivery of genetic materials in comparison to viral vectors, for treating diseases such as pancreatic cancer, hereditary transthyretin amyloidosis, *etc*. Due to their qualities, including ease of production, functionalization with various moieties, low immunogenicity and toxicity, high loading capacities, and the absence of unexpected gene integrations, NPs have emerged as one of the most dependable and fascinating advancements in biomedical research for gene therapy as a carrier. A few restrictions affecting the effectiveness of transfections of pDNA or siRNAs can be effectively overcome using functionalized NPs [46]. Recently, methods have been developed to introduce therapeutic nucleic acids into cells, such as Antisense Oligonucleotides (ASO), plasmid DNA, miRNA, and siRNA, using more coherent and biocompatible transfection systems [47]. Even though the benefits of using NPs in gene delivery are immense, there are still issues with the diagnostic gene therapy using nanoparticles, including cellular internalization, endosomal escape, non-specific adsorption by undesirable tissues, biodegradation, biocompatibility, and aggravation in body fluids.

Inorganic NP

Inorganic nanoparticles have shown strong applications as adaptable and effective nanocarriers for gene delivery in recent times. In addition, inorganic nanoparticles have a huge range of beneficial applications, such as scalability in the synthesis procedure, facile functionalization that improves interactions with biomolecules by chemical and thermal stability. Some commonly used methods for modifying the inorganic NPs for gene delivery: i)integrating the genetic material on the inorganic NPs directly using a reactive linker ii)forming a complex with negatively charged genetic material using positively charged inorganic NPs, and iii)using a cationic amphiphilic polymer generated from the inorganic NPs to induce the complexation of the genetic material with the NPs [48]. Some significant forms of inorganic materials that are used for gene therapy are SPION, AuNPs, and IONP. The particles are drawn in the case of IONP to an external magnetic field, which modifies the particle distribution inside the organism [46]. The efficiency of DNA transfer is improved when NPs are transported through cell compartments by means of a magnetic field. As a result, magnetic iron nanoparticles carrying DNA were used in mitochondrial treatment to interfere with the transfer of mitochondrial proteins and cause cell death [46, 49]. The small size and variable functionalization of siRNA make the development of iron NPs feasible, which further leads to a net positive charge on the surface that enhances the activity of siRNA. Recently, Fe3O4-synthesis NPs were used to target BCL2 in Ca9-22 oral cancer cells; when magnetotherapy was added, the gene silencing effect was enhanced [46, 50]. There has been an increased use of

AuNPs in both *in vivo* and *in vitro* gene therapy uses owing to their low toxicity, rapid endosomal escape, accelerated uptake, and high payload. For instance, AuNPs were used by Ryou and his colleagues to deliver RNA aptamers specific to the β-catenin gene into the cancer cells' nucleus [51]. By inhibiting β-catenin's ability to perform transcription in the nucleus of lung cancer cells, this technique successfully caused apoptosis. Additionally, siRNA, which binds with its target extremely selectively and produces a silencing complex without requiring genome integration, has been delivered by AuNPs.

Furthermore, siRNA delivery can be enhanced using different forms of functionalization, such as cationic quaternary ammonium or cationic lipid bilayer [52]. Vector delivery using CNTs has shown effective results due to its ability to move past plasma membranes and its high aspect ratio. Additionally, the properties of the nanoneedle protect the gene delivery from enzymatic breakdown and promote their penetration into the cytosol [48]. Taghavi *et al.* [53] created single-walled CNTs filled with PEG and PEI that had been altered by alkyl carboxylation to increase lipophilicity for better internalization. These results demonstrated that nanocarriers could thus increase the gene transport of shRNA to MCF7 cells.

Furthermore, the silanol group on the silica-based NPs' surface offers a net positive charge that is utilized for nucleic acid functionalization. Silica nanoparticles were employed for gene transfer in *in vitro* cellular models to improve both the sedimentation of NPs and the incorporation of genetic material. Mixing silica with different materials, such as polymers, lipids, or inorganic particles, helped in enhancing its capabilities as a nanocarrier [48, 54, 55].

Organic NPs

One of the most common organic methods is the interaction between nucleic acids that are negatively charged and cationic polymers/lipids. These are among the most appealing non-viral vectors that are used for delivering genes in gene therapies since the FDA and EMA have approved multiple formulations of lipid-based delivery of drugs. Lipid NPs have been widely accepted as delivery vectors since the current success of the SARS-CoV-2 vaccinations [56]. Due to their low positive charge pH, the ionizable lipids that comprise these spherical vesicles allow for endosomal escape after internalization by cells and interaction with nucleic acids *via* electrostatic forces. In addition to this, these lipids are neutral at physiological pH and thus less immunogenic and toxic. In order to achieve meaningful levels of genome editing *in vivo*, lipid nanoparticle processes can be used to deliver CRISPR/Cas9 components.

Using polymer-based methods for gene therapy delivery has gained a lot of attention from researchers in recent times. Both synthetic and natural polymers can be used for gene transfection. While creating NPs, biodegradable and biocompatible polymers must be selected meticulously [57, 58]. Another added advantage of this is the controlled breakdown of these biodegradable polymers. The breakdown of the polymer results in the release of the plasmid of the cell into the cytoplasm after the nanosystem reaches the cell.

Additionally, polymeric NPs protect nucleic acids from nuclease degradation. The cationic nature of the nanoparticle allows the nucleic acid to bind to it [48]. NPs called polyplexes are produced when negatively charged nucleic acids interact with positively charged polymers such as chitosan or PEI. Both lipoplexes and polyplexes exhibit high transfection efficiency in vitro. However, they cannot be used *in vivo* due to their toxicity and immunogenicity [57, 59]. Dendrimers in combination with surface groups that are positively charged have been used to study antisense oligonucleotides, gene transport, and siRNA delivery. Since the interaction between the dendrimer and–gene is often electrostatic, sequence specificity is not present. Gene transfection commonly uses a type of dendrimer called PAMAM, which is are spherical, nanoscale polymer [60].

Functionalization of NPs

In order to enhance active endocytosis, the NP's surface needs to be suitably modified using recognition molecules and also be rendered inactive using methods such as carbodiimide and glutaraldehyde. The most commonly used recognition molecule is mAbs. Another option is to utilize scFv, which are smaller and have the same target characteristic. In vivo experiments have demonstrated that tumour development can be inhibited in breast cancer using NPs functionalized with scFv against HER2. It is difficult to employ Mabs or scFv due to their high cost, which makes large-scale production methods tough.

Role of CRISPR-Cas9 in Genome Editing

CRISPR/Cas9, a groundbreaking gene-editing technology, is recognized for its transformative potential in genome editing [61]. In 2020, the Nobel Prize was awarded to Emmanuelle Charpentier and Jennifer Doudna for their innovative work in this field. Despite its promise, the primary challenge for CRISPR/Cas9 therapy lies in achieving safe and efficient *in vivo* delivery. Advancements in delivery systems based on nanotechnology are addressing this hurdle, particularly in cancer gene editing and immunotherapy [61, 62]. For instance, Liu *et al.* developed an MDNP with a core–shell structure [63]. The core, composed of PEI nanoparticles modified with PBA, was bound to a plasmid encoding dCas9 and sgRNA. They also introduced DLNPs with a CRISPR/Cas13a core, designed to target PD-L1 mRNA in specific tumor cells, where Cas13a is activated upon specific recognition. Additionally, Li *et al.* engineered exosomes by combining HuR with the CD9 C-terminus, offering promising methods for targeted CRISPR/dCas9 delivery in disease treatment [64]. Clinical trials have further explored polymer and lipid-based delivery systems for the application of CRISPR/Cas9, demonstrating their potential in treating various disorders.

Cell-Penetrating Peptides Applications

In physiological settings, CPPs provide viable methods for improving the functionality and cellular absorption of NPs. These peptides, typically cationic, are capable of crossing cell membranes and delivering attached therapeutic agents into cells [65]. For example, gelatin-silica NPs have been functionalized with CPPs, such as influenza hemagglutinin A2 and a fusogenic peptide derived from Tat, allowing for the effective transportation of plasmid DNA with endosomal escape and nuclear targeting characteristics [66]. Additionally, NPs containing siRNA targeting doxorubicin and vascular endothelial growth factor have been modified by tumor-responsive CPPs triggered by acidic pH and matrix metalloproteinase 2, which successfully inhibit angiogenesis and induce tumor cell death [67, 68]

Clinical Translation of Nanoparticle-Based Gene Therapies

The clinical use of gene treatments mediated by NP has advanced significantly. CALAA-01, one of the prototypes, was tested in a cancer clinical study [69]. This strategy employs a transferrin-targeting ligand to bind transferrin receptors that are overexpressed in cancer cells, a cyclodextrin-based polymer for transport, PEG for stability, and siRNA to target the M2 component of RRM2. Recent efforts have focused on lipid-based NP formulations, as well as integrating gene therapies with treatments like chemotherapy, radiation, photodynamic therapy, and immunotherapy. For instance, a phase 1 trial evaluated GEN-1—an IL-12 plasmid formulated with a PEG-PEI-cholesterol lipopolymer—administered intraperitoneally alongside standard chemotherapy for peritoneal and ovarian cancers. Similarly, a phase 2 study is underway to assess SGT-53, a P53 gene therapy, along with oral temozolomide used for treating recurrent glioblastoma, supported by SynerGene Therapeutics [70].

The Application of Nanomedicine in Tissue Engineering

The method for tissue as well as organ reconstruction first appeared 30 years ago [71]. Tissue engineering is explained as a multidisciplinary field that deals with engineering principles in bioscience for the expansion of biotic reserves that focus on restoring, conserving, or developing the function of tissue. These three basic methods are utilized in the biomedical domain for the regeneration of new tissues: scaffolds, cells, and growth factors [71, 72].

Integrating nanomedicine with the engineering methods of tissue to develop the best of both domains, which has an important effect on the treatment of patients [73]. Functional tissue as well as organ replacement requires accurate spatial as well as temporal control over biological processes. Essential methods to maintain as well as monitor these modified tissues involve the careful presentation as well as regulated delivery of bioactive components (growth factors, chemokines, inhibitors, genes, cytokines, *etc.*). As a result of this requirement, NP-based techniques have been utilized in tissue engineering scaffolds to regulate several growth agents, also allowing imaging contrast and controlling the properties of scaffolds. Based on the specific applications, materials like polymers, metals, ceramics, and their amalgam can be utilized to develop nanoparticles [74]. In addition, the ECM that is present around the cells of tissues is composed of a naturally occurring matrix of nanofibers organized hierarchically. Recent expansion of nanotechnology allows the design and creation of biomimetic microenvironments at the nanoscale, which serve as analogs to the natural ECM. These mechanisms have been specifically employed to develop nanostructured scaffolds as well as nano topographic surfaces, also to capture drugs as well as adjust their spatiotemporal release, including growth factors. As a result, these nanodevices provide a means to regulate various cellular processes, including cell adhesion and gene expression [75].

Advanced Properties of NPs that Promote Tissue Engineering

Nanoparticles in tissue engineering have highly developed properties that are effective in several implementations. Also altering their electrical, biological, and mechanical features, these NPs can be used to duplicate the unique microenvironment of given tissues [76]. Moreover, they can bring about various delivery obstacles, allowing the delivery drug to the targeted tissue [77]. Additionally, engineered nanoparticles can be tuned to achieve specific performance requirements across various engineering implementations, thanks to their vast range of physicochemical effects such as magnetic, electronic, vibrational, mechanical, thermal, optical, as well as surface properties [78]. Furthermore, bioceramics, biomedical polymers, and other inorganic materials have been combined to obtain a superior quality that mimics the natural structure of tissues. The mixture of polymer and inorganic nanoparticles can perform as a scaffold for tissue-engineered bone. By comparison with traditional polymer composites, nanoparticle-filled polymers provide many more advantages, including increased durability, reduced weight, enriched mechanical qualities, as well as a bioactive interface - a major component for the effective and lifelong use of prostheses. These data represent that nanostructured composites can imitate the surface as well as chemical properties of bone as well as cartilage, thereby facilitating better regeneration [79].

Improved Biological Characteristics

Tissue engineering depends mainly on the advanced biotic properties of NPs. NPs provide so many advantages in tissue engineering, which include the quality of contrast agents, decreased toxicity, and scalable features. A lot of substances like polymers, ceramics, fullerenes, quantum dots, carbon nanotubes, and graphene can be utilized to make NPs [80, 81]. Additionally, it was observed that GNPs with a range of 30 nm to 50 nm were more advantageous and systematic in enhancing the activity of human ADSCs. At the same time, in another study, it was reported that MC3T3-E1 osteoblast-like cells showed a preference for GNPs with a diameter range of 20 nm to 40 nm [82].

Nano Printing of Both Three and Four-Dimensional

The improvement of 3D bioprinting systems has allowed the creation of pre-programmed synthetic tissues that show specific geometries along with regulated cellular composition as well as spatial distribution. Also has the ability to enhance results, new bioinks having electroconductive characteristics are capable to guide for the repair of various types of tissues like heart, nerve tissue, and bone by regulating cellular destinies as well as functions [83]. Additionally, polymeric hydrogels have been extensively investigated for their role as ink materials in 3D and 4D bioprinting due to their capacity to be printed into scaffolds with a hierarchical structure and intrinsic properties similar to those of the extracellular matrix of the original tissue. By integrating nanoscale additives like nanoparticles into the composition of ink, it's now possible to significantly regulate the physicochemical, biological, mechanical, and structural characteristics of the material during as well as after printing [84].

Selective Cell Attachment

HA, PEG, or glycocalyx can chemically modify the surface of the scaffold. They can also be treated by antibacterial coatings, which comprise silver or N-alkylated poly(vinylpyridine), bioadhesive coatings comprise RGD peptides, plasma etching, growth factor binding, decoration, which include other groups of bioactive molecules, as well as there are some different ways to reach expected cell adhesion while preventing undesired attachments [79].

Developed Nanocomposite in Tissue Engineering

Organ physiology involves complicated biological systems that usually develop the procedure of new alternative medicine that is completely challenging, as these procedures have to follow a more holistic approach to manage the demands of precise medicine imposed. Organ-on-a-chip technology is almost a new field that originates from the mixture of chemical, engineering, and biological advancements to develop a structure that looks miniature structure that mimics the native tissue microenvironment. The main concept of organ-on-a-chip technology revolves around integrating microfluidic chips within a polymeric frame, which enables the manipulation of cell behaviour and resembles the physiological processes at a small scale. As silicon is the main material used in microchips, organ-on-a-chip devices can be classified as nanocomposites [84].

Smart Scaffolds Preparation

A basic function of living systems is their ability to respond to stimuli. Research experts have started to develop tissue engineering scaffolds that react to various external factors, such as temperature, light, pH, magnetic field, electric field, ionic strength, and chemicals, by incorporating characteristics found in natural biological systems. Examples of these types of responses include structure, shape or position, surface features, actuation (secretion), solubility, integrated sensing, the improvement of a complex molecular self-assembly, and a sol-to-gel transition [79].

The Application of Nanomedicine for the Development of a Vaccine

Vaccines serve as a backbone for the health of people, greatly reducing morbidity and mortality rates associated with infectious diseases. However, corresponding to another medical expansion, vaccines have several restrictions, such as rapid degradation, suboptimal immunogenicity, and non-specific delivery, all of which can delay the efficacy of vaccines [85]. The area of Nanomedicine provides a strategic way to direct and overcome these restrictions and obtain optimal vaccination techniques. NPs can be used to capture antigens of vaccines, which enhances their stability and enables selected delivery to immune cells. This targeted delivery improves antigen presentation as well as stimulates the immune response, potentially resulting in more effective vaccines [86].

Encapsulation as Well as Defense of Vaccine Antigens

Regular vaccines usually contain inactivated pathogens or weak or purified protein antigens. These antigens are liable to enzyme breakdown in harsh physiological environments before they reach immune cells [87]. NPs can be developed with a biocompatible shell that captures these antigens, shielding them from degradation and early release. This enables the sustained and targeted delivery to the proper immune compartment [88].

CHALLENGES AND FUTURE PERSPECTIVES

Nanomaterials play an important role in the TE, as they contribute to an exclusive advantage for the enhancement of the mechanical, electrical, and biological characteristics, as well as offering anti-microbial impacts, permitting delivery of genes, and enabling the formation of engineered artificial tissues. However, considering all aspects of advancements, one of the major aspects of challenges is the use of nanomaterials for the applications of therapeutic applications, the necessity of robust tools, and the process to analyze the safety profiles. The maximum of the NPs shows a well-enhanced safety profile and fewer side effects, as it may have multifaceted relations with the biological system, and its carcinogenicity, teratogenicity, and toxicity must be evaluated thoroughly. Current studies have emphasized the exposure and the dose-dependent toxicity of nanoparticles that highlight the critical need for thorough risk valuation [89, 90]. However, on increasing the prevalence of the products consisting of nanoparticles, there persist scientific and methodological gaps in the assessment of our precise risks linked with various nanoparticles [82]. Thus, for discovering better safety assessment methods, there is a need for improvement in the nano-toxicological research, such as the modification of *in vitro* and *in vivo* models on various accurate acquaintance scenarios, and to judge the performance of nanoparticles in the biological environments [19, 91].

Along with the development of nanomaterials at the industrial level for therapeutic usages, there must be a relied on long-term effects of chronic exposure to nanoparticles and continuous exposure to NPs raised concerned about the potential health benefits and cumulative toxicity [89, 90]. Addressing all these challenges required an effort to form a uniform protocol for evaluating the chronic impacts of NPs and creating an appropriate parameter for their use in a clinical manner [92]. In this context, establishing a robust governing framework is crucial to ensuring the safe incorporation of nanomaterials into clinical applications. Cooperative efforts between researchers, industry stakeholders are essential to bridge knowledge holes and create identical safety strategies.

CONCLUSION

Nanomaterials play a substantial role in the progress of medical and biological usages in the current generation. It enables the understanding of previously unexplained mechanisms underlying seemingly intolerable therapies by providing better biocompatibility, a controlled drug release profile, precise targeting capabilities, and a larger surface area for interaction with biological systems. Mainly, the area of theranostics is rolling quickly along with the incorporation of nanotechnology. Moving forward, it is essential to overcome the remaining barrier of the clinical transformation of nanomedicine, along with addressing the toxicity effects related to nanomaterials. Therefore, by performing all these, we can fully influence the varied properties of nanoparticles that are discussed in this chapter with advancement in the field of biomedical and healthcare technologies.

REFERENCES

[1] Haleem A, Javaid M, Singh RP, Rab S, Suman R. Applications of nanotechnology in medical field: a brief review. Glob Health J 2023; 7(2): 70-7. [http://dx.doi.org/10.1016/j.glohj.2023.02.008]

[2] Rehan F, Zhang M, Fang J, Greish K. Therapeutic applications of nanomedicine: recent developments and future perspectives. Molecules 2024; 29(9): 2073. [http://dx.doi.org/10.3390/molecules29092073] [PMID: 38731563]

[3] Greish K. Recent and future advances in anticancer drug delivery: an interview with Khaled Greish. Ther Deliv 2018; 9(6): 409-12. [http://dx.doi.org/10.4155/tde-2018-0019] [PMID: 29722635]

[4] Ramos AP, Cruz MAE, Tovani CB, Ciancaglini P. Biomedical applications of nanotechnology. Biophys Rev 2017; 9(2): 79-89. [http://dx.doi.org/10.1007/s12551-016-0246-2] [PMID: 28510082]

[5] Park W, Heo YJ, Han DK. New opportunities for nanoparticles in cancer immunotherapy. Biomater Res 2018; 22(1): 24. [http://dx.doi.org/10.1186/s40824-018-0133-y] [PMID: 30275967]

[6] Debele TA, Yeh CF, Su WP. Cancer immunotherapy and application of nanoparticles in cancers immunotherapy as the delivery of immunotherapeutic agents and as the immunomodulators. Cancers (Basel) 2020; 12(12): 3773. [http://dx.doi.org/10.3390/cancers12123773] [PMID: 33333816]

[7] Matsumura Y, Maeda H. A new concept for macromolecular therapeutics in cancer chemotherapy: mechanism of tumoritropic accumulation of proteins and the antitumor agent smancs. Cancer Res 1986; 46(12 Pt 1): 6387-92. [PMID: 2946403]

[8] Ding Y, Xu Y, Yang W, *et al.* Investigating the EPR effect of nanomedicines in human renal tumors *via* ex vivo perfusion strategy. Nano Today 2020; 35: 100970. [http://dx.doi.org/10.1016/j.nantod.2020.100970]

[9] Lee H, Shields AF, Siegel BA, *et al.* 64Cu-MM-302 positron emission tomography quantifies variability of enhanced permeability and retention of nanoparticles in relation to treatment response in patients with metastatic breast cancer. Clin Cancer Res 2017; 23(15): 4190-202. [http://dx.doi.org/10.1158/1078-0432.CCR-16-3193] [PMID: 28298546]

[10] Maeda H, Sawa T, Konno T. Mechanism of tumor-targeted delivery of macromolecular drugs, including the EPR effect in solid tumor and clinical overview of the prototype polymeric drug SMANCS. J Control Release 2001; 74(1-3): 47-61. [http://dx.doi.org/10.1016/S0168-3659(01)00309-1] [PMID: 11489482]

[11] Fang J, Islam W, Maeda H. Exploiting the dynamics of the EPR effect and strategies to improve the therapeutic effects of nanomedicines by using EPR effect enhancers. Advanced drug delivery reviews. 2020; 157: 142-60.

[12] Islam R, Maeda H, Fang J. Factors affecting the dynamics and heterogeneity of the EPR effect: Pathophysiological and pathoanatomic features, drug formulations and physicochemical factors. Expert Opin Drug Deliv 2022; 19(2): 199-212.

[13] Maeda H. Toward a full understanding of the EPR effect in primary and metastatic tumors as well as issues related to its heterogeneity. Adv Drug Deliv Rev 2015; 91: 3-6. [http://dx.doi.org/10.1016/j.addr.2015.01.002] [PMID: 25579058]

[14] Cross R. Without these lipid shells, there would be no mRNA vaccines for COVID-19. Chem Eng News 2021; 99(8): 144.

[15] Amaravadi RK, Kimmelman AC, Debnath J. Targeting autophagy in cancer: recent advances and future directions. Cancer Discov 2019; 9(9): 1167-81. [http://dx.doi.org/10.1158/2159-8290.CD-19-0292] [PMID: 31434711]

[16] Zhang J, Jiang C, Figueiró Longo JP, Azevedo RB, Zhang H, Muehlmann LA. An updated overview on the development of new photosensitizers for anticancer photodynamic therapy. Acta Pharm Sin B 2018; 8(2): 137-46. [http://dx.doi.org/10.1016/j.apsb.2017.09.003] [PMID: 29719775]

[17] Alsaab HO, Alghamdi MS, Alotaibi AS, *et al.* Progress in clinical trials of photodynamic therapy for solid tumors and the role of nanomedicine. Cancers (Basel) 2020; 12(10): 2793. [http://dx.doi.org/10.3390/cancers12102793] [PMID: 33003374]

[18] Lin L, Song X, Dong X, Li B. Nano-photosensitizers for enhanced photodynamic therapy. Photodiagn Photodyn Ther 2021; 36: 102597. [http://dx.doi.org/10.1016/j.pdpdt.2021.102597] [PMID: 34699982]

[19] Pham TC, Nguyen VN, Choi Y, Lee S, Yoon J. Recent strategies to develop innovative photosensitizers for enhanced photodynamic therapy. Chem Rev 2021; 121(21): 13454-619. [http://dx.doi.org/10.1021/acs.chemrev.1c00381] [PMID: 34582186]

[20] Islam R, Kotalík K, Šubr V, *et al.* HPMA copolymer conjugated 5-aminolevulinic acid exhibits superior efficacy for photodynamic therapy with tumor-responsive and targeting properties. Nanomedicine 2023; 48: 102636. [http://dx.doi.org/10.1016/j.nano.2022.102636] [PMID: 36549553]

[21] Xiang Y, Zheng S, Yuan S, Wang J, Wu Y, Zhu X. Near-infrared mediated orthogonal bioimaging and intracellular tracking of upconversion nanophotosensitizers. Mikrochim Acta 2022; 189(3): 120. [http://dx.doi.org/10.1007/s00604-022-05218-4] [PMID: 35201432]

[22] van Doeveren TEM, Karakullukçu MB, van Veen RLP, Lopez-Yurda M, Schreuder WH, Tan IB. Adjuvant photodynamic therapy in head and neck cancer after tumor-positive resection margins. Laryngoscope 2018; 128(3): 657-63. [http://dx.doi.org/10.1002/lary.26792] [PMID: 28786113]

[23] León D, Buchegger K, Silva R, *et al.* Epigallocatechin gallate enhances MAL-PDT cytotoxic effect on PDT-resistant skin cancer squamous cells. Int J Mol Sci 2020; 21(9): 3327. [http://dx.doi.org/10.3390/ijms21093327] [PMID: 32397263]

[24] Banerjee SM, MacRobert AJ, Mosse CA, Periera B, Bown SG, Keshtgar MRS. Photodynamic therapy: Inception to application in breast cancer. Breast 2017; 31: 105-13. [http://dx.doi.org/10.1016/j.breast.2016.09.016] [PMID: 27833041]

[25] Qiao L, Yang H, Shao X, Yin Q, Fu XJ, Wei Q. Research progress on nanoplatforms and nanotherapeutic strategies in treating glioma. Mol Pharm 2022; 19(7): 1927-51. [http://dx.doi.org/10.1021/acs.molpharmaceut.1c00856] [PMID: 35499303]

[26] Liao S, Cai M, Zhu R, *et al.* Antitumor effect of photodynamic therapy/sonodynamic therapy/sono-photodynamic therapy of chlorin e6 and other applications. Mol Pharm 2023; 20(2): 875-85. [http://dx.doi.org/10.1021/acs.molpharmaceut.2c00824] [PMID: 36689197]

[27] Xin J, Wang S, Wang J, Fu L, Zhang Z, Yao C. A Nucleus-Targeted Nanosystem Integrated with Photodynamic Therapy and Chemotherapy. J Biomed Nanotechnol 2022; 18(3): 837-48. [http://dx.doi.org/10.1166/jbn.2022.3286] [PMID: 35715898]

[28] Babič A, Herceg V, Bastien E, Lassalle HP, Bezdetnaya L, Lange N. 5-Aminolevulinic acid-squalenenanoassemblies for tumor photodetection and therapy: *in vitro* studies. Nanoscale Res Lett 2018; 13(1): 10. [http://dx.doi.org/10.1186/s11671-017-2408-y] [PMID: 29327259]

[29] Guan Q, Li YA, Li WY, Dong YB. Photodynamic therapy based on nanoscale metal–organic frameworks: from material design to cancer nanotherapeutics. Chem Asian J 2018; 13(21): 3122-49. [http://dx.doi.org/10.1002/asia.201801221] [PMID: 30183134]

[30] Sun B, Hyun H, Li L, Wang AZ. Harnessing nanomedicine to overcome the immunosuppressive tumor microenvironment. Acta Pharmacol Sin 2020; 41(7): 970-85. [http://dx.doi.org/10.1038/s41401-020-0424-4] [PMID: 32424240]

[31] Lu Q, Kou D, Lou S, *et al.* Nanoparticles in tumor microenvironment remodeling and cancer immunotherapy. J Hematol Oncol 2024; 17(1): 16. [http://dx.doi.org/10.1186/s13045-024-01535-8] [PMID: 38566199]

[32] Xu T, Liu Z, Huang L, Jing J, Liu X. Modulating the tumor immune microenvironment with nanoparticles: A sword for improving the efficiency of ovarian cancer immunotherapy. Front Immunol 2022; 13: 1057850. [http://dx.doi.org/10.3389/fimmu.2022.1057850] [PMID: 36532066]

[33] Saeed M, Gao J, Shi Y, Lammers T, Yu H. Engineering nanoparticles to reprogram the tumor immune microenvironment for improved cancer immunotherapy. Theranostics 2019; 9(26): 7981-8000. [http://dx.doi.org/10.7150/thno.37568] [PMID: 31754376]

[34] Chao PH, Chan V, Li SD. Nanomedicines modulate the tumor immune microenvironment for cancer therapy. Expert Opin Drug Deliv 2024; 21(12): 1719-33. [http://dx.doi.org/10.1080/17425247.2024.2412245] [PMID: 39354745]

[35] Simon B, Harrer DC, Schuler-Thurner B, *et al.* The siRNA-mediated downregulation of PD-1 alone or simultaneously with CTLA-4 shows enhanced *in vitro* CAR-T-cell functionality for further clinical development towards the potential use in immunotherapy of melanoma. Exp Dermatol 2018; 27(7): 769-78. [http://dx.doi.org/10.1111/exd.13678] [PMID: 29704887]

[36] Yu X, Fang C, Zhang K, Su C. Recent advances in nanoparticles-based platforms targeting the PD-1/PD-L1 pathway for cancer treatment. Pharmaceutics 2022; 14(8): 1581. [http://dx.doi.org/10.3390/pharmaceutics14081581] [PMID: 36015206]

[37] Murugan D, Murugesan V, Panchapakesan B, Rangasamy L. Nanoparticle Enhancement of Natural Killer (NK) Cell-Based Immunotherapy. Cancers 2022, 14, 5438, 2022.

[38] Kiaie SH, Salehi-Shadkami H, Sanaei MJ, *et al.* Nano-immunotherapy: overcoming delivery challenge of immune checkpoint therapy. J Nanobiotechnology 2023; 21(1): 339. [http://dx.doi.org/10.1186/s12951-023-02083-y] [PMID: 37735656]

[39] Zhang J, Wang S, Zhang D, *et al.* Nanoparticle-based drug delivery systems to enhance cancer immunotherapy in solid tumors. Front Immunol 2023; 14: 1230893. [http://dx.doi.org/10.3389/fimmu.2023.1230893] [PMID: 37600822]

[40] Zhao H, Li Y, Wei D, Luo H. The application of nanoparticle-based drug delivery systems in checkpoint blockade cancer immunotherapy. J Immunol Res 2018; 2018(1): 1-13. [http://dx.doi.org/10.1155/2018/3673295] [PMID: 30406152]

[41] Yang W, Cao J, Cheng H, *et al.* Nanoformulations targeting immune cells for cancer therapy: mRNA therapeutics. Bioact Mater 2023; 23: 438-70. [http://dx.doi.org/10.1016/j.bioactmat.2022.11.014] [PMID: 36471724]

[42] Gonçalves GAR, Paiva RMA. Gene therapy: advances, challenges and perspectives. Einstein (Sao Paulo) 2017; 15(3): 369-75.
[http://dx.doi.org/10.1590/s1679-45082017rb4024] [PMID: 29091160]

[43] Wong CH, Li D, Wang N, Gruber J, Lo AW, Conti RM. The estimated annual financial impact of gene therapy in the United States. Gene Ther 2023; 30(10-11): 761-73.
[http://dx.doi.org/10.1038/s41434-023-00419-9] [PMID: 37935855]

[44] Scheller EL, Krebsbach PH. Gene therapy: design and prospects for craniofacial regeneration. Journal of dental research. 2009 Jul;88(7):585-96.

[45] Rehan F, Zhang M, Fang J, Greish K. Therapeutic applications of nanomedicine: recent developments and future perspectives. Molecules 2024; 29(9): 2073.
[PMID: 38731563]

[46] Roma-Rodrigues C, Rivas-García L, Baptista PV, Fernandes AR. Gene therapy in cancer treatment: why go nano? Pharmaceutics 2020; 12(3): 233.
[http://dx.doi.org/10.3390/pharmaceutics12030233] [PMID: 32151052]

[47] Huang Y, Zhan Q, Wu C, *et al.* Trends and hotspots in nanoparticles for the targeted delivery of nucleic acids: a ten-year bibliometric study. Front Pharmacol 2022; 13: 868398.
[http://dx.doi.org/10.3389/fphar.2022.868398] [PMID: 35600858]

[48] Hamimed S, Jabberi M, Chatti A. Nanotechnology in drug and gene delivery. Naunyn Schmiedebergs Arch Pharmacol 2022; 395(7): 769-87.
[http://dx.doi.org/10.1007/s00210-022-02245-z] [PMID: 35505234]

[49] McBain SC, Yiu HH, Dobson J. Magnetic nanoparticles for gene and drug delivery. International journal of nanomedicine. 2008 Dec 1;3(2):169-80. Biochem Biophys Res Commun 2011; 416(1-2): 178-83.
[PMID: 22093830]

[50] Jin L, Wang Q, Chen J, Wang Z, Xin H, Zhang D. Efficient delivery of therapeutic siRNA by Fe3O4 magnetic nanoparticles into oral cancer cells. Pharmaceutics. 2019 Nov 17;11(11):615.

[51] Ryou SM, Kim JM, Yeom JH, Hyun S, Kim S, Han MS, Kim SW, Bae J, Rhee S, Lee K. Gold nanoparticle-assisted delivery of small, highly structured RNA into the nuclei of human cells. Biochem Biophys Res Commun 2011; 416(1-2): 178-83.

[52] Lee JM, Yoon TJ, Cho YS. Recent developments in nanoparticle-based siRNA delivery for cancer therapy. BioMed Res Int 2013; 2013(1): 1-10.
[http://dx.doi.org/10.1155/2013/782041] [PMID: 23844368]

[53] Taghavi S, Nia AH, Abnous K, Ramezani M. Polyethylenimine-functionalized carbon nanotubes tagged with AS1411 aptamer for combination gene and drug delivery into human gastric cancer cells. Int J Pharm 2017; 516(1-2): 301-12.
[http://dx.doi.org/10.1016/j.ijpharm.2016.11.027] [PMID: 27840158]

[54] Bhakta G, Sharma RK, Gupta N, Cool S, Nurcombe V, Maitra A. Multifunctional silica nanoparticles with potentials of imaging and gene delivery. Nanomedicine 2011; 7(4): 472-9.
[http://dx.doi.org/10.1016/j.nano.2010.12.008] [PMID: 21215332]

[55] Carvalho AM, Cordeiro RA, Faneca H. Silica-based gene delivery systems: From design to therapeutic applications. Pharmaceutics 2020; 12(7): 649.
[http://dx.doi.org/10.3390/pharmaceutics12070649] [PMID: 32660110]

[56] Polack FP, Thomas SJ, Kitchin N, *et al.* Safety and efficacy of the BNT162b2 mRNA Covid-19 vaccine. N Engl J Med 2020; 383(27): 2603-15.
[http://dx.doi.org/10.1056/NEJMoa2034577] [PMID: 33301246]

[57] Mirón-Barroso S, Domènech EB, Trigueros S. Nanotechnology-based strategies to overcome current barriers in gene delivery. Int J Mol Sci 2021; 22(16): 8537.

[http://dx.doi.org/10.3390/ijms22168537] [PMID: 34445243]

[58] Cheraghi R, Nazari M, Alipour M, Majidi A, Hosseinkhani S. Development of a targeted anti-HER2 scFv chimeric peptide for gene delivery into HER2-positive breast cancer cells. Int J Pharm 2016; 515(1-2): 632-43.
[http://dx.doi.org/10.1016/j.ijpharm.2016.11.008] [PMID: 27825868]

[59] Jiang Z, Thayumanavan S. Noncationic material design for nucleic acid delivery. Adv Ther (Weinh) 2020; 3(3): 1900206.
[http://dx.doi.org/10.1002/adtp.201900206] [PMID: 34164572]

[60] Choi YS, Lee MY, David AE, Park YS. Nanoparticles for gene delivery: therapeutic and toxic effects. Mol Cell Toxicol 2014; 10(1): 1-8.
[http://dx.doi.org/10.1007/s13273-014-0001-3]

[61] Xu X, Liu C, Wang Y, *et al.* Nanotechnology-based delivery of CRISPR/Cas9 for cancer treatment. Adv Drug Deliv Rev 2021; 176: 113891.
[http://dx.doi.org/10.1016/j.addr.2021.113891] [PMID: 34324887]

[62] Li T, Yang Y, Qi H, *et al.* CRISPR/Cas9 therapeutics: progress and prospects. Signal Transduct Target Ther 2023; 8(1): 36.
[http://dx.doi.org/10.1038/s41392-023-01309-7] [PMID: 36646687]

[63] Liu Q, Zhao K, Wang C, *et al.* Multistage delivery nanoparticle facilitates efficient CRISPR/dCas9 activation and tumor growth suppression in vivo. Adv Sci (Weinh) 2019; 6(1): 1801423.
[http://dx.doi.org/10.1002/advs.201801423] [PMID: 30643726]

[64] Li Z, Zhou X, Wei M, *et al.* *In vitro* and *in vivo* RNA inhibition by CD9-HuR functionalized exosomes encapsulated with miRNA or CRISPR/dCas9. Nano Lett 2019; 19(1): 19-28.
[http://dx.doi.org/10.1021/acs.nanolett.8b02689] [PMID: 30517011]

[65] Gessner I, Neundorf I. Nanoparticles modified with cell-penetrating peptides: Conjugation mechanisms, physicochemical properties, and application in cancer diagnosis and therapy. Int J Mol Sci 2020; 21(7): 2536.
[http://dx.doi.org/10.3390/ijms21072536] [PMID: 32268473]

[66] Ye S, Tian M, Wang T, *et al.* Synergistic effects of cell-penetrating peptide Tat and fusogenic peptide HA2-enhanced cellular internalization and gene transduction of organosilica nanoparticles. Nanomedicine 2012; 8(6): 833-41.
[http://dx.doi.org/10.1016/j.nano.2011.10.003] [PMID: 22033082]

[67] Taylor RE, Zahid M. Cell penetrating peptides, novel vectors for gene therapy. Pharmaceutics 2020; 12(3): 225.
[http://dx.doi.org/10.3390/pharmaceutics12030225] [PMID: 32138146]

[68] Huang S, Shao K, Liu Y, *et al.* Tumor-targeting and microenvironment-responsive smart nanoparticles for combination therapy of antiangiogenesis and apoptosis. ACS Nano 2013; 7(3): 2860-71.
[http://dx.doi.org/10.1021/nn400548g] [PMID: 23451830]

[69] Davis ME, Zuckerman JE, Choi CHJ, *et al.* Evidence of RNAi in humans from systemically administered siRNA *via* targeted nanoparticles. Nature 2010; 464(7291): 1067-70.
[http://dx.doi.org/10.1038/nature08956] [PMID: 20305636]

[70] Chen J, Guo Z, Tian H, Chen X. Production and clinical development of nanoparticles for gene delivery. Mol Ther Methods Clin Dev 2016; 3: 16023.
[http://dx.doi.org/10.1038/mtm.2016.23] [PMID: 27088105]

[71] Ikada Y. Challenges in tissue engineering. J R Soc Interface 2006; 3(10): 589-601.
[http://dx.doi.org/10.1098/rsif.2006.0124] [PMID: 16971328]

[72] Olson JL, Atala A, Yoo JJ. Tissue engineering: current strategies and future directions. Chonnam Med J 2011; 47(1): 1-13.
[http://dx.doi.org/10.4068/cmj.2011.47.1.1] [PMID: 22111050]

[73] Rehan F, Zhang M, Fang J, Greish K. Therapeutic applications of nanomedicine: recent developments and future perspectives. Molecules 2024; 29(9): 2073.
[http://dx.doi.org/10.3390/molecules29092073] [PMID: 38731563]

[74] Fathi-Achachelouei M, Knopf-Marques H, Ribeiro da Silva CE, *et al.* Use of nanoparticles in tissue engineering and regenerative medicine. Front Bioeng Biotechnol 2019; 7: 113.
[http://dx.doi.org/10.3389/fbioe.2019.00113] [PMID: 31179276]

[75] Shi J, Votruba AR, Farokhzad OC, Langer R. Nanotechnology in drug delivery and tissue engineering: from discovery to applications. Nano Lett 2010; 10(9): 3223-30.
[http://dx.doi.org/10.1021/nl102184c] [PMID: 20726522]

[76] Borzenkov M, Chirico G, Collini M, Pallavicini P. Gold nanoparticles for tissue engineering. Environmental Nanotechnology: Volume 1. 2018:343-90.

[77] Mitchell MJ, Billingsley MM, Haley RM, Wechsler ME, Peppas NA, Langer R. Engineering precision nanoparticles for drug delivery. Nat Rev Drug Discov 2021; 20(2): 101-24.
[PMID: 33277608]

[78] Buyukhatipoglu K, Chang R, Sun W, Clyne AM. Bioprinted nanoparticles for tissue engineering. 2009.
[http://dx.doi.org/10.1109/CIMSA.2009.5069956]

[79] Bianchi E, Vigani B, Viseras C, Ferrari F, Rossi S, Sandri G. Inorganic nanomaterials in tissue engineering. Pharmaceutics. 2022 May 26;14(6):1127.

[80] Rehan F, Zhang M, Fang J, Greish K. Therapeutic applications of nanomedicine: recent developments and future perspectives. Molecules 2024; 29(9): 2073.
[PMID: 38731563].

[81] Sharma K, Tharmatt A, Chawla PA, Shah K, Chawla V, Sapra B, Bedi N. An Insight into Advanced Nanoparticles as Multifunctional Biomimetic Systems in Tissue Engineering. InNanopharmaceuticals in Regenerative Medicine 2022 May 9 (pp. 1-19). CRC Press.
[http://dx.doi.org/10.1201/9781003153504-1]

[82] Hasan A, Morshed M, Memic A, Hassan S, Webster TJ, Marei HE. Nanoparticles in tissue engineering: applications, challenges and prospects. Int J Nanomedicine 2018; 13: 5637-55.
[PMID: 30288038]

[83] Alizadeh P, Soltani M, Tutar R, *et al.* Use of electroconductive biomaterials for engineering tissues by 3D printing and 3D bioprinting. Essays Biochem 2021; 65(3): 441-66.
[http://dx.doi.org/10.1042/EBC20210003] [PMID: 34296738]

[84] Loukelis K, Helal ZA, Mikos AG, Chatzinikolaidou M. Nanocomposite bioprinting for tissue engineering applications. Gels. 2023 Jan 24;9(2):103.

[85] Plotkin S. History of vaccination. Proc Natl Acad Sci USA 2014; 111(34): 12283-7.
[PMID: 25136134]

[86] Bezbaruah R, Chavda VP, Nongrang L, *et al.* Nanoparticle-based delivery systems for vaccines. Vaccines (Basel) 2022; 10(11): 1946.
[http://dx.doi.org/10.3390/vaccines10111946] [PMID: 36423041]

[87] Vela Ramirez JE, Sharpe LA, Peppas NA. Current state and challenges in developing oral vaccines. Adv Drug Deliv Rev 2017; 114: 116-31.
[http://dx.doi.org/10.1016/j.addr.2017.04.008] [PMID: 28438674]

[88] Yusuf A, Almotairy ARZ, Henidi H, Alshehri OY, Aldughaim MS. Nanoparticles as drug delivery systems: a review of the implication of nanoparticles' physicochemical properties on responses in biological systems. Polymers (Basel) 2023; 15(7): 1596.
[http://dx.doi.org/10.3390/polym15071596] [PMID: 37050210]

[89] Linkov I, Satterstrom FK, Corey LM. Nanotoxicology and nanomedicine: making hard decisions.

Nanomedicine 2008; 4(2): 167-71.
[http://dx.doi.org/10.1016/j.nano.2008.01.001] [PMID: 18329962]

[90] Miller MR, Poland CA. Nanotoxicology: the need for a human touch? Small 2020; 16(36): 2001516.
[http://dx.doi.org/10.1002/smll.202001516] [PMID: 32697439]

[91] Forest V. Experimental and computational nanotoxicology—Complementary approaches for nanomaterial hazard assessment. Nanomaterials (Basel) 2022; 12(8): 1346.
[http://dx.doi.org/10.3390/nano12081346] [PMID: 35458054]

[92] Domingues C, Santos A, Alvarez-Lorenzo C, Concheiro A, Jarak I, Veiga F, et al. Where Is It Headed. A Review of Nanomedicine and the Dilemma of Nanotoxicology. 2022; 16:9994-10041.

CHAPTER 4

Nanomaterials in Diagnostic Applications

Abhishek Mohanta[1], **Sohini Chatterjee**[1], **Mousumi Tudu**[1], **Suparna Garai**[1], **Arnab De**[2], **Pranab Naskar**[1] and **Amalesh Samanta**[1,*]

[1] *Division of Microbiology & Pharmaceutical Biotechnology, Department of Pharmaceutical Technology, Jadavpur University, Kolkata, India*

[2] *Department of Pharmaceutics, Bharat Technology, Uluberia, Howrah, West Bengal, India*

Abstract: In the past few years, nanomaterials have emerged tremendously for applications in the field of diagnosis and medicine. They have gained attention due to their extremely small size and mouldable characteristics. This chapter focuses on the different nanomaterials developed for use in diagnostics, treatment, and also as potent drug carriers. These nanomaterials, being very small in size, easily enter circulation to provide the desired therapeutic efficacy or facilitate faster diagnosis. Different nanomaterials, including nanoparticles, nanowires, nanoconjugates, and nanorods, have paved new dimensions in diagnosis and treatment. Not only do they facilitate the detection of diseases by serving as biomarkers, but they also bring to the forefront areas of medicine that were previously difficult to treat or detect using primitive and traditional analytical techniques.

Keywords: Nanomedicine, Nanotubes, Nanofilms, Nanofibers, Nanomembranes, Targeted Drug Delivery.

INTRODUCTION

The presence of several pathogenic viruses, along with microbes and their mutations, and the bacterial resistance towards antibiotics, diseases like cancer, diabetes, and other genetic disorders, poses a severe challenge to the medical system and also humanity. In order to treat such cases, it is very important to make an initial diagnosis and arrest the infection. In this regard, the recent development in the field of nanotechnology has paved the way to solve such crises in medicine and healthcare [1, 2].

Nanotechnology involves the use of nanomaterials, which are very tiny in size, ranging from 1-100 nm, but possess a bigger surface area. Nanomaterials are tested to have outstanding thermal, chemical, and optical properties, making

* **Corresponding author Amalesh Samanta:** Division of Microbiology & Pharmaceutical Biotechnology, Department of Pharmaceutical Technology, Jadavpur University, Kolkata, India; E-mail: amalesh.samanta@jadavpuruniversity.in

Soumik Podder & Amalesh Samanta (Eds.)

them a potential candidate in the biomedical field of research and development. Based on dimensions, nanomaterials can be zero-dimensional [nanoparticles; NPs], one-dimensional [nanorods, nanotubes], and two-dimensional [nanofilms, nanolayers] [3].

The ultra-small size and good surface area, prominent mechanical properties, and optical and magnetic behaviour have made nanoparticles a widely accepted nanomaterial for biomedical applications. The nanodevice should be easily synthesized and biocompatible with the human body. Nanodevices smaller than 500 Angstroms easily penetrate cell barriers, whereas thr ones that are nearly 200 Angstroms can circulate throughout the body, escaping blood vessels. Hence, they can interact with the body both extracellularly and intracellularly. Nanodevices can be used to detect and monitor cell abnormalities in regions that were previously not reachable, since they can reach all parts of the body [4].

The small size of these materials causes atoms and molecules to be mostly located at their surface, providing them with distinct physicochemical properties from those of bulk. Due to this arrangement of surface atoms, they tend to possess low binding energy and low melting point. The smaller size of nanomaterials leads to increased surface area per unit mass, thereby enhancing their chemical properties [5].

The process of nanomaterial engineering involves two different approaches, namely, top-down and bottom-up. In the case of the top-down method, larger pieces of material are broken down to the required size of the nanostructure. In the bottom-up procedure, single atoms and molecules are clustered to form a nanostructure. This is done with the help of supramolecular chemistry, biotechnology, and scanning probes. Both approaches are important in their own ways of nanomaterial synthesis, of which the bottom-up approach finds greater application [6].

Nanomaterials have combined several disciplines, including biotechnology, chemistry, molecular biology, and medicine, to develop newer approaches for medical diagnosis. They also offer high sensitivity toward detecting even very low concentrations of parasites, antibodies, or any other microbes in blood samples. This, in turn, helps to detect a disease at a very early stage, helping in providing better treatment facilities by healthcare professionals [7].

Nanotechnology also plays a crucial role in detecting cancer and its treatment, along with other diseases like gastrointestinal, antibacterial, antifungal, cardiovascular, neural, inflammatory, infectious, and autoimmune disorders, *etc* [8].

This book chapter focuses on the benefits of nanomaterials in biological sciences and their future in the medical field, particularly in diagnosis and treatment. We have elaborated the role of nanoparticles, quantum dots, one and two-dimensional nanomaterials, composites, carbon nanotubes, and others in diagnostic applications.

Different Types of Nanomedicine

A comparatively recent area of research and development, termed nanotechnology, has produced creative solutions for numerous medical problems. The term "nanomedicine" refers to the combination of its uses in illness screening, diagnosis, and treatment. This is an emerging discipline that could transform the entire healthcare system [9]. While particles between 1 and 100 nm in size are traditionally referred to as being in the nanomaterial's domain, those smaller than one μm are also sometimes recognized. The main target of these nanomaterials is to contribute at the molecular level in the pharmaceutical as well as medical fields [10]. Nanomedicines provide better therapeutic activity by improving target specificity, pharmacokinetic parameters, and minimizing side effects by enabling the delivery of lesser amount of dose with high effectiveness [11].

Nanoparticles: Nanoparticles refer to tiny particles having exterior diameters ranging from 1-100nm. Various methods can be employed for the preparation of nanoparticles, such as hydrothermal synthesis, chemical reduction, coprecipitation, seeding, microemulsion, and son electrodeposition [12]. The energy levels of atoms present on the surface significantly influence the characteristics of nanoparticles, such as electromagnetism, optical properties, *etc.*, because they have a far larger surface-to-mass proportion than conventional materials. Due to these special qualities, nanoparticles are very desirable for multiple applications, such as medical fields, solar power, petroleum, and electrical power storage, *etc.* (Fig. **1**) [13].

2D Materials: A variety of self-supporting, membrane-like nanomaterials with a significant diagonal shape to thickness proportion are known as 2D [two-dimensional] materials. The two-dimensional nanomaterials are a family of laminated materials that are extremely fine and have a linear, distinctly anisotropic design. Two-dimensional nanomaterials with linear texture have strong activity, a high surface-to-volume ratio, superior mechanical qualities, and intrinsic optical activity that makes them suitable for a range of biological applications [14]. In general, two-dimensional nanoparticles can be divided into three main groups: inorganic, organic, and hybrid. 2D nanomaterials provide a distinctive connection for nano- and micro-range systems by binding with cells at the nanoscale and by offering broad surfaces for association. Particular 2D nanoparticles are involved for the purpose of drug delivery, regenerative medicine, cell culture, biosensing, electrochemical sensing, biosensing, and diagnostic imaging [15].

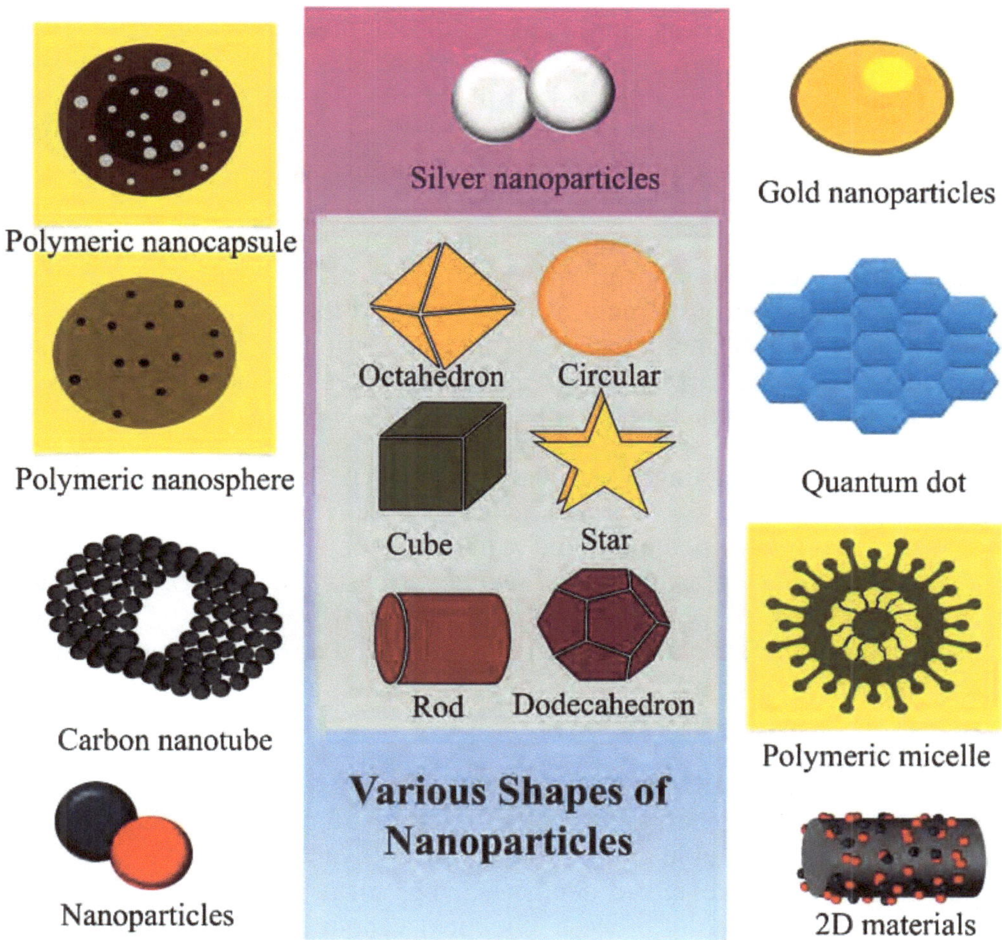

Fig. (1). Different types of NPs and their shapes [5].

Quantum Dots: Matter with a size range smaller than the exciton Bohr diameter is known as Quantum Dots [QDs], which are crystals of semiconductors at the nanoscale scale made of classes II–VI or III–V elements [16]. It has discrete, narrow optical line spectra and is made up of about 100–10000 atoms. For this reason, Quantum dots are frequently referred to as artificial atoms. Rod-shaped, tetrapod, and spherical quantum dots are possible to prepare. Although particularly spherical-shaped quantum dots are preferable in biomedical fields [17].

Nanofiber: Nanofibers are polymeric fibres having a size range from 1nm to 1μm. Fibers are classified as continuous or discontinuous/short fibres based on their lengths [18]. Although electrospinning, phase separation, and self-assembly methods [19] are commonly followed for the preparation of nanofibers, CO_2 laser supersonic drawing, solution blow spinning, electrohydrodynamic direct writing, plasma-induced synthesis, and centrifugal jet spinning are several methods used for nanofiber preparation. All these methods are emerging because the electrospinning method has several limitations, including the need for equipment, targets that are electrically transmissible, and high electrical potential. Nanofibers can be arranged into porous structures like biological tissue that can be applied in various biological applications such as tissue engineering, wound healing dressing preparation, *etc*. As the surface energy and surface area of a nanofiber are higher, it allows for better cell attachment [18].

Nanowire: Semiconducting nanowires are one of the most effective nanomaterials available for therapeutic uses. Electrical detection of different species can be done immediately and without labeling by using this nanowire [20]. Nanowires can be prepared by following various methods such as alternating current electrodeposition, heat evaporation, Chemical Vapor Deposition (CVD), and laser ablation [21]. Nanowires are mainly used in various fields such as electronics, energy storage, biosensing, medical gadget preparation, and drug/gene/protein delivery systems [22].

Nanorods: Nanorods are nanostructured rod-shaped materials prepared by electrospinning or hydrothermal process. Preferably, the hydrothermal process is used because it is affordable and time-saving [23]. Nanorods can be synthesised by various methods like electrodeposition, chemical vapour deposition, seed capping, vapour liquid solid process, chemical vapour deposition, biomolecular template synthesis, *etc.* These nanoparticles are potential candidates for drug or gene delivery, biosensing, biomedical imaging, *etc* [24].

Carbon Nanotubes: Carbon nanotubes were first discovered by Sumio Iijima in the year 1991. These are tubular, structured, straight fiber-like materials made of carbon [25]. There are two types of nanotubes, single-walled nanotubes and multi-walled nanotubes, depending on the distribution of the graphene tube. Nanotubes are prepared by chemical vapour deposition [CVD] method, electric arc discharge method, and laser ablation method [26]. These nanotubes are potentially useful for various biomedical purposes such as biosensing, targeted delivery of drugs, genes, proteins, and tissue engineering. There are some disadvantages of these nanotubes due to their hydrophobicity [27].

Nanodispersions: Nanodispersions are formulations consisting of nanosized components stabilized by surface-active agents. Nanodispersions widely cover nanosuspension, nanoemulsion, nanoliposomes, as well as swelling micelles, vesicles, and cubosomes [28]. Nanosuspensions are mainly developed to overcome the solubility and bioavailability issues of lipophilic drugs with poor water solubility, thereby improving their therapeutic effectiveness [29]. This preparation follows two major methods, the top-down process and the bottom-up process, respectively. These two methods include homogenization, precipitation, milling, supercritical fluid process, *etc* [30]. Nanosuspension technique helps to prepare various drug delivery systems, *e.g.*, carbamazepine, insulin, griseofulvin for oral drug delivery, hydrocortisone, prednisolone for ophthalmic drug delivery, clofazimine, paclitaxel for parenteral delivery, silver for topical delivery, *etc* [31]. Nanoemulsions consist of nanosized droplets ranging from approximately 20 to 500 nm. Due to their small droplet size, they provide remarkable qualities, including superior stability and flow properties, suitable for a wide range of medical and pharmaceutical fields, as well as the cosmetic field [32]. Nanoliposomes consist of nanosized bilayer lipid vesicles with enhanced stability, shelf life, and bioavailability. Nanoliposomes are used as a carrier for drug delivery, protein delivery, and gene delivery [33].

Nanocomposites: The term "nanocomposites" now refers to a wide range of systems, including one, two, three-dimensional, and amorphous substances that are blended at the nanoscale range and composed of distinguishable elements [34]. Depending on the matrix component, nanocomposites can be categorised as polymer matrix nanocomposites (PMNC), ceramic matrix nanocomposites (CMNC), and metal matrix nanocomposites (MMNC). PMNCs are referred to as materials where nano-sized particles are incorporated in a polymeric matrix.

CMNCs consist of several ceramic component layers, which enhance their chemical, thermal stability, and durability. MMNCs are multilayered materials made of a flexible or alloy metal matrix with a small amount of nano-strengthening materials embedded in it [35].

Membranes: Nanomembranes refer to the materials or structures having a thickness lower than 100 nm with a larger surface area, along with a size-t--thickness aspect ratio higher than 10^6. Nano membranes are made up of inorganic and organic materials, as well as hybrid or composite materials. In the case of inorganic nanomembrane preparation, commonly metals and their oxides are used, such as gold (Au), titanium oxide (TiO_2), and zinc oxide (ZnO). Organic nanomembranes consist of polyvinyl chloride (PVC), polyacrylonitrile, *etc.*, and hybrid nanomaterials are composed of polymers along with nanofillers [36].

Polymers: Nano polymers include both synthetic and natural polymers. According to their source, these can be categorized as natural inorganic nanopolymer, *e.g.*, graphite, natural organic nanopolymer, *e.g.*, polysaccharide, and synthetic nanopolymer, *e.g.*, concrete. Nanopolymers can be prepared by vapour condensation, vacuum evaporation, and the electrospinning process [37]. Nano polymers are biodegradable and biocompatible; this quality makes them suitable for various drug delivery systems, *e.g.*, nanotubes, nano cells, polymersomes, *etc* [38].

Diagnostic Applications of Nanomaterials: Nanomaterials play a vital role in biomedicine, and many nanomaterials have been developed in the last few decades to achieve the greatest outcomes in the field of medical diagnostics. Nanomaterials provide minimal surface heterogenic responsiveness, which allows the biomarkers to bind easily to their surfaces, and surface modification of nanomaterials also provides good adsorbing ability for the biomarkers. Different types of interactions occur between the nanomaterials and biomarkers, like Vander Waals, hydrogen bonds, covalent and non-covalent bonding, electrostatic forces, *etc* [39]. In this chapter, we will briefly discuss the diagnostic applications of the various nanomaterials.

Diagnostic Applications of Nanoparticles

Nanoparticles play a vital role in diagnostic applications because of their size at the nanoscale. Computed Tomography (CT), Magnetic Resonance Imaging (MRI), optical imaging, and numerous other imaging techniques utilise nanoparticles [40]. Modified and well-designed nanoparticles can increase the contrast in these imaging sense modalities so that tissues, organs, and even individual cells can be more clearly seen. Nanoparticles in drug delivery systems play a crucial role as active drug carriers because of their small size, specific target area, excellent surface properties, ability to decrease side effects, and ability to enhance the efficacy of drug molecules. They also functionalize with biomolecules like DNA, enzymes, antibodies, *etc* [41], by creating biosensors, and these biosensors can detect biological samples with higher specificity, for example, sensing cancer biomarkers, environmental pollutants, various pathogens, *etc.* Nanoparticles are used in point-of-care testing devices because they are capable of amplifying signals and improving the sensitivity of the devices, which can detect various types of infectious diseases, *etc* [41]. It can deliver diagnostic agents like drug molecules, genes, *etc.* Personalised medication can be given to patients in the targeted area. Nanoparticles are also used in environmental monitoring, like detecting heavy metals, toxins, environmental pollutants, and pathogens. In molecular diagnosis, nanoparticles play an important role (Fig. **2**) [42]. It also increases specificity and sensing quality, improves signal amplification, single-molecule detection of nucleic acid sequencing, and Polymerase Chain Reaction (PCR) [43 - 46].

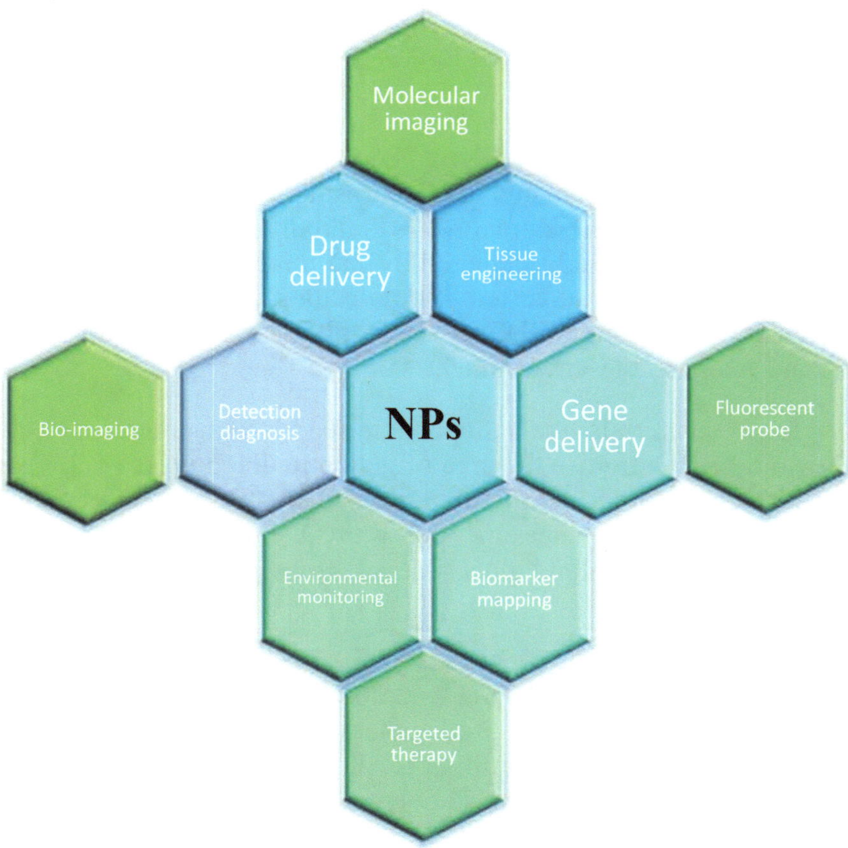

Fig. (2). Diagnostic applications of nanomaterials.

Diagnostic Application of 2D Materials: 2D materials like graphene and other nanomaterials play a significant role in the healthcare system. Several domains are being explored for the use of 2D materials in diagnostics, including 2D materials that are capable of detecting biomarkers for several diseases, like infectious diseases and cancer. It can be integrated into medical devices to get accurate measurement and detection of sensitive biomolecules in body fluids [47].

2D Materials have their own unique optical, mechanical, and electrical properties. It can be used to develop sophisticated, highly sensitive biosensors. For example, graphene can detect pathogens or some specific biomolecules by measuring the surface with receptors that can bind with targeting biomolecules. The shift in values in the case of conductivity and fluorescence can be easily detected by these [48].

Two-dimensional materials like graphene oxide provide unique optical characteristics that render them suitable contrast agents, enabling high-resolution imaging in the biomedical domain [49]. Toxins and pollutants from the environment can be effectively detected by 2D materials because of their large surface area and sensitivity to certain biomolecules. Detection of environmental hazardous materials through 2D materials plays a crucial role in reducing emissions and keeping the environment safe.

The ability for 2D materials like nanopores to read DNA sequencing quickly and accurately would revolutionise the area of genomic diagnostics [47]. Overall, 2D materials also play an important role in point-of-care testing, as wearable sensors, *etc.*, by which they can measure the human body's many physiological parameters, like heart rate, blood glucose level, blood pressure measurement, *etc.*

Quantum Dots

Overpopulation, pollution, rapid aging, and unhealthy lifestyles may lead to many neurological diseases, like neurodegenerative diseases, brain tumours, cerebrovascular disease, *etc.* Quantum dots can be used for non-invasive vascular visualisation and continuous monitoring because of their several advantages, like high tissue penetrability, good resolution, fluorescence imaging capabilities, and quick data gathering. Additionally, it can sensitise other fluorescent nanomaterials, enhancing their luminescence impact [50]. In cases of ischemic stroke, imaging of cerebral vascular structure, or traumatic brain injury, the probe can be used. It is also expected that it can be helpful for early detection of ischemic stroke, in hospital monitoring, *etc.* (Fig. **3**) [51].

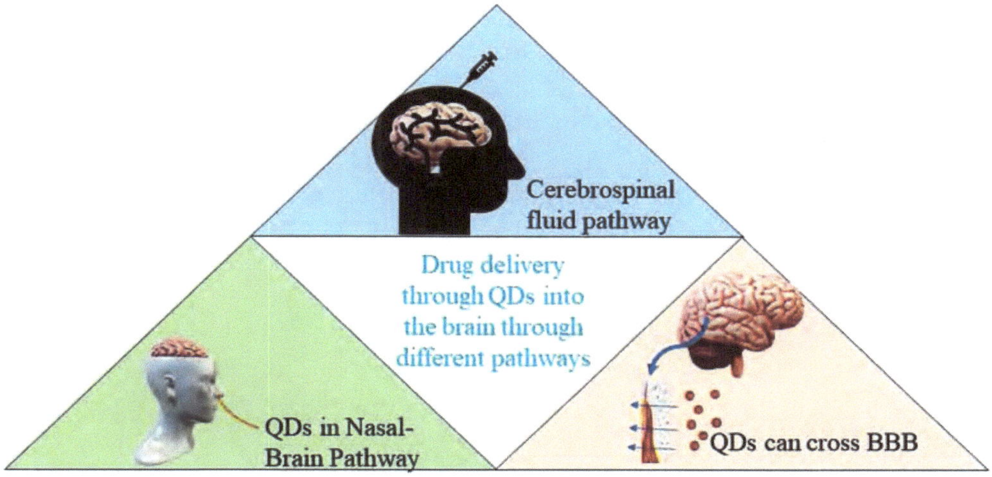

Fig. (3). Diagnostic application of quantum dots [68].

Nanofibre: They are porous nanostructures that allow them to interact freely with biomolecules. The interactions make it easier to detect body fluids, enzymes, and antibiotics, increasing the sensitivity of biosensors. They also allow target-oriented time-dependent drug release. They are also involved in disease detection, immunoassays, and in separation of pathogens from biological samples [52].

Nanowire: Nowadays, nanowire is a trending and innovative technology for the fabrication of nanofiber-based biosensors in health monitoring systems. It can detect exosomes, Circulating Tumour Cells (CTCs) from a blood sample, and plays a vital role in early cancer detection. Nanowires have a high surface area, and they can be used as a biosensing component. It can detect a single biomolecule with low concentration. Nanowire-based highly sensitive materials can detect specific viral or bacterial pathogens. It can offer more accurate, advanced technologies for health care diagnostic purposes [53].

Nanorods: Nanorods belong to a category of nanomaterials that have unique optical and electrical properties along with a high surface area to volume ratio and a size-dependent behaviour. The scope of nanorods in biomedical fields is huge, including their use as biosensors, targeted drug delivery, molecular detection, imaging, and theranostics. Nanorods find such profound use in disease diagnostics (cancer, cardiovascular, genetic disorders, *etc.*) due to their versatility, accuracy, and sensitivity [54].

Carbon Nanotubes – Carbon nanotubes (CNTs) are extensively used as a potential diagnostic material due to their characteristic physical, chemical, and electrical features. Some diagnostic applications of CNTs are:

- Carbon nanotubes have good electrical conductivity, which is why it is widely used as electrochemical biosensors to detect numerous biomolecules like DNA, cholesterol, glucose, *etc.* It is also used as an optical biosensor and can detect some specific molecules, like cancer biomarkers, *etc.* CNTs are used in a label-free detection system, which has a large surface area, so it can increase the sensitivity and detect target molecules at low concentrations [55].
- CNTs are applied as a contrasting substance for imaging purposes in Computed Tomography (CT), Magnetic Resonance Imaging (MRI), *etc.* (Fig. **4**). They are capable of detecting specific sequences of DNA or RNA by incorporating them into nanoscale devices. CNTs are incorporated into small or mini-sized portable devices for the detection of diseases on the spot, in a short period of time.
- It is also used to analyse blood samples, detect pathogenic microorganisms with accuracy in very short periods of time. CNTs are used in developing wearable devices that are light in weight and can monitor human physiological parameters like heart rate, blood pressure, and glucose level accurately [56].
- CNTs have some unique features; they are biocompatible, they are an electrically conductive material, they provide good sensitivity, and are versatile in nature, so they can detect a wide range of molecules [55].

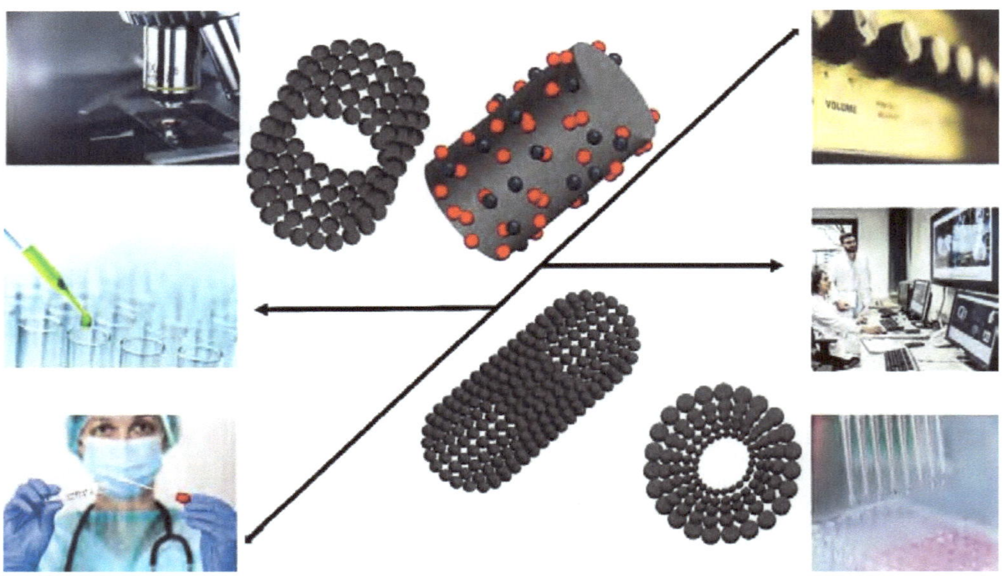

Fig. (4). Nanomaterials in various diagnostic fields.

Nano-dispersion: In diagnostic applications, nano-dispersion plays a key role and acts as an accurate diagnostic tool. When nanoparticles are dispersed uniformly within a liquid medium, that is called Nano-dispersion materials. For diagnostic purposes, like a contrast agent to enhance imaging in MRI, CT scan, *etc.* Mainly gold nanoparticles or ion oxide nanoparticles are used for this imaging purpose [57].

It also increases the sensitivity and performance of biosensors to detect biomarkers at minimum concentration. They also used it as a Point-of-Care (POC) diagnostic tool to get the result quickly with accuracy. In a pregnancy test kit, COVID-19 test kit nano-dispersed materials are used as probes to get authentic and faster results (Fig. **4**). It also plays a vital role in drug delivery for diagnosis. Nanoparticles loaded with drug molecules are used for targeted drug delivery in case of noncommunicable diseases (NCDs) like cancer, stroke, *etc* [58]. It can be used in *in-vitro* diagnosis as a diagnostic kit to analyse and monitor biological samples (blood, urine, *etc.*).

Nanocomposites in Diagnostic Applications

Nanocomposites are materials that are mainly composed of nanoparticles studded in a matrix that play a pivotal role in biomedical and diagnostic applications. Nanocomposites provide good mechanical strength, optical characteristics, and good electrical conductivity, making them beneficial for diagnostic purposes. In this chapter, we will discuss briefly how nanocomposites are used for diagnostic purposes:

- Nanocomposites are used as biosensors, and they can amplify signals and are capable of enhancing the sensitivity by which they can detect biomolecules accurately. Nanocomposites of gold nanoparticles or silver nanoparticles, which contain conductive polymers, are more efficient for electron transfer, and they can detect biomolecules like cholesterol, glucose, and DNA due to their sensitive detection. Fluorescent nanoparticle-containing nanocomposites play a pivotal role in optical biosensors [59]. They can generate highly sensitive real-time optical signals and detect target analytes like toxins, pathogens, *etc.* Cancer and critical cardiac conditions can be detected with the help of immunosensors produced from nanocomposites by enhancing the antigen-antibody reactions and detection of trace amounts of biomarkers that are associated with the disease [60].
- **Nanocomposites** are also used in fluorescent imaging and optical diagnostic purposes, by which live cell imaging and cancer detection are possible. It is also used as a colorimetric sensor by which the detection of heavy metals, pathogens, toxins, and environmental monitoring is possible [60].

Nanomembranes in Diagnostic Applications

Nanomembranes are biocompatible and highly sensitive components appropriate for analysing biomolecules and detecting biomarkers. Nanomembranes are incorporated into biosensors to enhance selectivity, sensitivity, and reduce the detection time of specific biomarkers and pathogens. In an electrochemical biosensor, it plays a crucial role by detecting diseases like cancer, diabetes (by monitoring glucose level), *etc* [61].

- Nanomembranes are capable of separating out the cells, bacteria, or viruses from the biological fluids like saliva, blood, *etc.* It can capture target cells like circulating tumour cells from the blood sample, which is helpful to detect cancer at an early stage.
    - Nanomembranes are incorporated into wearable sensors to detect and analyse interstitial fluids, sweat, or other biological fluids to detect diagnostic information and continuous monitoring of the patient's health condition [62].
- Nanomembranes are also used in DNA/RNA extraction from biological samples to diagnose infectious diseases and genetic disorders. It is highly effective in the separation and filtration process by which blood purification, isolation of exosomes, and nanoparticle separation are done [63].
- Nanomembranes are used to detect specific biomarkers like proteins, antibodies, antigens, *etc.* It can be functionalized with a specific antibody to bind with a selective antigen present in the sample to detect infectious or autoimmune disorders.
- Nanomembranes are highly sensitive, rapid, responsive, and biocompatible, with an accurate selectivity component that is relatively easy to manufacture on an industrial scale for the huge production of diagnostic devices. But maintaining its structural integrity and durability over time is challenging, and the manufacturing cost, its implementation in diagnostic devices is challenging and costly [61].

Polymers in Diagnostic Applications: Nano-polymer plays an important role in our daily lives. Nano-polymers are innovative components playing a significant role in biomedical and diagnostic applications. They are unique in having specific physical, chemical, and biological properties. In industry, nano-polymers are used to produce building materials, fibres, adhesives, concrete, liquid crystal, apparel, plastics, ceramics, *etc.* Their nano-scale size improves surface area, increases the interactions with biological targets, and makes them suitable for *in vivo* interactions [64]. Here are some diagnostic applications of nano-polymers:

- Nano-polymer increases the sensitivity and selectivity when incorporated into a biosensor. They create a sophisticated detection platform of specific biomolecules like antibodies or enzymes. Nano-polymers play a remarkable role in the detection of various pathogens, like bacteria, viruses, glucose level monitoring in diabetic patients, and other medical diagnostic purposes [37].
- Nano-polymers can transmit fluorescent dyes in a specific wavelength, thereby emitting light at an excited state. Nano-polymers are widely used in *in vivo* imaging, cancer diagnosis, and fluorescence resonance energy transfer. Targeted nanopolymers can detect cancer cells by enhancing the contrast of images, and they are capable of accumulating tumour tissues. It can help to visualize molecular interactions in living organisms, tissues, and cells with high definition. Nano-polymers are also used in Fluorescence Resonance Energy Transfer (FRET) in molecular biology research, new drug discovery, *etc* [65].
- Nano-polymers can release drug molecules in the targeted area, and they are responsive according to the changes of the physiological environment, like pH, temperature, *etc*. It is also capable of delivering drug molecules to the desired site and can monitor the treatment efficacy by imaging or sensing. Detection of diagnosis of infectious diseases through nanopolymer offering in minutes, not in days, and the technique is well known as lab-on-a-chip technology. It can bind with specific proteins and amino acids and plays a vital role in the detection of DNA and proteins [66, 67].

Future Perspective: Biomaterials are a prospective component in biotechnology, nanotechnology, and material science. They play a pivotal role in regenerative medicine, medical devices and equipment, drug delivery, tissue engineering, and many other healthcare sectors. They can change their properties like stiffness, shape, drug release, and response to external stimuli like pH, temperature, *etc*. They are self-healing materials, can mimic the biological environment and play a vital role in tissue engineering and wound healing. Personalized biomaterials like patient-specific implants, scaffolds, self-healing hydrogel, biopolymeric hydrogel films, *etc*., could significantly improve patient safety, and in the future, they will play a crucial role in diagnostic purposes. With continuous research and development, further innovation on biomaterials may help to develop artificial organs like the liver, kidneys, and heart that can mimic the human organ's functionalities. In summary, biomaterials will play a transformative role in immunotechnology, 3D bioprinting, biosensors, nano-scale drug delivery, cancer, immunotherapy, implantable biosensors, health monitoring, and smart medical devices to enhance the quality of life.

CONCLUSION

Nanomaterials enhance the functionality and versatility in medical science by providing the quality of accurate diagnosis. These materials have their own unique properties like flexibility, high surface area, and biocompatibility. Nanomaterials have significant potential in imaging, biosensing, and detection of biomolecules, for example, gold nanoparticles, magnetic nanoparticles, quantum dots, nanomembranes, and nanopolymers are revolutionizing diagnostic materials, allowing for to detection of highly sensitive molecules as biomarkers, targeting drug therapy and disease monitoring, and disease progression. Despite these advantages, drawbacks remain, like toxicity, long-term stability, long-term biocompatibility, widespread clinical trials to evaluate safety and efficacy, *etc.* In conclusion, nanomaterials enable point-of-care diagnosis, introduce advanced technologies in medical devices to detect diseases early and quickly. Diagnostic application of nanomaterials is still sprouting, and it will play a leading role in modern medical science.

REFERENCES

[1] Abd Elkodous M, El-Sayyad GS, Nasser HA, *et al.* Engineered nanomaterials as potential candidates for HIV treatment: between opportunities and challenges. J Cluster Sci 2019; 30(3): 531-40. [http://dx.doi.org/10.1007/s10876-019-01533-8]

[2] Liu Y, Miyoshi H, Nakamura M. Nanomedicine for drug delivery and imaging: A promising avenue for cancer therapy and diagnosis using targeted functional nanoparticles. Int J Cancer 2007; 120(12): 2527-37. [http://dx.doi.org/10.1002/ijc.22709] [PMID: 17390371]

[3] Chen S, Zhu J, Wu X, Han Q, Wang X. Graphene oxide--MnO2 nanocomposites for supercapacitors. ACS Nano 2010; 4(5): 2822-30. [http://dx.doi.org/10.1021/nn901311t] [PMID: 20384318]

[4] Wang Y, Iqbal H, Ur-Rehman U, *et al.* Albumin-based nanodevices for breast cancer diagnosis and therapy. J Drug Deliv Sci Technol 2023; 79: 104072. [http://dx.doi.org/10.1016/j.jddst.2022.104072]

[5] Roduner E. Size matters: why nanomaterials are different. Chem Soc Rev 2006; 35(7): 583-92. [http://dx.doi.org/10.1039/b502142c] [PMID: 16791330]

[6] Arole V, Munde S. Fabrication of nanomaterials by top-down and bottom-up approachesan overview. J Mater Sci 2014; 1: 89-93.

[7] de la Escosura-Muñiz A, Baptista-Pires L, Serrano L, *et al.* Magnetic bead/gold nanoparticle double□labeled primers for electrochemical detection of isothermal amplified Leishmania DNA. Small 2016; 12(2): 205-13. [http://dx.doi.org/10.1002/smll.201502350] [PMID: 26578391]

[8] Kundu S, Abdullah MF, Das A, *et al.* Antifungal ouzo nanoparticles from guar gum propionate. RSC Advances 2016; 6(108): 106563-71. [http://dx.doi.org/10.1039/C6RA19658F]

[9] Zhang L, Gu FX, Chan JM, Wang AZ, Langer RS, Farokhzad OC. Nanoparticles in medicine: therapeutic applications and developments. Clin Pharmacol Ther 2008; 83(5): 761-9. [http://dx.doi.org/10.1038/sj.clpt.6100400] [PMID: 17957183]

[10] Boulaiz H, Alvarez PJ, Ramirez A, *et al.* Nanomedicine: application areas and development prospects. Int J Mol Sci 2011; 12(5): 3303-21.
[http://dx.doi.org/10.3390/ijms12053303] [PMID: 21686186]

[11] Zarbin MA, Montemagno C, Leary JF, Ritch R. Nanotechnology in ophthalmology. Can J Ophthalmol 2010; 45(5): 457-76.
[http://dx.doi.org/10.3129/i10-090] [PMID: 20871642]

[12] Nam NH, Luong NH. Nanoparticles: Synthesis and applications. Materials for biomedical engineering. Elsevier 2019; pp. 211-40.
[http://dx.doi.org/10.1016/B978-0-08-102814-8.00008-1]

[13] Modena MM, Rühle B, Burg TP, Wuttke S. Nanoparticle characterization: what to measure? Adv Mater 2019; 31(32): 1901556.
[http://dx.doi.org/10.1002/adma.201901556] [PMID: 31148285]

[14] Murali A, Lokhande G, Deo KA, Brokesh A, Gaharwar AK. Emerging 2D nanomaterials for biomedical applications. Mater Today 2021; 50: 276-302.
[http://dx.doi.org/10.1016/j.mattod.2021.04.020] [PMID: 34970073]

[15] Chimene D, Alge DL, Gaharwar AK. Two-dimensional nanomaterials for biomedical applications: emerging trends and future prospects. Adv Mater 2015; 27(45): 7261-84.
[http://dx.doi.org/10.1002/adma.201502422] [PMID: 26459239]

[16] Jamieson T, Bakhshi R, Petrova D, Pocock R, Imani M, Seifalian AM. Biological applications of quantum dots. Biomaterials 2007; 28(31): 4717-32.
[http://dx.doi.org/10.1016/j.biomaterials.2007.07.014] [PMID: 17686516]

[17] Bailey RE, Smith AM, Nie S. Quantum dots in biology and medicine. Physica E 2004; 25(1): 1-12.
[http://dx.doi.org/10.1016/j.physe.2004.07.013]

[18] Rasouli R, Barhoum A, Bechelany M, Dufresne A. Nanofibers for biomedical and healthcare applications. Macromol Biosci 2019; 19(2): 1800256.
[http://dx.doi.org/10.1002/mabi.201800256] [PMID: 30485660]

[19] Eatemadi A, Daraee H, Zarghami N, Melat Yar H, Akbarzadeh A. Nanofiber: Synthesis and biomedical applications. Artif Cells Nanomed Biotechnol 2016; 44(1): 111-21.
[http://dx.doi.org/10.3109/21691401.2014.922568] [PMID: 24905339]

[20] Patolsky F, Zheng G, Lieber CM. Nanowire sensors for medicine and the life sciences. Nanomedicine (Lond) 2006; 1(1): 51-65.
[http://dx.doi.org/10.2217/17435889.1.1.51] [PMID: 17716209]

[21] Mahbub T, Hoque ME. Introduction to nanomaterials and nanomanufacturing for nanosensors. Nanofabrication for smart nanosensor applications. Elsevier 2020; pp. 1-20.
[http://dx.doi.org/10.1016/B978-0-12-820702-4.00001-5]

[22] Felton EJ, Reich DH. Biological applications of multifunctional magnetic nanowires. Biomedical Applications of Nanotechnology. 2007; pp. 1-22.

[23] Naidu KCB, Kumar NS, Banerjee P, Reddy BVS. A review on the origin of nanofibers/nanorods structures and applications. J Mater Sci Mater Med 2021; 32(6): 68.
[http://dx.doi.org/10.1007/s10856-021-06541-7] [PMID: 34117944]

[24] Pearce ME, Melanko JB, Salem AK. Multifunctional nanorods for biomedical applications. Pharm Res 2007; 24(12): 2335-52.
[http://dx.doi.org/10.1007/s11095-007-9380-7] [PMID: 17684708]

[25] Ajayan PM, Zhou OZ. Applications of carbon nanotubes. Carbon nanotubes: synthesis, structure, properties, and applications 2001; 391-425.
[http://dx.doi.org/10.1007/3-540-39947-X_14]

[26] Popov V. Carbon nanotubes: properties and application. Mater Sci Eng Rep 2004; 43(3): 61-102.

[http://dx.doi.org/10.1016/j.mser.2003.10.001]

[27] Simon J, Flahaut E, Golzio M. Overview of carbon nanotubes for biomedical applications. Materials (Basel) 2019; 12(4): 624.
[http://dx.doi.org/10.3390/ma12040624] [PMID: 30791507]

[28] Sethuraman V, Ramesh A, Janakiraman K, Balakrishnan N. Nanodispersions for drug delivery applications: a special focus toward cancer therapeutics. J Nanopart Res 2024; 26(6): 116.
[http://dx.doi.org/10.1007/s11051-024-06026-y]

[29] Agrawal YK, Patel VR. Nanosuspension: An approach to enhance solubility of drugs. J Adv Pharm Technol Res 2011; 2(2): 81-7.
[http://dx.doi.org/10.4103/2231-4040.82950] [PMID: 22171298]

[30] Geetha G, Poojitha U, Khan KAA. Various techniques for preparation of nanosuspensiona review. Int J Pharma Res Rev 2014; 3(9): 30-7.

[31] Chingunpituk J. Nanosuspension technology for drug delivery. Walailak J Sci Technol 2007; 4(2): 139-53.

[32] Sghier K, Mur M, Veiga F, Paiva-Santos AC, Pires PC. Novel therapeutic hybrid systems using hydrogels and nanotechnology: a focus on nanoemulgels for the treatment of skin diseases. Gels 2024; 10(1): 45.
[http://dx.doi.org/10.3390/gels10010045] [PMID: 38247768]

[33] Panahi Y, Farshbaf M, Mohammadhosseini M, *et al.* Recent advances on liposomal nanoparticles: synthesis, characterization and biomedical applications. Artif Cells Nanomed Biotechnol 2017; 45(4): 788-99.
[http://dx.doi.org/10.1080/21691401.2017.1282496] [PMID: 28278586]

[34] Okpala CC. Nanocomposites–an overview. International Journal of Engineering Research and Development 2013; 8(11): 17-23.

[35] Al-Mutairi NH, Mehdi AH, Kadhim BJ. Nanocomposites materials definitions, types and some of their applications: A review. European Journal of Research Development and Sustainability 2022; 3(2): 102-8.

[36] Ciganė U, Palevičius A, Janušas G. Review of nanomembranes: materials, fabrications and applications in tissue engineering (bone and skin) and drug delivery systems. J Mater Sci 2021; 56(24): 13479-98.
[http://dx.doi.org/10.1007/s10853-021-06164-x]

[37] Saiyad M, Shah N. Nanopolymers in drug delivery system. Mater Today Proc 2022; 67: 25-30.
[http://dx.doi.org/10.1016/j.matpr.2022.05.019]

[38] Abuzreda A. Nanopolymers Types, Classification, Properties, and uses. Adv Env was Man Rec 2023; 6(2): 402-8.

[39] Baetke SC, Lammers T, Kiessling F. Applications of nanoparticles for diagnosis and therapy of cancer. Br J Radiol 2015; 88(1054): 20150207.
[http://dx.doi.org/10.1259/bjr.20150207] [PMID: 25969868]

[40] Padmanabhan P, Kumar A, Kumar S, Chaudhary RK, Gulyás B. Nanoparticles in practice for molecular-imaging applications: An overview. Acta Biomater 2016; 41: 1-16.
[http://dx.doi.org/10.1016/j.actbio.2016.06.003] [PMID: 27265153]

[41] Rarokar N, Yadav S, Saoji S, *et al.* Magnetic nanosystem a tool for targeted delivery and diagnostic application: Current challenges and recent advancement. Int J Pharm X 2024; 7: 100231.
[http://dx.doi.org/10.1016/j.ijpx.2024.100231] [PMID: 38322276]

[42] Nayak AK, Bera H, Hasnain MS, De A, Pal D, Samanta A. Gellan gum-based nanomaterials in drug delivery applications. Biopolymer-Based Nanomaterials in Drug Delivery and Biomedical Applications. Elsevier 2021; pp. 313-36.

[http://dx.doi.org/10.1016/B978-0-12-820874-8.00004-X]

[43] Oliveira BB, Ferreira D, Fernandes AR, Baptista PV. Engineering gold nanoparticles for molecular diagnostics and biosensing. Wiley Interdiscip Rev Nanomed Nanobiotechnol 2023; 15(1): e1836. [http://dx.doi.org/10.1002/wnan.1836] [PMID: 35932114]

[44] Tabatabaei MS, Islam R, Ahmed M. Applications of gold nanoparticles in ELISA, PCR, and immuno-PCR assays: A review. Anal Chim Acta 2021; 1143: 250-66. [http://dx.doi.org/10.1016/j.aca.2020.08.030] [PMID: 33384122]

[45] Singh A, Amiji MM. Application of nanotechnology in medical diagnosis and imaging. Curr Opin Biotechnol 2022; 74: 241-6. [http://dx.doi.org/10.1016/j.copbio.2021.12.011] [PMID: 34995920]

[46] Hazra A, Tudu M, Mohanta A, Samanta A. Gum odina prebiotic induced gut modulation for the treatment of colon cancer on Swiss albino mice: By using capecitabine loaded biopolymeric microsphere. Int J Biol Macromol 2024; 267(Pt 2): 131410. [http://dx.doi.org/10.1016/j.ijbiomac.2024.131410] [PMID: 38582484]

[47] Mukherjee S, Mukherjee A, Bytesnikova Z, Ashrafi AM, Richtera L, Adam V. 2D graphene-based advanced nanoarchitectonics for electrochemical biosensors: Applications in cancer biomarker detection. Biosens Bioelectron 2024; 250: 116050. [http://dx.doi.org/10.1016/j.bios.2024.116050] [PMID: 38301543]

[48] Lu B, Xia Y, Ren Y, *et al.* When Machine Learning Meets 2D Materials: A Review. Adv Sci (Weinh) 2024; 11(13): 2305277. [http://dx.doi.org/10.1002/advs.202305277] [PMID: 38279508]

[49] Younis M, Kumar Digra S, Gupta A, Anand V, Kumar P. Potential of 2D Materials: Novel Insights and Applications in Colorectal Cancer Research. Two-dimensional Hybrid Composites: Synthesis, Properties and Applications. Springer 2024; pp. 351-73. [http://dx.doi.org/10.1007/978-981-99-8010-9_13]

[50] Wang ZG, Wan LS, Liu ZM, Huang XJ, Xu ZK. Enzyme immobilization on electrospun polymer nanofibers: An overview. J Mol Catal, B Enzym 2009; 56(4): 189-95. [http://dx.doi.org/10.1016/j.molcatb.2008.05.005]

[51] Soldado A, Barrio LC, Díaz-Gonzalez M, de la Escosura-Muñiz A, Costa-Fernandez JM. Advances in quantum dots as diagnostic tools. Adv Clin Chem 2022; 107: 1-40. [http://dx.doi.org/10.1016/bs.acc.2021.07.001] [PMID: 35337601]

[52] Rezaei Z, Mahmoudifard M. Pivotal role of electrospun nanofibers in microfluidic diagnostic systems – a review. J Mater Chem B Mater Biol Med 2019; 7(30): 4602-19. [http://dx.doi.org/10.1039/C9TB00682F] [PMID: 31364667]

[53] Ambhorkar P, Wang Z, Ko H, *et al.* Nanowire-based biosensors: from growth to applications. Micromachines (Basel) 2018; 9(12): 679. [http://dx.doi.org/10.3390/mi9120679] [PMID: 30572645]

[54] Kim MJ, Jung DH, Lee CY, Hong S, Heo JH, Lee JH. Structurally engineered silica shells on gold nanorods for biomedical applications. Small Struct 2023; 4(9): 2300047. [http://dx.doi.org/10.1002/sstr.202300047]

[55] Zhang Y, Guo J, Tang Z, *et al.* Recent developments and trends of biosensors based on carbon nanotubes for biomedical diagnosis applications: A review. Biosens Bioelectron 2023; X: 100424.

[56] Barani M, Khatami M, Behnam B, Rajendram R, Kesharwani P, Sahebkar A. Aptamerconjugated carbon nanotubes or graphene for targeted cancer therapy and diagnosis. Aptamers engineered nanocarriers for cancer therapy. Elsevier 2023; pp. 277-94. [http://dx.doi.org/10.1016/B978-0-323-85881-6.00018-X]

[57] Ma WW, Zhu M, Lam ET, *et al.* A phase I pharmacokinetic and safety study of Paclitaxel Injection Concentrate for Nano-dispersion (PICN) alone and in combination with carboplatin in patients with

advanced solid malignancies and biliary tract cancers. Cancer Chemother Pharmacol 2021; 87(6): 779-88.
[http://dx.doi.org/10.1007/s00280-021-04235-z] [PMID: 33634324]

[58] Kumar M, Hilles AR, Almurisi SHA, Bhatia A, Mahmood S. Micro and nano-carriersbased pulmonary drug delivery system: Their current updates, challenges, and limitations– A review. JCIS Open. 2023; p. 100095.

[59] Andoh V, Ocansey D, Naveed H, *et al.* The Advancing Role of Nanocomposites in Cancer Diagnosis and Treatment. Int J Nanomedicine 2024; 19: 6099-126.
[http://dx.doi.org/10.2147/IJN.S471360] [PMID: 38911500]

[60] Ali MA, Singh C, Srivastava S, *et al.* Graphene oxide–metal nanocomposites for cancer biomarker detection. RSC Advances 2017; 7(57): 35982-91.
[http://dx.doi.org/10.1039/C7RA05491B]

[61] Zanghelini F, Frías IAM, Rêgo MJBM, *et al.* Biosensing breast cancer cells based on a three-dimensional TIO_2 nanomembrane transducer. Biosens Bioelectron 2017; 92: 313-20.
[http://dx.doi.org/10.1016/j.bios.2016.11.006] [PMID: 27840037]

[62] Welch EC, Powell JM, Clevinger TB, Fairman AE, Shukla A. Advances in biosensors and diagnostic technologies using nanostructures and nanomaterials. Adv Funct Mater 2021; 31(44): 2104126.
[http://dx.doi.org/10.1002/adfm.202104126]

[63] Senapati S, Basuray S, Slouka Z, Cheng LJ, Chang HC. A nanomembrane-based nucleic acid sensing platform for portable diagnostics. In: Lin B, Ed. Microfluidics. Topics in Current Chemistry. Berlin, Heidelberg: Springer 2011; 304: pp. 153-69.
[http://dx.doi.org/10.1007/128_2011_142]

[64] Hazra A, Chatterjee S, Mohanta A, Paul P, Samanta A. A review on fungal pullulan as a natural polymer focusing on targeted therapy for colon cancer and other pharmaceutical applications. Polym Adv Technol 2023; 34(10): 3183-92.
[http://dx.doi.org/10.1002/pat.6139]

[65] De A, Das S, Ghosh S, *et al.* Theranostic nanovesicles. Applications of Nanovesicular Drug Delivery. Elsevier 2022; pp. 39-51.
[http://dx.doi.org/10.1016/B978-0-323-91865-7.00001-8]

[66] Tudu M, Hazra A, Paul P, Mohanta A, Chatterjee S, Samanta A. Effect of Different Ratios of Polyvinyl Alcohol-Gum Odina for the Preparation and Characterization of Biodegradable Composite Films. Biopolymers 2025; 16(1): e23630.
[http://dx.doi.org/10.1002/bip.23630]

[67] Ojha D, Mukherjee H, Mondal S, *et al.* Anti-inflammatory activity of Odina wodier Roxb, an Indian folk remedy, through inhibition of toll-like receptor 4 signaling pathway. PLoS One 2014; 9(8): e104939.
[http://dx.doi.org/10.1371/journal.pone.0104939] [PMID: 25153081]

[68] Hu Y, Wang X, Niu Y, He K, Tang M. Application of quantum dots in brain diseases and their neurotoxic mechanism. Nanoscale Adv 2024; 6(15): 3733-46.
[http://dx.doi.org/10.1039/D4NA00028E] [PMID: 39050959]

CHAPTER 5

Nanomedicine for Conjugated Therapy and Diagnosis in Cancer Treatment

Panchanan Sahoo[1,2,*], **Mandira Das**[2], **Subham Adhikari**[2], **Abhishek Mukherjee**[3] and **Chandan Kumar Ghosh**[2,*]

[1] *Division of Biochemistry, ICMR-National Institute for Research in Bacterial Infections, Kolkata, West Bengal, India*

[2] *School of Materials Science and Nanotechnology, Jadavpur University, Kolkata, India*

[3] *Agricultural and Ecological Research Unit, Biological Science Division, Indian Statistical Institute, Giridih, Jharkhand, India*

Abstract: Cancer remains a leading cause of mortality worldwide, necessitating continuous innovation in its diagnosis and treatment. Traditional therapies, including chemotherapy and radiotherapy, face significant limitations such as systemic toxicity, poor selectivity, and drug resistance. Nanomedicine has emerged as a transformative strategy that integrates diagnosis and therapy (theranostics) within a single nanoplatform, enabling targeted drug delivery, stimuli-responsive controlled release of payload, multimodal therapy, and real-time treatment monitoring. This chapter reviews the evolution and applications of various nanomedicine modalities, including polymeric nanoparticles, lipid-based carriers, metallic and silica-based nanoparticles, quantum dots, and Prussian blue nanoparticles, among others. It explores their mechanism of action through both passive and active targeting strategies, discusses the integration of multimodal therapeutic functionalities, and addresses the challenges related to the tumor microenvironment, immune interactions, and clinical translation. Through an analysis of recent advancements and clinical evaluations, this chapter provides a comprehensive understanding of how nanomedicine is redefining cancer care and outlines the prospects and limitations for its widespread implementation in personalized oncology.

Keywords: Active and Passive Targeting, Clinical Translation, Multimodal Theranostics, Personalized Oncology, Stimuli-responsive Release.

* **Corresponding author Panchanan Sahoo and Chandan Kumar Ghosh:** Division of Biochemistry, ICMR-National Institute for Research in Bacterial Infections, Kolkata, West Bengal, India; E-mail: panchanansahoo288 @gmail.com School of Materials Science and Nanotechnology, Jadavpur University, Kolkata, India; E-mail: chandan.kghosh @jadavpuruniversity.in

Soumik Podder & Amalesh Samanta (Eds.)

INTRODUCTION

Cancer is a major global health concern, responsible for approximately 19.3 million new cases and 10.0 million deaths annually [1]. Its rising incidence and mortality rates pose a substantial challenge to increasing life expectancy worldwide. Although developed nations have experienced gradual improvements in cancer-survival rates due to advances in tumor biology, diagnostic innovations, and therapeutic strategies, the overall disease burden remains significant [2]. Addressing these growing challenges requires innovative approaches, continuous advancements, and optimized implementation of current cancer management strategies. Traditional cancer therapies, including chemotherapy, radiotherapy, and surgery, remain the basis of treatment, often used in combination to manage malignancies. Surgery remains essential for localized solid tumors, while systemic therapies are crucial to address metastatic conditions [3]. Radiotherapy is also a key modality in cancer care. However, its associated acute and long-term toxicities present substantial limitations [4]. Similarly, conventional chemotherapy faces obstacles such as drug instability, poor solubility, resistance, systemic toxicity, and collateral tissue damage [5]. Nanomedicine has revolutionized the field of drug delivery and therapeutics by offering innovative solutions to overcome the limitations of conventional therapies. By leveraging the unique properties of nanoplatforms, they provide intrinsic theranostic capabilities-combining enhanced precision, targeted delivery, and controlled release of therapeutic agents. These nanoplatforms can mitigate challenges such as poor drug solubility, rapid clearance, and systemic toxicity, leading to more effective and safer treatment outcomes [6]. A key advantage of nanomedicine lies in its ability to exploit the Enhanced Permeability and Retention (EPR) effect, which allows preferential accumulation in tumor tissues [7]. However, passive targeting alone is often insufficient due to physiological barriers and tumor heterogeneity [8]. To address these limitations, advanced nanomedicine designs now incorporate active targeting, stimuli-responsive approaches, and multifunctional capabilities to improve theranostic outcomes. Recent advancements in nanotechnologies emphasize the integration of diagnosis and therapy, co-delivery of multiple therapeutic agents, and responsiveness to tumor microenvironmental or external stimuli in a single nanoplatform. Multifunctional nanomedicine that combines these features holds immense potential for treating cancer. They not only improve drug efficacy and safety profiles but also enable real-time monitoring of therapeutic responses, paving the way toward truly personalized medicine.

This chapter explores the evolution of nanomedicine systems, focusing on their applications in overcoming current challenges in conventional cancer treatment (Fig. **1**). A special emphasis is placed on highlighting the recent advances of each type of nanomedicine in cancer clinical care, including upconversion nanoparticles, plasmonic nanoparticles, magnetic nanoparticles, quantum dots, carbon nanoparticles, prussian blue nanoparticles, mesoporous silica nanoparticles, lipid-based nanocarriers, and polymeric nanoparticles. Finally, the prospects and challenges of nanomedicine in clinical care are outlined.

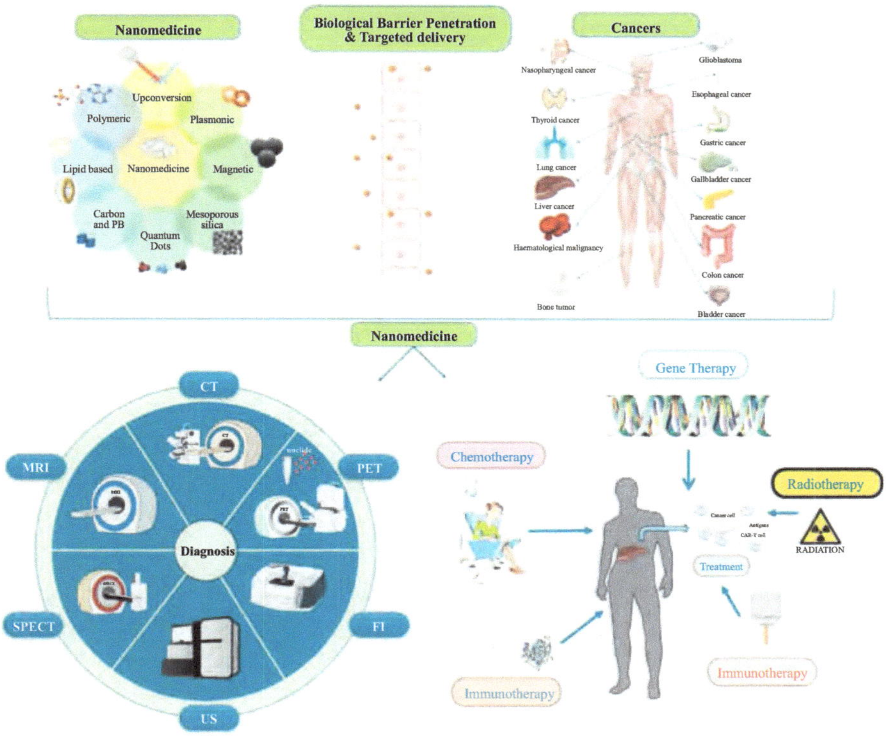

Fig. (1). Schematic representation of various types of nanomedicine used in multimodal targeted cancer theranostic applications.

KEY PRINCIPLES OF NANOMEDICINE

The introduction of nanomedicine for cancer therapy is motivated by the shortcomings of the traditional treatment methods and the transformative promise of nanotechnology-based approaches.

Requirement of Nanomedicine

Limitations of Conventional Cancer Treatments

Cancer treatment has traditionally relied on surgery, chemotherapy, radiotherapy, and immunotherapy. While these therapeutic approaches have significantly improved survival rates, they come with notable limitations. Chemotherapeutic agents, such as doxorubicin and cisplatin, act on rapidly dividing cells [9]. While effective against tumor cells, they also harm healthy dividing cells in tissues like bone marrow, the gastrointestinal tract, and hair follicles. This nonspecific action leads to adverse effects, including immunosuppression, nausea, and alopecia [10]. Doxorubicin is effective in treating breast and ovarian cancers but causes cardiotoxicity due to its accumulation in cardiac tissues. Additionally, many anticancer drugs, such as paclitaxel, have poor solubility in water, resulting in limited bioavailability [11]. To address this, toxic solvents like Cremophor EL are often required, but they induce hypersensitivity reactions, further complicating treatment. Another challenge is the development of drug resistance, where cancer cells adapt by increasing drug efflux or enhancing DNA repair mechanisms, rendering treatments like doxorubicin less effective. Systemic drug delivery also suffers from poor tumor targeting, as only a small fraction of the administered drug reaches the tumor site. For instance, the Blood-Brain Barrier (BBB) poses a significant hurdle in delivering chemotherapeutics to brain tumors. Furthermore, rapid drug metabolism and clearance reduce circulation time, necessitating frequent high-dose administrations that amplify toxicity and burden patients. Conventional cancer diagnostics have limitations, including low sensitivity and specificity, which hinder early detection. Imaging techniques like Computed Tomography (CT) scans and mammograms may miss small or dense tumors, while repeated exposure to ionizing radiation increases the risk of secondary cancers [12]. The use of gadolinium-based Magnetic Resonance Imaging (MRI) contrast agents in clinical practice poses toxicity risks due to Gd retention in tissues and may cause Nephrogenic Systemic Fibrosis (NSF) in patients with renal impairment. High production costs, short circulation half-life, nonspecificity, and limited biocompatibility further challenge their widespread adoption. Moreover, these diagnostic methods often fail to provide real-time monitoring of treatment response and can be invasive in the case of biopsies, which may cause discomfort and infection risk [13].

Advantages of Nanomedicine in Cancer Theranostics

Nanomedicine offers innovative solutions to these challenges, revolutionizing both cancer therapy and diagnosis (Fig. **2**). One key advantage is targeted drug delivery, where Nanoparticles (NPs) can be functionalized to recognize specific cancer biomarkers, thereby minimizing off-target effects. For instance, HER2-targeted liposomal doxorubicin selectively delivers the drug to HER2-positive breast cancer cells, significantly reducing cardiotoxicity [14]. Nanoplatforms also enhance the solubility and stability of hydrophobic drugs, eliminating the need for toxic solvents. Abraxane®, an albumin-bound form of paclitaxel, exemplifies improved drug tolerability and safety. By co-delivering drugs with resistance inhibitors, nanoplatforms can overcome multidrug resistance mechanisms [15].

Polymeric NPs, for example, deliver doxorubicin alongside siRNA to suppress P-glycoprotein-mediated resistance in breast cancer cells. Nanomedicine also exploits the Enhanced Permeability and Retention (EPR) effect, which allows them to accumulate preferentially in tumors due to their leaky vasculature (detailed in the section below) [16]. Additionally, sustained and controlled drug release extends circulation time and reduces dosing frequency, as demonstrated by liposomal formulations of cisplatin, which improve patient compliance and minimize nephrotoxicity. Nanoplatforms also facilitate combination therapies, integrating Photothermal Therapy (PTT), Photodynamic Therapy (PDT), Chemodynamic Therapy (CDT), Chemotherapy (CT), gene therapy, *etc.*, for synergistic effects. For instance, gold nanoparticles can co-deliver chemotherapy drugs and photosensitizers for combined chemotherapy and photothermal therapy [17].

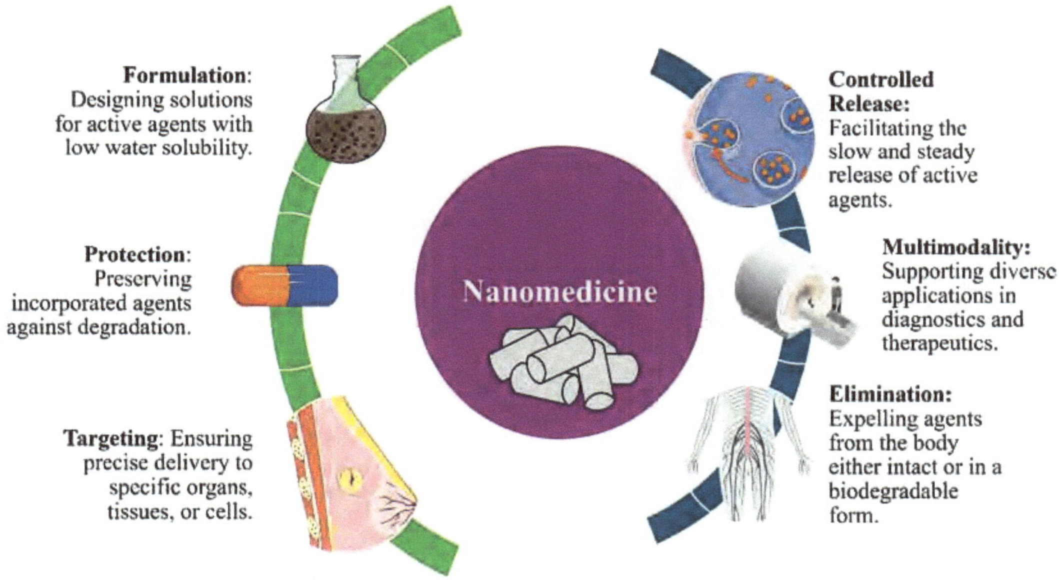

Fig. (2). Advancements of nanomedicines in cancer theranostic applications.

In diagnostics, nanomedicine enables highly sensitive and specific detection of cancer biomarkers, allowing earlier and more accurate diagnosis. For example, antibody-conjugated gold nanoparticles can detect Prostate-Specific Antigen (PSA) at very low concentrations (pM). Nanoplatform also improve imaging resolution in various diagnostic techniques like MRI, CT, and Positron Emission Tomography (PET), Single-Photon Emission Computed Tomography (SPECT), fluorescence imaging, upconversion imaging, *etc* [18]. For instance, Superparamagnetic Iron Oxide Nanoparticles (SPIONPs) enhance T_2 -T--weighted MRI contrast for tumor detection. By integrating therapeutic and diagnostic capabilities, nanoplatform enable real-time monitoring of drug delivery and treatment efficacy. For example, Quantum dots provide simultaneous tumor imaging and therapy tracking. Furthermore, nanomedicine-based diagnostics reduce radiation exposure by enhancing imaging efficiency, as seen in nanoplatform-enhanced PET scans that require lower tracer doses. Emerging nanosensors, such as paper-based platforms for biomarker detection, offer affordable and portable diagnostic solutions, making cancer detection more accessible in resource-limited settings [19]. Thus, nanomedicine addresses these challenges by providing targeted, efficient, and minimally invasive solutions, transforming cancer management, and paving the way for improved patient care (Tables **1** and **2**).

Table 1. Characteristics of different nanoparticles.

Different Types of Nanoparticles (NPs)		Advantages	Disadvantages
Inorganic NPs	Upconversion NPs	UCNPs, when excited with lower-energy light, emit higher-energy light, making them suitable for bioimaging and biosensor applications. UCNPs are highly resistant to photobleaching and photodegradation	Long-term exposure can cause systemic DNA toxicity.
	Plasmonic NPs	Chemically stable and biocompatible, they can be used as effective photothermal agents for localized destruction of cancer cells. They exhibit a strong nonlinear optical effect, making them useful for biomedical imaging applications as well. They act as effective chemical reactants, making them useful for energy applications and environmental remediation.	Precise size and shape synthesis is complex and lacks scalability. High cost.
	Magnetic NPs	High surface area-to-volume ratio, can be functionalised easily with ligands, tunable to various sizes, which makes it efficient for drug delivery, highly sensitive to magnetic fields, and helps in biosensing and diagnostic purposes.	Potential toxicity and gets aggregated in tissues.
	Mesoporous silica NPs	High surface area and porosity, which make it suitable for application in drug loading, catalysis, and sensing	High cost, low stability, and prone to aggregation.
	Calcium Phosphate NPs	Biocompatible and biodegradable, it is safe for use in biomedical applications such as drug delivery, bone tissue engineering, and imaging.	Limited stability and risk of overaccumulation in Organs

(Table 1) cont.....

Different Types of Nanoparticles (NPs)		Advantages	Disadvantages
	Carbon NPs	Biocompatible, excellent high surface area, can be easily functionalized, excellent electrical and thermal conductivity.	Some environmental issues and difficulty in controlled drug release.
	Quantum Dots	Tunable optical properties which help in biosensing, highly photostable, high surface area for functionalization, and emits different color which helps in bioimaging.	Toxic to cells and organisms, not very stable, and can cause environmental contamination.
	Prussian Blue NPs	Highly biocompatible, easily functionalized, its magnetic properties make it suitable for use in Magnetic Resonance Imaging, and can be made into different sizes, which makes it effective for drug delivery and bioimaging.	Limited large-scale productions
Organic NPs	Liposome	Biocompatible, can encapsulate hydrophilic and hydrophobic drugs, targeted drug delivery, and sustained drug release.	Limited stability and high manufacturing costs.
	Solid Lipid NPs	Biocompatible, improves the shelf life of drugs, controlled and sustained release of encapsulated drugs, safe for long-term use in drug delivery and gene therapy.	Limited drug loading capacity and limited stability, prone to agglomeration.
	Nanostructured Lipid Carriers	Easily prepared and easier for targeted drug delivery	Less versatile for delivering hydrophilic drugs.
	Polymeric NPs	Biocompatible, it can be synthesized in a wide range of sizes and shapes, thereby improving tissue penetration.	Low stable and limited penetration to specific tissues.

Table 2. A list of nanomedicines authorized by regulatory agencies and under clinical trials.

Product	Nanomedicine	Drug	Application	Approval/Phase Trial
Doxil	Pegylated Liposome	DOX	Breast cancer, ovarian cancer, multiple myeloma, Kaposi's sarcoma	Approved 11/17/1995 FDA50718
Abraxane	Albumin nanoparticle	Paclitaxel	Applied intravenously in various cancers	USA (2005)
Feridex I.V	Iron oxide NP coated dextran	-	MRI contrast agent	Approved by the US-FDA in 1996
Myocet	Non-pegylated liposome	DOX	Breast Cancer	Approved in Europe
NanoTherm	Iron Oxide Np	-	Intratumoral application to cancers	Europe (2010)

(Table 2) cont.....

Product	Nanomedicine	Drug	Application	Approval/Phase Trial
ThermoDox	Heat-activated liposome	DOX	Breast cancer and primary liver cancer	Approved 2014
DaunoXome	Lipid NPs	Daunorubicin	HIV associated Kaposi's Sarcoma	USA
Oncaspar	Pegylated nanoparticles	Asparaginase in	Leukemia	Approved 2006
Rexin G	Micro RNA 122 tagged in protein phospholipid	Micro RNA 122	Sarcoma, pancreatic cancer	Approved in PHILIPPINE
Caelyx	PEGylated liposome	DOX	Metastatic breast, Kaposi's sarcoma, multiple myeloma	USA 1996
Eligard	Polymeric micelles	Leuprolide	Prostate cancer	USA 2002
Lipusu	Liposomes	Paclitaxel	Ovarian cancer, metastatic gastric cancer	China 2003
Oncaspar	Polymeric micelles	Pegaspargase	Acute lymphoblastic leukemia	USA 1994
Lipodox	Liposome	DOX	Kaposi's sarcoma, ovarian cancer, multiple myeloma, metastatic pancreatic cancer	China 2013
Nanoxel	Polymeric micelles	Paclitaxel	Breast cancer, ovarian cancer	India 2007
ThermoDox	Liposome	DOX	Liver cancer	Phase 1
Nano-QUIT	PLGA-PEG-NPs	Quercetin	Oral Cancer	Phase 1
Docetaxel-PM	Polymeric micelles	Docetaxel	Esophagus cell carcinoma, metastatic cancer	Phase 2
Genexol PM	Polymeric micelles	Paclitaxel	Bladder cancer	Phase2
Abraxane	Albumin	Paclitaxel	Pancreatic cancer	Phase 2
Cetiximab nanoparticles	Ethylcellulose nanoparticles	Cetuximab	Colon Cancer	Phase 1
mRNA-NP vaccine	Liposome	mRNA	Melanoma	Phase 1
LipoVNB	Liposome	Vinorelbine tartrate	Advanced malignancy	Phase1/2
Cri-PEC	Polymeric micelles	Docetaxel	Ovarian cancer	Phase 2
ABT-888	PEGylated Liposomes	DOX	Ovarian cancer	Phase 2

(Table 2) cont.....

Product	Nanomedicine	Drug	Application	Approval/Phase Trial
KM1	virus	Carboplatin	Ovarian cancer	Phase 1
Bind-014	Polymeric micelles	Docetaxel	KRAS-positive non-small cell lung cancer	Phase 2
Nab Paclitaxel	Albumin	Paclitaxel	Non-small cell lung cancer	Phase 2

Progress and Challenges towards Targeted Delivery of Nanomedicine Passive Targeting and EPR Effect

The clinical translation of passively targeted Nanomedicine (NMs) began over two decades ago with the approval of PEGylated liposomal doxorubicin (Doxil™) [20]. This approach in cancer theranostics relies on natural physiological differences between healthy and tumor tissues to direct nanomedicine to cancer sites without the need for specific ligands. This strategy capitalizes on the EPR effect, a phenomenon where tumor vasculature exhibits leaky blood vessels and poor lymphatic drainage, allowing nanoplatforms of suitable size to accumulate and reduce systemic toxicity [21]. It also offers a more straightforward, cost-effective design for delivering a wide range of theranostic agents. Several passively targeted NMs, including Abraxane™, Doxil™, Onivyde™, Marqibo™, Mepact™, Myocet™, SMANCS™, and Genexol-PM™, are in clinical use worldwide, while others, such as EndoTAG-1, CPX-1, and AZD2811, are demonstrating safety and efficacy in clinical evaluations [22, 23]. While most passively targeted nanomedicines improve pharmacokinetics, drug solubility, or toxicity profiles, only a few have demonstrated significant theranostic advantages by enabling tumor-specific imaging and real-time monitoring of therapeutic efficacy. For instance, in phase III trials for metastatic breast cancer, for example, AbraxaneTM (nab-paclitaxel) showed higher response rates than paclitaxel, while CPX-351 (VyxeosTM), an FDA-approved liposomal formulation of cytarabine-daunorubicin, significantly improved survival in patients with high-risk acute myeloid leukemia [24]. Similarly, SPIONPs were used clinically as a T_2-weighted MR contrast agent, while gold nanoparticles are in clinical trials as a CT contrast agent [25, 26]. The heterogeneity of the EPR effect across tumors significantly influences the therapeutic outcomes of nanomedicine. Variations in endothelial gaps (~10 nm to 100 nm) lead to inconsistent nanomedicines extravasation. Although theoretical models suggest that they should extravasate more in tumor cores due to hypoxic conditions, experimental evidence often contradicts this. Additionally, factors such as tumor perfusion, which varies both spatially and temporally, further complicate their distribution. The tumor interstitial matrices also pose diffusion barriers, limiting penetration. Importantly, reducing particle size can minimize diffusional resistance, enhancing percolation into the interstitial matrix. For instance, Wong and team introduced a multistage strategy in which gelatin nanoparticles (100 nm) degrade into small fragments (~10 nm) *via* tumor-associated Matrix Metalloproteinases (MMPs) after extravasation into tumor tissue [27]. While promising, this approach has yet to undergo clinical evaluation. Physicochemical properties, including size, shape, elasticity, and surface charge, critically influence nanoplatform interactions with physiological barriers. For example, silica nanoconjugates (~ 50 nm) demonstrate enhanced tumor penetration, cellular uptake, and prolonged retention compared to other sizes, resulting in superior accumulation and therapeutic efficacy against both primary and metastatic tumors *in vivo* [28]. Similarly, softer nanoparticles (~10 kPa elasticity) demonstrate longer circulation compared to stiffer counterparts (~3000 kPa) [29]. However, tumor-specific optimization of these properties is essential to maximize theranostic efficacy, as demonstrated by studies correlating NPs characteristics with tumor pathophysiology. The limited translational relevance of preclinical tumor models, such as subcutaneous xenografts, necessitates improved methodologies. High-EPR tumor models often exaggerate therapeutic benefits, highlighting the need for preclinical systems that better reflect human tumor biology [30]. Advanced imaging modalities, including functional ultrasound and PET/CT, have been employed to assess EPR heterogeneity and predict their accumulation in tumors, facilitating patient stratification for improved clinical outcomes [31]. Despite these challenges, nanomedicine-based platforms still offer superior drug-delivery efficiency compared to conventional formulations, with a median of 0.7% of the Injected Dose (ID) reaching tumors, significantly outperforming free-drug formulations [32]. Enhancing the EPR effects through methods such as vasodilation or Injectable Nanoparticle Generators (iNPGs) represents a promising avenue [33]. Additionally, cell-mediated delivery systems leveraging immune or tumor-homing cells have shown improved accumulation and therapeutic efficacy in low-EPR tumors and metastases. These approaches, still in development, underscore the potential of nanomedicines in personalized cancer therapy. Continued investigation into the EPR phenomenon, development of advanced preclinical models, and exploration of alternative targeting mechanisms are critical to overcoming the current limitations and optimizing nanomedicine-based cancer therapies.

Active Targeting and Challenges

Active targeting, a complement of passive targeting, enhances tumor localization of nanomedicines by improving targeting efficiency and retention at the desired site. However, Kirpotin and team demonstrated that although incorporating targeting ligands on the nanoplatform surface enhances targeted cellular internalization, it does not necessarily increase overall tumor localization [34].

Similarly, Schmidt and Wittrup created a mechanistic model illustrating that active targeting does not substantially improve tumor localization compared to non-targeted nanomedicine (diameters ≥50 nm), which contrasts with the behavior of antibodies and small molecules [35]. Ligand-conjugated nanomedicines facilitate the transport of high-molecular-weight biomolecules like DNA, proteins, and RNA, that are susceptible to enzymatic degradation and unable to cross cell membranes. However, the active targeting approach encounters several physiological barriers, particularly in escaping the endocytic pathway. Internalized nanoplatforms often undergo intracellular trafficking to subcellular compartments, which can limit their theranostic potential. For instance, nanoplatforms internalized *via* clathrin-mediated endocytosis, such as those targeting the transferrin receptor, may follow a degradative pathway leading to lysosomal degradation. Effective *in vivo* endosomal escape remains difficult to achieve, despite efforts involving pore-forming peptides, pH-buffering substances (proton sponge effect), and fusogenic nanoplatforms [36]. Endosome recycling further complicates this process. Sahay *et al.* reported that 70% of siRNA-containing Lipid Nanoparticles (LNPs) underwent exocytosis after internalization. Gilleron *et al.* explored the intracellular destiny of siRNA-loaded LNPs, revealing that endosomal escape in hepatocytes takes place at a low efficiency (1-2%) and only within specific compartments with early and late endosome characteristics [37]. These findings underscore the need to deepen our understanding of endosomal escape mechanisms across cell types to enhance delivery efficiency, reduce off-target effects, and improve therapeutic outcomes. Traditional active targeting relies on conventional disease markers like CD19 for B-cell malignancies or HER2 for breast cancer. While effective for monoclonal antibodies, these markers may not facilitate efficient nanoplatforms internalization or endosomal escape, particularly for intracellular therapeutics like nucleic acids. Therefore, target selection should involve evaluating expression levels, internalization potential, and endosomal escape capability. Designing effective nanomedicine requires consideration of architecture, ligand choice, and conjugation chemistry, making the process highly complex. Tumor heterogeneity and the presence of supportive stromal cells, such as tumor-associated macrophages and fibroblasts, further complicate active targeting. Most cell-specific nanomedicine targets a single receptor type on tumor cells, overlooking the heterogeneity of tumors and enabling resistant clones to thrive. This often leads to partial or transient treatment responses, followed by resistant tumor relapse. Developing nanomedicine with versatile targeting moieties or combining multiple nanomedicines with different targeting ligands is crucial for improving efficacy. Conjugating targeting ligands involves complex chemical synthesis and purification steps. Although this has not been a primary barrier to clinical translation, it increases production costs, time, and quality control requirements.

Kedmi and team proposed a solution to simplify this process by utilizing a lipidated single-chain Fv-based linker platform that self-assembles into lipid-based nanomedicines and binds IgGs of specific isotypes [38]. This approach eliminates the need for chemical conjugation and unbound antibody removal. Moreover, linkers capable of binding diverse targeting moieties could enable the development of a versatile nanoplatform, which can be redirected to different cellular targets by simply mixing with specific targeting agents. Such innovations could address challenges posed by tumor heterogeneity while simplifying the manufacturing process, thereby paving the way for breakthroughs in active targeting.

An Immune Barrier due to Protein Corona

In this context, the targeting efficiency of nanomedicine is influenced by several factors, including administration route and protein corona formation, a coating of serum proteins and opsonins that forms on the nanomedicine surface. These factors significantly affect not only the release patterns of encapsulated therapeutics but also elimination by the Mononuclear Phagocyte System (MPS), immunogenicity, and overall therapeutic efficacy [39, 40]. This corona can alter nanomedicine properties such as size, stability, surface characteristics, and pharmacokinetics, ultimately impacting cellular uptake, toxicity, intracellular trafficking, and biodistribution [41]. Moreover, it may also obscure targeting ligands, thereby reducing the targeting capabilities. Although nanomedicine-protein interactions have been extensively studied but their *in vitro* and *in vivo* effects remain underexplored. These interactions can shorten circulation times through opsonization and MPS recognition. However, in tumors with high blood flow, this requirement may be mitigated. Additionally, unfavourable interactions between nanomedicine and the immune system can lead to either immunostimulation or immunosuppression, such as activation of Toll-like Receptor (TLR) signalling by cationic nanomedicines [42]. Strategies to address these challenges include stealth coatings like PEG, which reduce immune recognition but may cause adverse effects like complement activation. Preclinical models are essential for predicting and minimizing these interactions. Recently, immune recognition has been a greater challenge for actively targeted nanomedicine. For instance, full-length IgG targeting moieties may be identified by the MPS *via* Fc receptors, which can be addressed by utilizing small antibody fragments, like Fab, scFv, or alternative homing molecules like aptamers or natural ligands [43, 44]. Another promising approach involves functionalizing nanomedicine with 'self' markers to reduce interactions with serum proteins and the immune system [45]. Additionally, nanomedicine-cell and nanomedicine-ECM interactions are also crucial in targeted delivery. Advancements in nano-bio interaction research are critical for refining nanomedicine design and enhancing therapeutic delivery. A deeper understanding of these interactions will enable more effective ways to improve targeting, reduce off-target effects, and address the complexities of active targeting.

Passive Targeting *Vs.* Active Targeting

Therefore, passive targeting *via* the EPR effect often falls short for effective tumor delivery, highlighting the need for systematic studies to address physiological barriers. Leveraging natural cell tropism and tumor-infiltrating lymphocytes can enhance nanomedicine accumulation. Advances such as ionizing lipids for endosomal escape and multi-layered nanomedicines for targeted delivery are addressing these challenges, alongside immune interaction evaluation tools like complement activation and cytokine assays to predict toxicity [46, 47].

Active targeting offers potential for treating disseminated malignancies but faces complexities in design, good manufacturing practice production, and costs. For instance, SGT-94, a TfR-targeting cationic liposome in Phase I trials, demonstrates progress. Success requires improved preclinical models that mimic human conditions and diagnostic methods, such as imaging technologies, to evaluate nanomedicine targeting [48]. Tailored patient selection can enhance outcomes, reduce adverse effects, and lower healthcare costs.

Design Parameters for Developing Actively Targeted Nanomedicine

When designing actively targeted nanomedicines, various biological and design parameters must be integrated alongside experimental models to assess their efficacy (Fig.**3**). For solid tumors, it is crucial to select models that closely mimic human tumor characteristics. The dimension and physicochemical properties of nanomedicines should correspond to tumor architecture and the extent of the EPR effect, and tools to quantify the EPR effect should be developed concurrently. For accessible tumors, local delivery routes may bypass the reliance on the EPR effect. Target receptor and targeting moiety selection should account for target exclusivity or overexpression, as well as the nature of nanoplatform cargo. For intracellular delivery (*e.g.*, nucleic acids or proteins), the receptor internalization pathway must avoid degradation by endocytic mechanisms. Receptor internalization can be influenced by nanomedicine design factors such as binding site, receptor clustering, and ligand density, necessitating systematic testing of various targeting moieties and densities. If the nanomedicine acts as a drug depot, non-internalizing strategies may enhance tumor retention. Understanding the interaction between the targeting moiety and receptor is essential, as excessive ligand density can induce receptor clustering, leading to adverse cellular effects, steric hindrance, or impaired drug release. Optimizing ligand density is therefore critical, as evidenced by Colombo *et al.*, who demonstrated that gold nanoparticles functionalized with either a single or dual antibody type showed reduced *in vivo* efficacy with the single antibody compared to dual-antibody formulations, despite better *in vitro* performance with the single antibody [49]. These results highlight the importance of optimizing targeting ligand density through imaging and efficacy studies in both *in vitro* and *in vivo* models. To fully leverage the benefits of actively targeted nanomedicines, systematic design approaches and advanced tools to control ligand density and investigate nanomedicine-receptor interactions are essential.

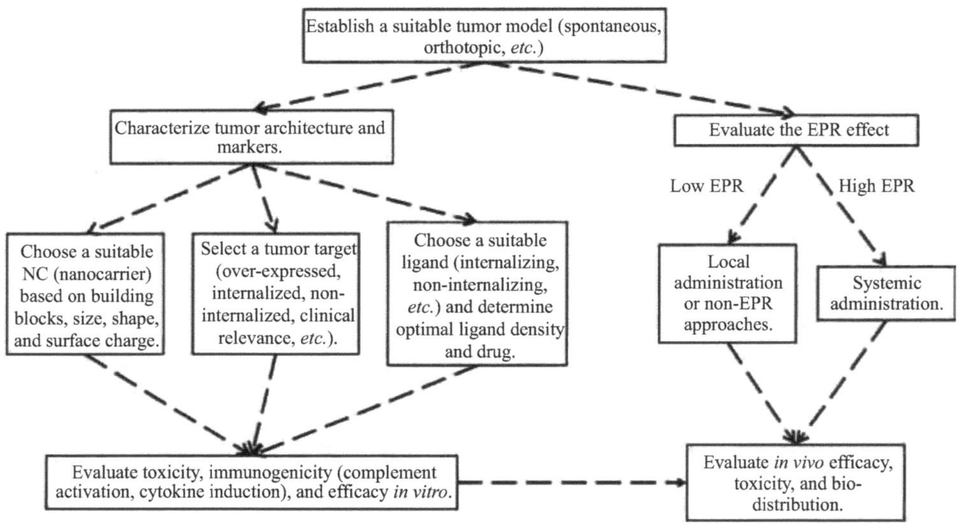

Fig. (3). Schematic representation of the workflow in the designing of an actively targeted nanoplatform.

Stimuli-Responsive Controlled Switch Nanomedicines

A significant challenge in the theranostic use of nanomedicine is the premature and non-specific release of encapsulating agents. Stimuli-responsive nanomedicines release therapeutics in response to specific microenvironments in a controlled, spatiotemporal manner, offering a promising solution. The concept originated in the late 1970s with temperature-sensitive liposomes designed for localized release of drugs *via* hyperthermia [50]. Since then, substantial advancements have been made in developing targeted stimuli-responsive nanomedicines for cancer theranostics. By modifying them to the tumor microenvironment, therapeutic release can be precisely controlled, thereby mitigating premature drug leakage during circulation. Such designs often employ biocompatible nanoplatforms capable of undergoing hydrolytic cleavage, protonation, or conformational changes triggered by intrinsic or extrinsic stimuli. These systems can range from simple to highly complex, depending on the selected stimulus and particle response. Despite the versatility offered by diverse stimuli and responsive nanomedicines, transitioning them from research to clinical practice remains a challenge. Complex chemistries can hinder pharmaceutical growth, development, and scalability, while variation in intrinsic stimuli (*e.g.*, pH, enzymatic activity, and reducing agents) between clinical and preclinical settings introduces additional hurdles (Fig. **4**). Extrinsic stimuli like heat, light, ultrasound, magnetic fields, and electric fields are more precisely controllable, making them the basis of clinically advanced stimuli-responsive NMs such as ThermoDox, NanoTherm, and MTC-DOX [51]. These systems share a common trait and simple design, facilitating their scalability and clinical translation. Despite their potential, extrinsic stimuli-based nanomedicines face challenges, including limited tissue penetration, precision in localization to avoid off-target effects, and the need for patient compliance in delivering the external stimulus (Fig. **4**). Biocompatibility also remains a critical consideration, especially when chemical synthesis is involved, necessitating rigorous toxicity assessments for regulatory approval. For successful clinical translation, stimuli-responsive NMs should prioritize simplicity, leverage readily available biomaterials, avoid extensive chemical modifications, and employ extrinsic stimuli for activation. Such approaches balance efficacy, scalability, and safety, making them viable for clinical applications.

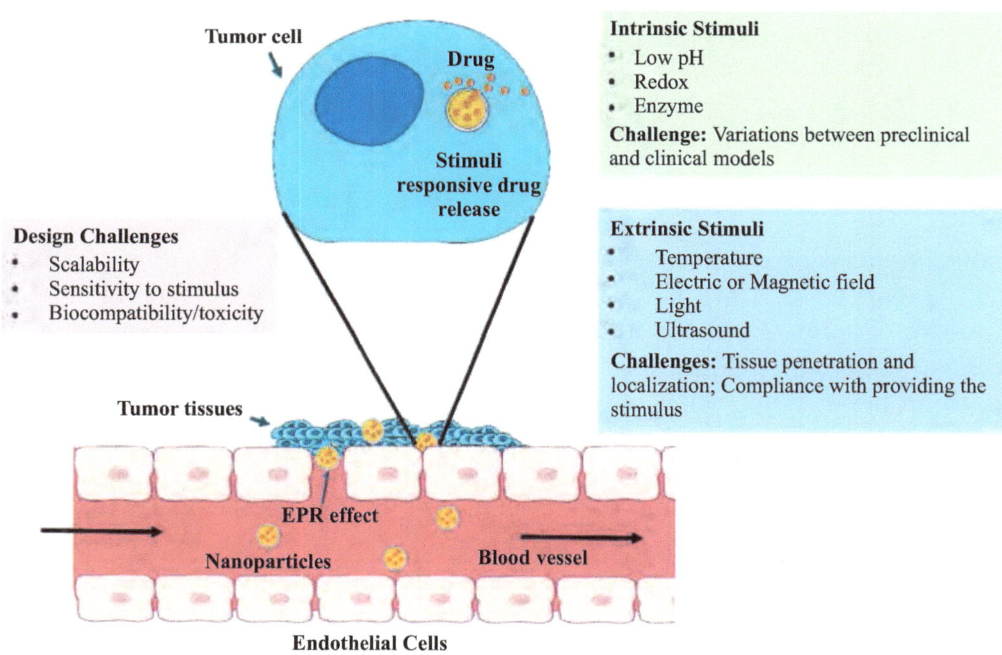

Fig. (4). Challenges of stimuli-responsive nanomedicines in clinical translation.

Integration of Multimodal Theranostics

The next generation of nanomedicine focuses on developing multimodal theranostic agents capable of performing multiple tasks simultaneously, such as co-delivering drugs for combinational therapies, targeting multiple molecular pathways, or integrating diagnostic and therapeutic modalities. In recent times, various proof-of-concept nanoplatforms incorporating multiple functional agents have shown great promise. For example, polymeric NPs co-loaded with doxorubicin and DNA demonstrated superior tumor suppression compared to single-drug delivery in preclinical studies [52]. Similarly, biodegradable polymersomes carrying both doxorubicin and paclitaxel outperformed free drugs, while PEGylated liposomes co-delivering tariquidar and paclitaxel effectively overcame tumor multidrug resistance [53, 54]. Advanced nanomedicine combines targeted delivery with stimuli-responsive mechanisms. For instance, drugs can be encapsulated within the hydrophobic core of polymeric micelles, while targeting ligands, such as folate-receptor molecules, are attached to their hydrophilic surface to enhance cellular uptake [55]. Drug release can also be precisely controlled using pH-sensitive linkers. In this context, our group also developed a dual-stimulus (pH and GSH) responsive Prussian blue-based nanoplatform carrying doxorubicin for targeted multimodal theranostic (PTT, PDT, chemotherapy, and MRI diagnosis) applications [56]. Further innovations involve nanoplatforms that integrate multiple targeting mechanisms and enable the simultaneous delivery of diverse chemotherapeutics, paving the way for highly sophisticated multifunctional nanomedicine.

VARIOUS NANOMEDICINES FOR CANCER CLINICAL CARE

Nanotechnology offers innovative approaches for developing safer and more effective cancer treatments. Recently, NPs have been utilized in various theranostic applications due to their intrinsic biological, transport, optical, electrical, magnetic, and thermal properties, which arise from their high surface area to volume ratio. As previously mentioned, the combination of many functional elements makes it easier to solubilize, prevent degradation, release over time, evade the immune system, penetrate tissue, image, target, and activate when prompted. Unlike conventional drugs, NPs exhibit distinct behaviour within the body [57, 58]. In this section, the applications of various selected nanomedicines, including both organic and inorganic nanoparticles, are broadly discussed (Fig. **5**). In addition to these bare NPs, integrating various counterparts enables multimodal theranostic approaches within a single nanoplatform.

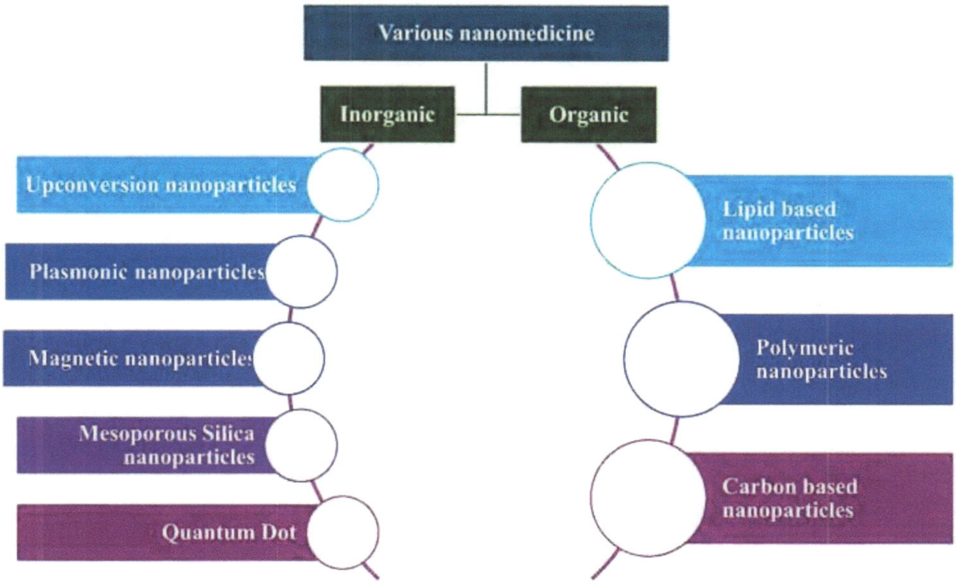

Fig. (5). Various nanomedicines for clinical cancer care.

Inorganic Nanoparticles for Cancer Theranostics

Inorganic nanoparticles have gained notable attention in cancer clinical care due to their exceptional physicochemical properties, including high stability, intrinsic optical and magnetic characteristics, and ease of surface functionalization. These nanosystems are developed to refine the diagnosis and treatment of various cancers by enabling precise interventions, like targeted drug delivery, hyperthermia, or oxidative-induced therapy, and advanced imaging modalities (Table **3**). The versatility of inorganic NPs makes them integral components in the development of innovative strategies for cancer theranostics, offering potential breakthroughs in personalized medicine. However, a major concern is the toxicity of heavy metals in inorganic NPs, which requires suitable surface functionalization (as discussed previously). Prior studies have revealed that some quantum dots containing heavy metals like Cd, Se, or Zn showed no adverse effect in an *in-vivo* model over a 90-day observation period [59]. Notably, the FDA mandates that inorganic NPs be cleared entirely from the human body within a reasonable timeframe, underscoring the need for innovative chemical designs to ensure their safe and efficient elimination. Moreover, inorganic NPs are also used as biosensors. For example, gold NPs are used in a pregnancy kit to detect hormones in a urine sample and confirm pregnancy. Additionally, silver NPs are widely used as antibacterial medicine [60]. Various inorganic NPs are discussed below.

Table 3. List of various inorganic NPs in combination therapy.

Inorganic Nanoparticles	Combination Therapy	Drug	Tumor Cells/Target	References
Upconversion NPs	PDT/chemotherapy PDT/immunotherapy	Lapatinib/cyclometalated iridium(III) Zinc phthalocyanine/Tm^{3+}-doped UCNPs/ tirapazamine	SKOV3 B16F10	[116, 117]
Plasmonic Nanoparticles	PTT/catalytic therapy/ chemotherapy Gene Therapy Colloidal gold	Gold nanorods with doxorubicin Dox Aurimune	HT-29 A375 Solid tumors	[118 - 120]
Mesoporous silica Nps	Chemotherapy/PTT PTT/immunotherapy Silica Nanoparticles	Doxorubicin Polydopamine Targeted SNP	CT-26 B-16-OVA Head and neck melanoma	[121 - 123]
Mg^{2+}-Catechin	Catechin Nanoformulations	Catechin and RNA	Bladder cancer	[124]
Zinc Oxide	SiRNA conjugated with irinotecan Doxorubicin-loaded ZnO NPs ZnO Quantum Dots ZnO NPx	- DOX Transferrin Isotretinoin	Breast cancer Cancer cell imaging In-Vivo application	[125 - 128]
Iron Oxide NPs	Chemotherapy various combinations Tagged with C595 monoclonal antibodies and conjugated with SPIONs Iron Oxide NPs Iron Oxide NPs	Doxorubicin and Curcumin Monoclonal Antibody Ferumoxytol Ferumoxtran-10	Cancer Ovarian Cancer and MRI MRI imaging on Prostate Cancer Head and Neck Cancer	[129 - 132]
MoS_2 nanosheet	Chemotherapy/hyperthermia	Doxoruboicin	Breast cancer	[133]
Hafnium oxide nanoparticle	-	NanoXray	Radiotherapy Solid tumor	[134]
Prussian Blue Nps	Mild Temperature PTT	lonidamine	Liver cancer cell line	[203]
Prussian Blue NPs	PTT and MRI imaging	-	HUVEC and HeLa cells	[204]
Prussian Blue NPs	GSH-induced drug release, PTT, PDT, MRI	Doxorubicin	TNBC cells	[205]
Prussian Blue NPs	PTT/Chemotherapy/MRI imaging	Curcumin	TNBC cells	[206]

Upconversion Nanoparticles

Upconversion Nanoparticles (UCNPs) have a high tissue-penetration depth and emit luminescence from Near-Infrared (NIR) light, making them ideal for bioimaging. They are generally guest-host systems in which lanthanide ions (such as Ho^{3+}, Er^{3+}, Tm^{3+}, Yb^{3+}, *etc.*) are embedded in a host lattice (*e.g.*, $NaGdF_4$, $NaYF_4$, *etc.*). Through the consecutive absorption of two or more low-energy NIR photons *via* long-lived intermediate states of lanthanides, the upconversion process, anti-Stokes mechanism, emits higher-energy photons in the visible or ultraviolet range. Unlike nonlinear multiphoton bioimaging, which requires high power densities and expensive ultrashort-pulsed lasers, upconversion can be achieved with low excitation irradiance ($\sim 10^{-1}$ $W \cdot cm^{-2}$) using affordable continuous-wave laser diodes or incoherent light sources. The unique electronic configurations of lanthanides, characterized by well-defined ladder-like energy levels shielded by outer 5s and 5p shells, ensure size and host-independent 4f–4f transitions, producing sharp, photostable luminescence resistant to photobleaching and photochemical degradation [61]. This property minimizes autofluorescence background noise and prevents blinking, offering superior imaging resolution compared to conventional fluorescent dyes or quantum dots [62, 63]. However, UCNPs synthesized with hydrophobic surfactants, such as oleic acid or oleate require surface modification to become biocompatible. Typically, their hydrophobic surfaces are functionalized with Polyethylene Glycol (PEG) or cancer-specific targeting molecules, enhancing their stability and selectivity for biological applications. Alternatively, the hydrophobic surfactants can be removed through HCl treatment to produce detergent-free UCNPs, making them suitable for bioimaging and therapeutic applications [64]. Most UCNPs are developed using core-shell or core-shell-shell structures, making them suitable for carrying various diagnostic or therapeutic payloads, such as chemotherapeutic drugs, genes, or photosensitizing agents, to achieve a multimodal theranostic approach. They are typically investigated as anti-cancer drug carriers using one of two main approaches, including physical adsorption onto a mesoporous silica shell or electrostatic attachment on their surface. Drug release from these systems may occur *via* simple diffusion or an NIR-triggered mechanism, enabling precise spatiotemporal control [65]. For example, Kuang and team developed $NaGdF_4:Tm^{3+}/Yb^{3+}$ core-shell UCNPs loaded with photoactivatable platinum(IV)-established poly-prodrugs and functionalized with siRNA (PUCNP@Pt@siPLK1) for trimodal theranostics, combining upconversion imaging, NIR-triggered drug release, and gene therapy, effectively reducing Plk1 levels and inducing apoptosis in A2780 ovarian cancer cells [66]. Moreover, to achieve UCNP-based targeted drug delivery, Zhao *et al.* developed lapatinib-functionalized photosensitizing nanocomplexes combined with $NaYF_4:Yb^{3+}/Tm^{3+}@NaYF_4$ core-shell UCNPs and co-loaded with polymeric micelles (PolyIrLa), effectively enhancing the system's precision and therapeutic efficacy [67]. In another study, Ding *et al.* designed biodegradable K_3ZrF_7:Yb/Er UCNPs (ZrNPs) that induced pyroptosis for an immunotherapy-based cancer treatment. ZrNPs dissolved within cancer cells, releasing K^+ and $[ZrF_7]^{3-}$ ions that disrupted intracellular osmolarity and homeostasis. Cytolysis occurred through reactive oxygen species (ROS) generation, caspase-1 activation, gasdermin D (GSDMD) cleavage, and interleukin-1β (IL-1β) maturation. ZrNP-induced pyroptosis improved dendritic cell maturity, enhanced effector-memory T cells activation, suppressed tumor growth, and reduced pulmonary metastasis *in vivo* (Fig. **6**) [68]. UCNPs were also incorporated in polymeric micelles for NIR-triggered PDT. The lapatinib-functionalized nanomedicine demonstrated specific targeting to reduce off-target toxicity and a dual role for lapatinib, inhibiting tyrosine kinase *via* the EGFR2 and HER2 pathways, resulting *in vitro* apoptosis of SKOV3 cells. *In vivo* results illustrated that PolyIrLa significantly inhibited tumor growth compared to non-targeted PolyIr, highlighting the efficacy of combining PDT with lapatinib for targeted cancer therapy. Additionally, Wu and team also developed an innovative cancer therapy platform combining PDT and optogenetics. They created a system that co-loaded Tirapazamine (TPZ), a hypoxia-activated prodrug, and zinc phthalocyanine (ZnPc), a photosensitizer, onto silica-based yolk-shell UCNPs (UCNP-YS@ZnPc@TPZ). To enhance therapeutic efficiency, they incorporated an optogenetically engineered bacterium [69]. The $NaYF_4$:Yb/Tm/Nd@$NaYF_4$:Nd UCNPs produced simultaneously blue and red emissions under 808 nm NIR light, generating ROS for PDT and activating interferon-gamma (IFN-γ) expression in modified bacteria through light-regulated pDawn plasmid. This system protected the engineered bacteria and enhanced the therapeutic environment by encapsulating both the UCNP-YS@ZnPc@TPZ and the specific bacteria with chitosans, which swelled in acidic conditions, synergistically triggering apoptosis and immunogenic cell death. Orally administered UCNP-YS@ZnPc@TPZ and engineered bacteria dramatically enhanced CD4+ and CD8+ T-cell populations in B16F10-xenografted mice, demonstrating strong immune activation. This combinational therapy demonstrated the most substantial tumor cell reduction without noticeable nanoparticle accumulation or body weight loss, confirming the nanoplatform's safety and efficacy. Importantly, RGD-modified UCNPs-based nanotechnology has been developed for advanced brain tumor imaging, specifically glioblastoma. These nanoprobes incorporate the MRI contrast agent Gd^{3+}–DOTA (1,4,7,10-tetraazacyclododecane-1,4,7,10-tetraacetic acid) to enable dual-modality imaging. Compared with traditional MRI agents, this nanoparticle-based formulation offers enhanced tumor contrast and targeted delivery through EPR effects and RGD ligand modifications. Remarkably, these NPs achieved clear tumor boundary delineation with a significantly reduced MRI agent dose-just one-eighth of the standard dose-while maintaining high imaging contrast and their potential for fluorescence-guided surgical resection of glioblastoma. This approach paves the way for more accurate and efficient tumor removal while minimizing damage to surrounding healthy tissues [70]. Importantly, doping of high-Z lanthanide elements like Lu^{3+} or Yb^{3+} enables substantial X-ray enfleeblement for CT imaging, while radionuclides like ^{18}F and ^{153}Sm in fluoride-based UCNPs facilitate PET and SPECT imaging, respectively [71, 72].

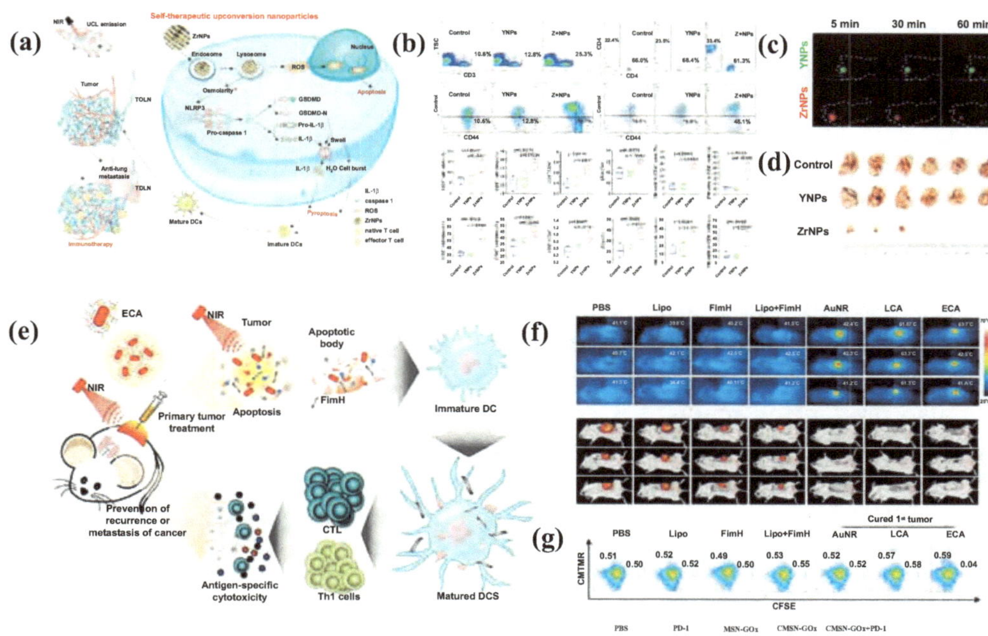

Fig. (6). (a) Schematic illustration of dissolution of ZrNPs inside cancer cells and release of ions that created a homeostasis imbalance, increased ROS, and induced pyroptosis. (b) Flow cytometric and population analysis of different parameters. (c) *In vivo* UCL imaging. (d) Electronic pictures of excised tumors. Reproduced from ref. 68 with permission from [ACS], copyright [2021]. (e) Schematic representation of ECA nanoparticles for combination therapy to4T1 tumor cells. (f) Photothermal images of CT-26-iRFP tumors *in vivo* models. (g)ECA nanoparticles led to lysis of CT-26 antigen-coated splenocytes. Reproduced with permission from [ACS], copyright [2022] [77].

Plasmonic Nanoparticles

Plasmonic Nanoparticles (PMNPs) are highly effective in converting light into localized heat when excited by external light due to the combined oscillation of electrons. The ability to tune the peak wavelengths of light that interact with these NPs depends on their size and material, allowing for versatility in theranostic applications. For example, Gold Nanoparticles (GNPs) and Copper Sulfide (CuS) NPs are commonly used for therapy like PTT, while GNPs can also be used as a fluorescence imaging agent to treat cancer. Importantly, multimodal therapeutic approaches can be achieved by incorporating PMNPs with chemotherapeutic, immunotherapeutic, or photosensitizing agents [73]. This multi-modal approach enhances the effectiveness of cancer treatment by targeting tumor cells through different mechanisms, leading to more comprehensive tumor destruction. Moreover, therapies activated by external stimuli, including light, offer the advantage of reducing off-target cytotoxicity [74 - 76]. For instance, Hwang and team developed a synergistic anticancer approach using PMNPs for PTT and immunotherapy. They synthesized *E. coli* membrane-coated Gold Nanorods (GNRs) (ECA-GNRs) and then functionalized them with FimH, which specifically targets N-glycans on epithelial tissue, thereby enhancing overall therapeutic efficiency in both *in vitro* and *in vivo* models. In an *in vitro* model using CT-26 cells, the ECA-GNRs induced apoptotic cell death under NIR (808 nm) light. Intravenous injection of ECA-GNRs in mice inhibited tumor growth and significantly improved the survival rate. After NIR-activated PTT, the nanoplatform enhanced immune response through Dendritic Cells (DC) maturation, an antigen-specific T-cell immunity, and production of IFN-γ and TNF-α, effectively preventing secondary cancer challenges and metastasis. By combining PTT with immunotherapy, this work demonstrates the potential of ECA as a dual-purpose therapeutic approach that can eliminate primary tumors while also preventing metastasis and recurrence of tumors (Fig. **6**) [77]. Maji *et al*. also developed a novel triple combination therapy using a hybrid nanoparticle system (GNR-ICG@rGO-DOX) for cancer treatment, integrating catalytic therapy, PTT, and chemotherapy. The system utilized GNRs as a base, loaded with Indocyanine Green (ICG), reduced Graphene Oxide (rGO), and the chemotherapeutic drug Doxorubicin (DOX). To improve stability and bioavailability, the GNRs were coated with polyethylene glycol (PEG) and mesoporous silica, ensuring effective loading of ICG and DOX on the exterior layer. The rGO present in the GNR-ICG@rGO-DOX nanoparticles exhibited peroxidase-like activity, generating ROS, which contributed to the catalytic therapy component. Under 808 nm NIR irradiation, both ICG and GNRs provided efficient heat conversion, significantly increasing cytotoxicity compared to controls. The study emphasized that ICG, with its high removal rate and low extinction coefficient in the NIR region, contributed to the enhanced heat conversion efficiency of the system. GNR-ICG@rGO-DOX was successfully used as an anticancer therapy when it was injected peritumorally into HT-29 cells and HT-29 tumor-bearing animals [78]. Gold nanoparticles (GNPs) are widely utilized as platforms for drug delivery due to their modifiable surface properties, which enable the binding of numerous therapeutic agents to enhance their ability to target tumors. For example, gold nanoparticles (GNPs) conjugated with eugenol showed significantly higher toxicity against the PC-3 prostate cancer cell line and the PANC-1 pancreatic duct adenocarcinoma cells compared to free eugenol, demonstrating the encapsulation of the clove-derived phytochemical into

GNPs, which enhanced its pharmacological potential and bioavailability [79]. Similarly, AuNPs conjugated to hyaluronic acid and a dendrimer were developed for tumor-targeted delivery of doxorubicin [80]. GNPs can also serve as dual delivery systems for chemotherapeutics and siRNA. For example, GNPs loaded with DOX and Bcl-2 siRNA demonstrated promising antitumor efficacy in triple-negative breast cancer cells. The co-loaded nanocarriers reduced the expression of Bcl-2 by 40% when treated with 50 nM siRNA. Furthermore, Dox-Bcl2-GNPs notably decreased cell proliferation and inhibited cell migration more effectively than free DOX, highlighting their potential for combinatorial cancer therapy [81]. Hen and team demonstrated the potential of PMNPs for gene therapy, specifically for CRISPR-Cas9 gene editing, using external-stimulus-responsive methods. They developed activatable CRISPR-Cas9 complexes (RNPs) loaded onto copper sulfide (CuS) NPs, with complementary DNA sequences surface-coated onto the sgRNA. These complexes could be heated by NIR light. The CuS-RNP complexes were further functionalized with Doxorubicin (DOX) using electrostatic interactions, resulting in CuS-RNP/DOX@PEI NPs. Upon 808 nm NIR irradiation, it facilitated endosomal escape, releasing Cas9 RNPs into the cytosol to knock out the target gene, as well as releasing DOX for chemotherapy. A second NIR irradiation cycle was observed to induce PTT, reducing tumor thermotolerance. *In vivo* experiments in A375 tumor-bearing mice showed that the CuS-RNP/DOX@PEI NPs significantly reduced tumor cell density and the expression of the target gene (Hsp90a). Overall, their study demonstrated the mutual effects of combining gene therapy, PTT, and chemotherapy in a single nanoplatform, achieving excellent antitumor efficacy [82].

Magnetic Nanoparticles

Magnetic nanoparticles (MNPs) exhibit superparamagnetic properties for which they are widely used as MRI contrast agents in various therapies. Superparamagnetic NPs, when exposed to an exterior magnetic field, generate a strong local magnetic field that significantly enhances the contrast in MRI scans. This makes MNPs ideal for improving the resolution and sensitivity of MRI, especially for imaging tumors, organs, and other tissues with high precision. The ability to fine-tune the size, surface properties, and magnetic characteristics of these NPs allows for specific targeting of cells or tissues, further enhancing their utility in diagnostic imaging and medical applications [83]. Considering their ease of manufacture, straightforward separation, and capacity to aggregate at certain areas, MNPs have been thoroughly investigated over the past 20 years for PTT, PDT, and drug delivery applications in addition to their usage in MRI. The controllable size, composition, and shape of MNPs make them highly versatile, and they can be synthesized using methods such as thermal decomposition, hydrothermal reactions, and co-precipitation. To improve theranostic performance, these NPs are often surface-coated with organic molecules (like surfactants or polymers) or inorganic materials (like silica or carbon) [84 - 86]. These NPs can be focused and held at locations by using an external magnetic field, allowing for accurate drug administration to the intended areas. Drug dosage can be optimized by using MRI to track its distribution. For instance, Liu *et al.* employed MRI to track the delivery of chemotherapy for illnesses of the central nervous system by combining targeted ultrasound with MNP-based delivery. In both *in vitro* and *in vivo* models, the combined application of magnetic targeting and focused ultrasound greatly increased NPs accumulation and tumor treatment efficacy, indicating the possibility of combining magnetic guidance with additional methods to increase drug delivery efficiency [87]. In 2013, Li *et al.* developed Fe_3O_4 NPs functionalized with polyethyleneimine (PEI) and folic acid-PEG (FA-PEG) as a T_2 MRI contrast agent [88]. Later in 2015, Zhang *et al.* developed polymer-coated bare NP as a core. They further encapsulated them with doxorubicin within the NPs and wrapped them with magnetic phenyl porous silicon NPs (M-phMSNs). Finally, the porous nanoplatform was sealed with acid-sensitive PED, which allowed DOX to be released in a slightly acidic environment, mimicking a cancer microenvironment. Additionally, the nanoplatform enabled the release of the fluorescently labelled drug, making it useful for both drug delivery and tracking [89]. Moreover, Yuan *et al.* developed a Fe_3O_4-based nanoplatform for MRI imaging of apoptotic tissues in mice, enabling real-time monitoring of cell death (Fig. **7**) [90]. The DOX-loaded FeNPs exhibited complete drug release in 4 days under *in vitro* conditions, with faster release at acidic pH. When compared to only DOX, these NPs showed 2.8 times higher cellular uptake in U251 glioma cells, which led to better *in vitro* cytotoxicity. Oncogenes TOP II, MiR-155, and Ku70 were markedly downregulated, while tumor suppressor genes p53, caspase 3, GAS5, and MEG3 were upregulated following nanoplatform treatment. Crucially, in the multidrug-resistant MDCK-MDR1–U251 co-culture paradigm, the use of an external magnetic field greatly improved the permeability and cytotoxicity of nanoparticles. Naked SPIONs tend to self-agglomerate due to high surface energy, strong electrostatic interactions, and oxidation sensitivity, which limits *in vivo* performance. Surface modification using surfactants is a crucial tactic to improve colloidal stability; however, too much surfactant can lead to particle agglomeration by bridging and neutralizing charges. Precisely adjusting surfactant levels can regulate particle size and improve dispersion. Additionally, SPIONs lead to quick opsonization and clearance by the RES, which hampers *in vivo* utility. To address this, PEG, PLA, PLGA, polycaprolactone, casein, and chitosan have been employed to coat FeNPs, providing stealth-like properties and immune system evasion [91 - 93]. Overexpression of the tyrosine kinase-like orphan receptor (ROR1) in TNBC cells encourages tumor growth, making it a viable target for gene therapy. Although small interfering RNA (siRNA)-based gene therapy against ROR1 offers potential, systemic delivery is challenging due to siRNA's susceptibility to degradation. Traditional viral vectors for gene delivery present risks like immunogenicity, inflammation, and insertional mutagenesis, prompting the development of nonviral systems such as lipid-, polymer-, and metal-based carriers. Superparamagnetic FeNPs facilitate organ-specific delivery under external magnetic fields. Silk sericin-coated FeNPs (SS-FeNPs) have recently been developed for TNBC therapy's tailored ROR1 siRNA delivery. The sericin coating mitigates FeNP toxicity and immune responses, while polyethyleneimine (PEI) coating imparts a positive charge for siRNA conjugation. *In vitro* studies demonstrated significantly higher apoptosis in TNBC cells treated with ROR1-siRNA-FeNPs compared to controls. Guided by an external magnetic field, the nanoplatform showed increased tumor accumulation and reduced tumor growth in BALB/c mice. This treatment also resulted in pronounced tumor necrosis, highlighting the potential of SS-FeNPs in targeted TNBC therapy [94].

Mesoporous Silica Nanoparticles

Mesoporous silica nanoparticles (MSNPs) are exceptionally effective drug delivery vehicles due to their adjustable mesoporous structure, high surface area, and enormous pore volume. They have been used to encapsulate and distribute a variety of therapeutic compounds, such as ibuprofen, cisplatin, camptothecin, doxorubicin, peptide medicines, alendronate, protein pharmaceuticals, and genes, since the first MSN-based drug delivery system was documented in 2001. These features make MSNs flexible platforms for targeted and controlled drug administration in various medical applications [95]. Mesoporous silica has also been applied as a coating material for other nanostructures to enhance drug delivery capabilities. For example, Zhang *et al.* created mesoporous silica-coated Gold nanorods equipped with DOX, which exhibited effective NIR-triggered drug release, resulting in an *in vitro* enhanced synergistic PTT and chemotherapeutic efficiency. Moreover, Lai *et al.* created mesoporous silica-coated multicolor upconversion nanoparticles (UCNPs) functionalized with zinc-dipicolyamine analogs and filled with polypeptide-wrapped chemotherapeutics, which allowed ATP-stimulated drug release by displacing the polypeptide. The potential for accurate and responsive drug delivery systems was demonstrated by measuring the luminescence energy transfer between the UCNPs and the loaded medicines in order to track real-time drug release [96]. Similarly, Xie *et al.* developed a combination therapy using GOx-loaded MSNs for immuno-combination and starvation. They created a hydrodynamic size of 100 nm (CMSN-GOx) by coating MSNs with lipids and proteins after extracting the membrane of B16F10 melanoma cancer cells. Through improved DC maturation, induced apoptosis, and passive and active targeting, GOx was safely delivered to tumor locations. In a mouse model, the combined therapy resulted in the best survival rate and reduced tumor volume (Fig. **7**(e-f)) [97].

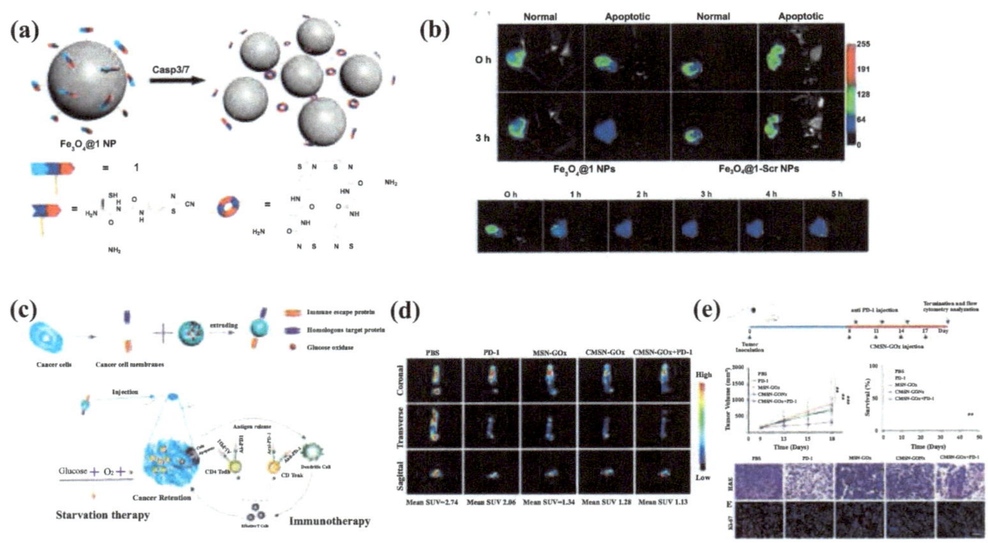

Fig. (7). (a) Schematic representation of Fe_3O_4 nanoparticles for MRI imaging of tumor apoptosis. (b) MRI images of different variations of Fe_2O_3 nanoparticles in saline-treated mice and doc-treated mice. Reproduced from ref. 90 with permission from (ACS), copyright (2016). (c) Schematic illustration of CMSN-GO--induced starvation and immunotherapy on the tumor model. (d) PET images of mice. (e) Tumor volume of the mice and H&E staining, and Ki67-stained images. Reproduced with permission from (ACS), copyright (2019) [97].

Other Inorganic Nanoparticles

Calcium Phosphate (CaP)

Calcium phosphate (CaP) NPs are biocompatible, biodegradable, biomimetic inorganic nanoparticles, utilized in combinational cancer therapy by loading with multiple payloads [98, 99]. High loading efficiency of enzymes and medications is made possible by the mild conditions under which CaPNPs are generated and functionalized (room temperature to 37 °C). Fu *et al.* showed how to target CD44-overexpressed tumors using cancer starvation therapy that uses glucose oxidase (GOx) and L-arginine (L-Arg) co-loaded with hyaluronic acid-functionalized CaPs (GCAH). Glucose oxidation by GOx produces H_2O_2, which helps produce nitric oxide (NO). Controlled NO release acts as a gas cancer therapy by converting ROS into toxic anions. In 4T1 tumor-bearing BALB/c mice, GCAH injections reduced tumor growth by 80%, with the use of both active and passive delivery methods. Additionally, cation-doped CaPs were also developed for chemodynamic starvation and PDT-chemodynamic starvation therapies [100].

Quantum dots (QDs)

Quantum dots (QDs) are NPs made of II-VI or III-V elements like sulfides, selenides, tellurides, and carbon. They emit light signals under laser exposure, offering advantages in light stability, long fluorescence lifetime, broad absorption spectrum, and simultaneous detection using a single light source [101]. For instance, Guo *et al.* created QDs with a Zn–Cu–In–S/ZnS core-shell structure and then modified their surface using small molecule cyclic peptides, showing promising potential for accurate tumor visualization [102]. Moreover, Sasaki *et al.* developed PbS QDs modified with antibodies and proteins, demonstrating targeted imaging and therapeutic applications [103]. Additionally, Rosal *et al.* reported the PbS QDs for tumor imaging, addressing issues like poor tissue permeability and stability of QDs *in vivo* mouse skin perfusion model [104]. Santos *et al.* also created Ag_2S QDs that greatly increased the photothermal effect by demonstrating substantial absorption at long wavelengths.

Prussian Blue Nanoparticles

Prussian blue nanoparticle (PBNP), a coordination polymer, has garnered a significant research interest in the biomedical field due to its exceptional physicochemical properties, including advanced multimodal imaging capabilities, catalytic potential, strong photothermal conversion efficiency, easy surface modifiability, stability, drug loading capacity, biocompatibility, and biodegradability. Owing to the ability to absorb NIR light through charge transfer between Fe^{3+} to Fe^{2+} *via* cyanide bridge, PBNPs have been explored as an innovative agent for laser-guided tumor ablation during PTT. In this context, PBNPs exhibit considerably greater molar extinction coefficient (1.09×10^9 M^{-1} cm^{-1}; 808 nm) compared to conventional photothermal (PT) agents such as $Cu_{2-x}Se$ (7.7×10^7 M^{-1} cm^{-1}; 808 nm) and carbon nanotubes (7.9×10^6 M^{-1} cm^{-1};808 nm), which endows PBNPs with a remarkable light-to-heat conversion efficiency. Furthermore, functionalized PBNPs exhibit exceptional photostability and dispersibility in both aqueous and biological mimic environments. As a result, they have gained widespread recognition as a potent agent for photothermal ablation in disease treatment. For instance, Cheng *et al.* successfully developed PEG-functionalized PBNPs, which not only enhanced their physiological stability but also facilitated their preferential accumulation within tumor tissues, leading to a notable improvement in the photothermal effectt (Fig. **8**). Their *in vivo* therapeutic efficiency demonstrated that the injection of PBNPs under laser irradiation results in complete tumor ablation (temp. rise ~ 60 °C), hence considerably prolonging the survival rate [105]. The effectiveness of PTT is contingent upon various factors, including the concentration, morphology, size, surface modification, and chemical composition of NPs. Li and colleagues devised a straightforward approach to confer PBNPs with tunable localized surface plasmon resonance (LSPR) and heightened PTT efficiency through the in situ doping of platinum (Pt) NPs onto PBNCs. Their findings have demonstrated that the coordination of Pt with cyanide in Pt-doped PBNCs has not only reduced the occurrence of $[Fe(CN)_6]$ vacancy but also expanded the routes for electron transitions, resulting in the red shift of absorption peak and an overall improvement in PTT efficiency (Fig. **8**) [106]. Similarly, our group has also reported that the incorporation of Gd^{3+} atoms in the lattice site of PBNPs significantly enhanced the photothermal conversion efficiency compared to bare PBNPs [107]. Additionally, tuneable absorption has led to the use of PBNPs in the biomedical field, particularly as a novel next-generation ROS and reactive nitrogen species (RNS)-mediated phototherapeutic agent. For instance, Zhou and colleagues recently published a study showcasing their findings on the remarkable capabilities of HA@PBNC on cancer theranostic applications. According to them, this nanoplatform has exhibited exceptional proficiency in generating $^1O_2$ and demonstrated a remarkable η value when exposed to NIR irradiation. Their investigations by both *in vitro* and *in vivo* studies confirm that this multifunctional nanoplatform not only possesses the ability to destroy CD44-overexpressing cancer cells but also effectively impedes tumor growth, which is primarily attributed to the synergistic effect of PTT and PDT, bolstered by target specificity [108]. Moreover, PBNPs are noted to decompose H_2O_2 into O_2, thus counteracting solid tumor hypoxia through nanoenzymatic activities including peroxidase (POD), catalase (CAT), and superoxide dismutase (SOD). *Zhang et al.* made a significant discovery that PBNPs possessed remarkable multienzyme-like activities, facilitated by their abundant redox potentials, thus functioning as efficient electron carriers [109]. Regarding drug delivery, one strategy involves creating HMPBNPs to enhance the surface area, resulting in the enhancement of drug loading capacity. For instance, Chen *et al.* developed a NIR responsive co-delivery system (PCM@HMPBNs) using 1-tetradecanol as a phase change molecule (PCM), which functioned as both a thermosensitive gatekeeper and a carrier for encapsulation of both hydrophilic doxorubicin and hydrophobic camptothecin drugs. The synthesized PCM@drugs@HMPBNs arrangement exhibits minimal release of both drugs, while precise drug delivery activation or deactivation has been enabled through different NIR light treatments to effectively induce cellular apoptosis against HeLa cancer cells [110]. An alternative strategy involves surface modification using organic or inorganic substances, as well as alternative cell membranes and metal-organic frameworks (MOFs). Peng *et al.* developed gelatin-stabilized PBNPs conjugated with DOX for synergistic PTT and chemotherapy [111].

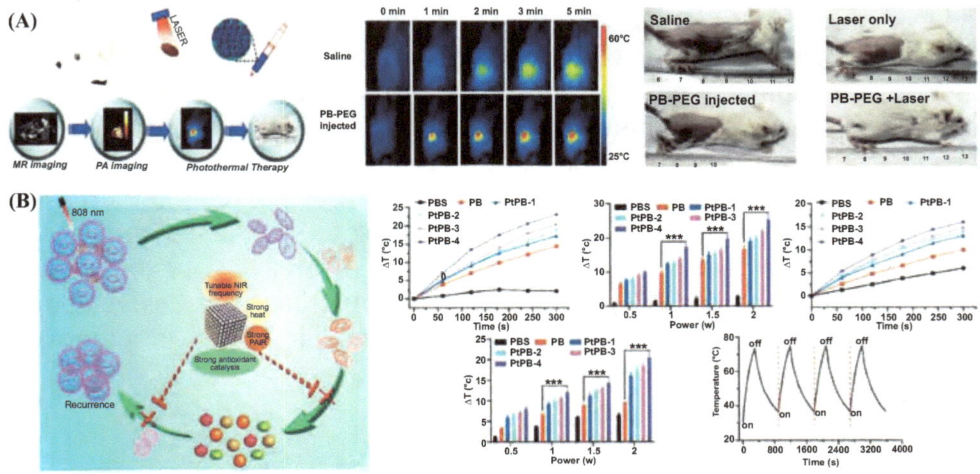

Fig. (8). (A)Schematic illustration of PBNPs used for PTT and bimodal imaging; its efficiency in *in vivo* PTT. (Copyright 2014. Reproduced with permission from *Biomaterials, Elsevier*).[105] (B) Schematic representation of PtPB nanoenzyme-mediated imaging-guided PTT with relief of inflammation and its *in vitro* PTT efficiency. Reproduced with permission from [*ACS nano*], copyright (2014) [106].

PBNPs also find extensive utility as contrast agents in PAI and T_1-T_2 weighted MRI due to their potent magnetic properties and distinct structure. In a pioneering study, Wang and colleagues skillfully fabricated PBNP@MIL-100 (Fe), a dual MOF-based nanocomposite, and utilized it as a T_1W-T_2W dual modal MRI CA for image-guided cancer treatment. The r1 and r2 values of the nanocomposite have been meticulously determined to be 1.313 and 22.258 $mM^{-1}s^{-1}$, respectively. More notably, after intravenous administration of these nanostructures into mice, a discernible enrichment has been observed in MRI, providing further evidence of the remarkable T_1W-T_2W MRI efficacy of PBNP@MIL-100 (Fe) nanocomposites [112]. In a separate study, Kim *et al.* effectively engineered poly-L-lysine-coated Prussian blue (PB-PLL) to serve as a biocompatible and effective PAI contrast agent, specifically tailored for labelling and tracking human mesenchymal stem cells (hMSCs). Upon implantation, the labeled hMSCs displayed robust photoacoustic contrast, exhibiting a linear response with an *in vivo* detection limit of 200 cells/μL. The photoacoustic contrast obtained from these labeled nanocomposites is both sensitive and enduring, enabling noninvasive and prolonged monitoring of engrafted hMSCs in living organisms for up to 14 days [113].

Extensive research has been conducted on PBNPs that boast multiple theranostic modes and excellent drug loading capacity. They have shown great promise in the realm of multimodal imaging-guided therapy and have proven to exhibit outstanding performance in various experiments [114]. For instance, Tian *et al.* introduced an innovative imaging-guided photothermal-chemotherapy approach for TNBC utilizing a periodic mesoporous organosilica-coated Prussian blue (PB@PMO) nanoplatform. The PB@PMOs exhibited remarkable features, including excellent photothermal conversion capability as well as proficiency in MR and PA imaging. *In vivo* tumor-bearing mouse model of MDA-MB-231-Luc, the combined photothermal-chemotherapy strategy was proven more effective in inhibiting TNBC compared to monotherapy, as evident from reduced bioluminescence intensity and tumor volume. Moreover, histopathological analysis demonstrated that the combination therapy induced extensive apoptosis and necrosis in the tumor without causing apparent side effects in major organs [115].

Organic Nanoparticle in Cancer Theranostics

Organic nanoparticles are clusters of organic molecules with diverse structures, offering potential for customization to meet specific application needs (Table **4**). Advances in *in silico* methods now aid in designing and synthesizing organic molecules with enhanced optical properties, streamlining the development process [135]. Organic nanoparticles are typically formed through noncovalent intermolecular interactions, making them more labile and facilitating clearance from the body. This inherent flexibility allows for potential shape or conformational changes in response to environmental stimuli [136]. Various organic nanoparticles and their utility in cancer care are discussed below.

Table 4. List of organic NPs used in cancer theranostic applications.

Nanoplatform	Formulations/Type of Treatments	Drug	Applications	References
Liposome(2B3-101)	Liposomal glutathione combination	Doxorubicin	Breast cancer	[173]
Liposome	Combination of chemotherapies	Irinotecan and cisplatin	Cancer	[174]
Liposome	Chemotherapy/gene therapy	Docetaxel and DNA	Hepatocellular carcinoma	[175]
Liposome	CPX-1 [Celator]	Irinotecan HCI/floxuridine	Colorectal Cancer	[176]
Liposome	EphA2 Targeting Liposomes [MD Anderson Cancer Center]	siRNA	Solid tumor	[177]

(Table 4) cont.....

Nanoplatform	Formulations/Type of Treatments	Drug	Applications	References
Liposome	Antibody Fragment (EGFR)	Doxorubicin	Solid Tumors	[3]
Liposome	Transferrin (transferrin receptor)	Oxaliplatin	Gastric cancer	[178]
Liposome	Human Antibody Fragment GAH (tumor antigen)	Doxorubicin	Gastric cancer	[179]
Liposome	scFv Antibody (transferrin receptor)	p53 plasmid DNA	Solid tumors	[180]
Liposome	Antibody (ErbB2/ErbB3)	Doxorubicin	ErbB2-positive breast cancer	[181]
Liposome	Anti-angiogenesis/chemotherapy	Combretastatin and doxorubicin	Melanoma	[182]
Liposome	RNA Therapy	Vorinostat and siRNA	Cervical Cancer	[183]
Liposome	Stimuvax (BLP25)	Anti-MUC1 cancer vaccine	Non-small-cell lung cancer	[184]
Liposome	OSI-7904L	Thymidylate synthase inhibitor	Colorectal cancer	[185]
Liposome	MBP-426	Oxaliplatin	PANC-1 Pancreas tumor	[186]
Liposome	-	Vinorelbine	Solid tumor	[187]
Liposome	-	Irinotecan	Recurrent glioma	[188]
Liposome	-	Vincristin	Non-Hodgkin lymphoma	[189]
Liposome	-	Lurtotecan	Small-cell lung cancer	[190]
Liposome	-	Mitomycin-C Prodrug	Solid tumor	[191]
Polymeric Nanoparticle	Chemotherapy/RNA therapy	Paclitaxel and siRNA	Breast cancer	[192]
Polymeric nanoparticle	DHAD-PBCA-NP	Mitoxantrone	Hepatocellular carcinoma	[193]
Polymeric micelle	-	Paclitaxel	Advanced breast cancer	[194]
Polymeric Nanoparticles	PEGylated micelles	SN-38	Solid tumors, small-cell lung cancer, breast cancer,	[195]
Polymeric Nanoparticles	pH-sensitive polymeric micelle	Epirubicin	Solid tumors	[196]

(Table 4) cont.....

Nanoplatform	Formulations/Type of Treatments	Drug	Applications	References
Polymeric Nanoparticles	miR-10b and miR-21 complex	Antisense oligonucleotides	Triple-negative breast cancer	[197]
Polymeric Nanoparticles	Chemotherapy/gene therapy	Paclitaxel and DNA	Breast cancer	[198]
Lipid Polymer Nanoparticle	Cytokine-induced therapy/chemotherapy	Doxorubicin	Breast cancer	[199]
Lipid polymer Nanoparticle	PDT/chemotherapy	Cisplatin and pyrolipid	Head and neck cancer	[200]
Albumin nanoparticle	Chemotherapy	Docetaxel	Prostate cancer	[201]
Carbon nanotube	RNA therapy	siRNA	Prostate cancer	[202]

Lipid-Based Nanocarriers

Considering various kinds of organic nanocarriers, lipid-based nanoplatforms are a widely studied type of nanocarrier in cancer therapy [137, 138]. Lipid-based drug carriers provide numerous benefits, including excellent biocompatibility, biodegradability, high bioavailability, the ability to encapsulate both hydrophilic and hydrophobic drugs with large loading capacities, controlled and sustained drug release, and customizable physical and chemical properties to regulate their biological behavior [138 - 140]. Lipid-based nanocarriers are classified into three main types based on their composition and physicochemical properties: liposomes, solid lipid nanoparticles (SLNs), and nanostructured lipid carriers (NLCs).

Liposomes

Liposomes are considered safe nanocarriers as they are primarily made of lipid moieties like cholesterol and phospholipids, which make them biocompatible and biodegradable. They possess a bilayer structure with an aqueous core, allowing the encapsulation of both hydrophilic and lipophilic drugs. Liposomes can be functionalized with various components to enhance circulation time, target selectivity, cellular uptake, and stimuli-responsive controlled drug release. These features have led to their successful clinical application, with several formulations in routine use and many others in clinical trials or pending approval [141, 142]. Despite the clinical success of liposomal formulations in cancer therapy, they remain under active investigation as multimodal induced nanocarriers. Conventional liposomes reduce the side effects of various chemotherapeutics by optimizing pharmacokinetics and biodistribution to enhance tumor-targeted delivery. Nevertheless, their therapeutic efficacy is restricted by rapid clearance from the body due to opsonization by plasma components and uptake by RES, primarily in the liver and spleen [143]. Liposome clearance begins with opsonin binding to their surface, as the RES recognizes opsonin-coated liposomes rather than the liposomes themselves. To counter this, stealth liposomes were developed using PEG and other polymers as steric stabilizers.

PEG coatings enhance liposome stability, as well as prevent gatherness and phagocytosis, thereby significantly extending systemic circulation time [144]. In a clinical study, one-third of the dose was cleared during the first distribution half-life (1–3 hours) of Doxil® (PEGylated Doxorubicin Liposomes), while the remaining dose was gradually cleared with an ultimate half-life of 42–46 hours. In comparison, free doxorubicin had an initial dispersion half-life of about 5 minutes and a terminal half-life of 25–30 hours. Liposome encapsulation significantly reduced the clearances and the volume of distribution of doxorubicin, resulting in a ~300-times increase in its area under the curve (AUC) compared to the free drug [145]. Liposome-based nanoplatforms have also been explored for theranostic applications. A multimodal drug delivery nanoplatform was developed using thermoresponsive liposomes co-encapsulating indocyanine green and doxorubicin, leveraging natural phase-change material. Additional modifications with folic acid and gadolinium enabled active tumor cancer targeting and imaging capabilities. These liposomes demonstrated NIR-triggered drug release and trimodal imaging (fluorescence, MRI, and photoacoustic) for guided combination therapies, including chemotherapy, PDT, and PTT. In a HeLa tumor xenograft mouse model, the formulation showed effective tumor accumulation and inhibition with no visible toxicity [146].

Solid- Lipid Nanoparticles (SLNs)

SLNs consist of a solid lipid core surrounded by an emulsifier layer, which improves stability in aqueous environments. Triglycerides (such as tripalmitin and tristearin), partial glycerides (such as glyceryl behenate), fatty acids (such as palmitic acid and stearic acid), steroids (such as cholesterol), and waxes are examples of lipid materials utilized in the manufacturing of SLN. Common surfactants include poloxamers, lecithin, sodium glycocholate, polysorbates, sorbitan esters, and various combinations thereof. Because core lipids and surfactants have a major impact on the size, charge, storage stability, drug loading, and drug release profiles of the nanoparticles, their selection is a critical factor during the SLN synthesis [147]. SLNs merge the advantages of polymeric nanoparticles, liposomes, and microemulsions, thereby revolutionizing drug delivery. The advantages of using SLN include simplified production, compatibility with both hydrophobic and hydrophilic drugs, enhanced storage stability, sterilization, suitability for large-scale manufacturing, controlled drug release, and minimal cytotoxicity. Numerous SLN-based nanoplatforms have shown increased effectiveness against different types of malignancies [148, 149]. Using cetyl esters, cetyl palmitate, or myristyl myristate as core lipids and Pluronic® F68 as a surfactant, linalool-containing SLN nanoplatforms were developed [150]. The spherical SLNs exhibited a restricted size distribution, near-neutral zeta potential (−4.0 mV), high encapsulation efficiency (>80%), and mean diameters between 90 and 130 nm. Among the nanoplatforms, the SLNs made with myristyl myristate showed higher *in vitro* cytotoxicity against HepG2 human hepatocellular carcinoma and A549 human lung adenocarcinoma cells in a dose-dependent manner. Additionally, SLN encapsulated with curcumin demonstrated higher cytotoxicity against SKBR3 human breast cancer cells compared to the free drug [151]. Similar to liposomes, SLNs have been conjugated with tumor-specific ligands for active targeting. For example, a pH-sensitive SLN formulation of doxorubicin was modified with an arginine–glycine–aspartic acid (RGD) peptide to overcome multidrug resistance in breast cancer. With a 98.5% encapsulation efficiency, the drug loading was 9.8%. With a 39% initial burst release in the first 8 hours and a sustained release for the next 96 hours, the *in vitro* drug release at pH 5 displayed a biphasic trend. Drug release was slower at physiological pH (pH 7.4) or at higher pH (pH 9). The AUC of the RGD-modified SLN formulation of doxorubicin was 5.58 times greater than that of the bare solution. Most significantly, compared with free doxorubicin or nontargeted SLNs, the targeted doxorubicin-loaded SLNs demonstrated higher tumor inhibition [152].

Nanostructured Lipid Carriers (NLCs)

Nanostructured lipid carriers (NLCs), a second-generation class of lipid NPs, were developed to overcome the drawbacks of solid lipid nanoparticles (SLNs), including low drug-loading capacity, polymorphic transitions, gradual lipid crystallization, and drug leakage during storage [153]. Solid and liquid lipids, surfactants, and other substances, including co-surfactants and counter-ions, are the usual constituents of NLCs. A liquid lipid phase has a distributed solid lipid matrix. The addition of liquid lipids disrupts the highly ordered crystalline structure of solid lipids, creating an irregular crystalline lattice that improves drug loading and prevents drug leakage [154]. Like SLNs, the solid lipids commonly used in NLCs include triglycerides, partial glycerides, fatty acids, steroids, and waxes. Liquid lipids often consist of digestible natural oils (*e.g.*, corn oil, soybean oil), medium-chain triglycerides (*e.g.*, glyceryl tricaprate), fatty acids (*e.g.*, oleic acid), and other substances such as Cetiol V, Miglyol 812, and squalene. A variety of surfactants and their mixtures are employed to enhance NLC stability in aqueous environments. Frequently used surfactants include Tween (*e.g.*, Tween 20, Tween 80), poloxamers (*e.g.*, Pluronic F68), and lecithins. Surfactant types significantly affect the stability, crystallinity, and toxicity of NLCs [155]. A previous investigation comparing the anticancer efficacy of liposomes and doxorubicin-encapsulated NLCs in an animal model of 4T1 breast cancer found no discernible differences in tumor volume between liposome-encapsulated and free doxorubicin. However, doxorubicin encapsulated in NLC demonstrated the highest tumor growth inhibition. Furthermore, both liposomes and NLCs were effective in delaying lung metastases [156]. NLCs have recently gained significant attention as a promising drug delivery system for cancer therapy. Resveratrol, a naturally occurring polyphenol, inhibits cancer cell expansion, metastasis, and invasion by interacting with several molecular targets such as P53, MAPK, caspases, VEGF, and MMP-2. However, its *in vivo* application is restricted by low aqueous solubility, poor photostability, and high first-pass metabolism. To overcome these challenges, an NLC-based parenteral formulation of resveratrol was developed to improve its conveyance to breast cancer cells [157 - 159].

Polymeric Nanoparticles

Polymeric nanocarriers have become a powerful approach for delivering chemotherapy drugs to specific tumors. Their advantages include high entrapment efficiency, improved physiological stability, simplicity in surface functionalization, scalability, and the ability to be produced using acceptable manufacturing techniques [160]. It is possible to modify the polymer's molar ratio and composition in polymeric nanoparticles to improve cellular absorption, regulate drug release, and maximize breakdown rates [161]. These nanoparticles have significant payload flexibility, allowing for the loading of hydrophobic and hydrophilic molecules, small and large molecules, as well as proteins, DNA, and RNA. Drug loading can occur *via* adsorption, encapsulation, or conjugation. Depending on the formulation procedure, the drug may be dispersed throughout the polymeric matrix or restricted to the particle's core [162]. PLGA, PLA, PGA, PCL, and PLGA-PEG are commonly used polymers in nanoparticle fabrication, along with natural polymers such as alginate, chitosan, gelatine, and albumin.

Owing to its sustained-release profile, low toxicity, biocompatibility, and biodegradability, PLGA is a FDA-approved polymer frequently utilized in biomedical applications [163, 164]. It is made up of different ratios of lactic acid and glycolic acid copolymers. The use of PLGA nanoparticles as drug carriers has been thoroughly investigated. For instance, PLGA nanoparticles encapsulating LY294002 (a PI3K/AKT signaling inhibitor) and docetaxel showed improved accumulation at tumor locations and regulated release of therapeutic drugs [165]. In both orthotopic and xenograft mouse models of gastric cancer, these nanoparticles demonstrated exceptional anticancer efficacy [166]. However, drug accumulation in tumor tissues is often limited by the inability of PLGA nanoparticles to interact directly with particular receptors or cell surface markers that are overexpressed on cancer cells. This was addressed by decorating PLGA nanoparticles with active-targeting ligand molecules. For instance, to treat lung cancer, RGD-conjugated PLGA nanoparticles (RGD-PLGA NPs) were created to administer cisplatin and UCNPs in a regulated and targeted manner [167]. Compared to the commercially available Ciszest-50 injectable, these nanoparticles demonstrated a 6.3-fold greater AUC and regulated drug release for up to 72 hours. Additionally, RGD-PLGA NPs showed improved biocompatibility, minimal lung tissue damage, and minimal systemic toxicity.

A major limitation of PLGA NPs is the high burst release of encapsulated drugs, which may lead to toxicity. Coating agents such as alginate and chitosan (CS) have been employed to solve this problem. For instance, chitosan and folic acid were applied to docetaxel-loaded PLGA NPs to boost drug delivery to cancer cells and improve the docetaxel release profile. The amount of chitosan and folic acid used, as well as the pH of the release medium, had an adverse effect on the *in vitro* release of docetaxel [168]. Compared to the free drug, the coated NPs exhibited enhanced cytotoxic effects. Because of its exceptional biocompatibility, biodegradability, nontoxicity, and low immunogenicity, chitosan is employed extensively in biomedical science, particularly in cancer therapy. Its solubility is increased by the many protonable amino groups throughout its backbone, which become protonated in acidic conditions [169]. Chemical modification of these amino groups can improve their solubility, biocompatibility, and targeting capacity. Chitosan NPs can achieve sustained doxorubicin release within the breast tumor microenvironment. The surface of the NPs was PEGylated to increase blood circulation time. To improve tumor targeting, anti-human mammaglobin (Anti-hMAM) and anti-human epidermal growth factor (Anti-HER2) antibodies were also encapsulated in the PEGylated nanoparticles. When compared to free doxorubicin, the antibody-conjugated PEGylated nanoparticles showed more cytotoxicity toward MCF-7 breast cancer cells [170]. In another study, dual-functionalized trimethyl chitosan nanoparticles (FTD NPs) were designed to carry doxorubicin and Survivin-targeting therapies, such as Survivin CRISPR/Cas9-expressing plasmid (sgSurvivin pDNA) or Survivin shRNA-expressing plasmid (iSur pDNA). Folic acid modification enhanced NPs uptake into cancer cells, while 2-(Diisopropylamino) ethyl methacrylate (DPA) conjugation introduced pH sensitivity, enabling rapid doxorubicin release in an acidic environment. Both RNAi-based treatments and nanoparticles containing CRISPR/Cas9 had similar antitumor efficacy. However, the combination of doxorubicin and sgSurvivin pDNA-loaded NPs produces stronger effects than either treatment alone or in other combinations, confirming their synergistic potential.

Carbon Nanomaterials

Nanomaterials containing carbon (CNPs), including carbon nanotubes (CNTs), fullerenes, and graphenes, have magnificent thermal, optical, and electrical properties. They are broadly used in bioassays, analysis, and oncology for drug delivery. CNPs absorb NIR light efficiently and are ideal for photothermal diagnostic reagents [171]. For example, Liang *et al.* synthesized nanomedicines based on single-layered CNTs for PTT, effectively inhibiting the rapid expansion of metastatic cancer cells. Another nanomedicine, SWNT@MS-PEG, was developed with CNTs as the inner layer and surface-modified molecules. This design incorporated with DOX within the pores of the nanotubes, coated with mesoporous silicon material and PEG. The coating reduced drug release in normal tissues, minimizing toxic side effects on healthy cells. Under 808 nm laser irradiation (0.5 W), the nanomedicine produced a significant PTT effect, raising the lesion site temperature by over 25°C within 10 minutes. In *in vivo* model, the nanomedicine effectively identified adriamycin-resistant cancer cells after tail vein injection, significantly inhibiting subcutaneous tumor growth. This work provided innovative strategies for addressing chemotherapy-resistant tumors through the synergy of photothermal therapy and drug delivery [172].

PROSPECTS AND CHALLENGES OF NANOMEDICINE IN CANCER TREATMENT

Prospects

Nanomedicine is a promising innovation in cancer theranostics. Leveraging the unique characteristics of tumors, like overexpressed receptors or ligands in cancer cells, researchers can design highly targeted nanocarriers. These nanoparticles enable precise tumor detection, facilitating early diagnosis and accurate localization of malignancies. Advances in materials science and computational technologies have led to the development of diverse nanovectors tailored for delivering chemotherapeutic agents, genes, and antibodies. These nanocomposites exhibit extended circulation times and can actively or passively target tumor sites, enhancing drug delivery efficiency while minimizing off-target effects. Tumor-specific microenvironments, with distinct biomarkers, can act as triggers for controlled drug release at the target site, enabling precision therapy with reduced side effects.

In addition to drug delivery, nanotechnology has broadened its applications to include photothermal-photodynamic therapy and immunotherapy. Utilizing nanocomposites, these therapies either generate heat/ROS to destroy tumor cells or stimulate the immune system to combat malignancies. However, considerations like tumor heterogeneity, pharmacokinetics, and *in vivo* toxicology must be meticulously addressed to optimize therapeutic outcomes [207]. Real-time monitoring of drug distribution remains a challenge but is critical for enhancing the efficacy and safety of nanomedicine-based treatments.

Challenges

Despite its promise, several obstacles hinder the full potential of nanomedicine in clinical applications. A key barrier is the tumor microenvironment (TME), which significantly impacts drug delivery and therapeutic outcomes [208, 209]. The malignant cells, immune cells, tumor-associated fibroblasts, and extracellular matrix (ECM) in TME often contribute to drug resistance through abnormal angiogenesis, desmoplasia, and hypoxia [210, 211]. Addressing these barriers requires strategies like vascular normalization and extracellular matrix modulation to improve nanomedicine delivery and therapeutic efficacy.

Another major challenge is the limited clinical translation of nanomedicine. Safety concerns in preclinical and clinical trials result in a low approval rate for new nano-drugs [212]. Nanoparticles can induce oxidative stress, inflammation, and physical damage due to incomplete biodegradation or accumulation in normal tissues. Generally, nanomedicine undergoes four key stages in *in vivo* application: absorption, circulation, metabolism, and excretion. Their metabolism and degradation predominantly occur in the liver and kidneys, with excretion occurring mainly *via* the kidneys (urine) and biliary tract (feces) [213]. However, recent studies suggest that some nanomedicines may resist breakdown or elimination, potentially persisting in the body over extended periods. Such prolonged retention in normal tissue can lead to physical damage, including microcirculation obstruction, resulting in cellular dysfunction and inflammatory responses [214, 215]. This damage is often attributed to nanomedicine's inability to biodegrade and its tendency to aggregate and migrate freely within tissues, posing significant challenges to its safe application. Therefore, developing biocompatible and biodegradable nanocarriers is a critical focus in recent times. Additionally, the lack of reliable preclinical models and standardized analytical methods for characterizing the nanocarrier further complicates the development process.

The ultimate goal of any nanomedicine is clinical translation, which requires meticulous optimization of surface characterization and its efficacy. However, the transition from preclinical studies to clinical application poses significant challenges, including the development of reliable pharmacokinetic replicas, effective formulations, and comprehensive evaluation of the biological properties. The precise design of nanomedicines' physicochemical characteristics is essential for achieving immune evasion, tumor penetration, cellular targeting, and controlled drug release [216]. Despite promising results in cellular and animal studies, clinical trials often reveal challenges due to the substantial physiological differences between humans and animal models. Moreover, biocompatibility remains a critical challenge in the clinical translation of nanotechnology-based drug delivery systems. As a common example, the EPR effect, a basis mechanism for nanoparticle tumor targeting in animal models, often shows limited relevance in human clinical studies [217]. This discrepancy underscores the need for innovative theories and techniques to bridge the gap between experimental models and clinical reality. Moreover, designing nanomedicines with optimized size, surface properties, drug-loading capacities, and controlled release mechanisms remains a complex task.

CONCLUSION

Nanomedicine represents a significant leap forward in the landscape of cancer theranostics, addressing critical limitations of conventional modalities. By exploiting tumor-specific features and enabling controlled and targeted delivery of therapeutics, nanomedicine offers enhanced efficacy, reduced systemic toxicity, and real-time monitoring capabilities. Passive and active targeting strategies, coupled with stimuli-responsive mechanisms, have been instrumental in advancing multifunctional theranostic systems. However, clinical translation remains hampered by challenges, including tumor heterogeneity, biological barriers, safety concerns, and discrepancies between animal models and human physiology. Moving forward, the development of more biocompatible, scalable, and tunable nanocarriers, along with improved preclinical models and regulatory frameworks, will be essential. Through sustained interdisciplinary collaboration and technological innovation, nanomedicine holds the potential to redefine cancer therapy, enabling safer, smarter, and more personalized treatment paradigms.

REFERENCES

[1] Duncan R, Gaspar R. Nanomedicine(s) under the Microscope. Mol Pharm 2011; 8(6): 2101-41. [http://dx.doi.org/10.1021/mp200394t] [PMID: 21974749]

[2] Lammers T, Kiessling F, Hennink WE, Storm G. Drug targeting to tumors: Principles, pitfalls and (pre-) clinical progress. J Control Release 2012; 161(2): 175-87. [http://dx.doi.org/10.1016/j.jconrel.2011.09.063] [PMID: 21945285]

[3] Mamot C, Ritschard R, Wicki A, *et al.* Tolerability, safety, pharmacokinetics, and efficacy of doxorubicin-loaded anti-EGFR immunoliposomes in advanced solid tumours: a phase 1 dose-escalation study. Lancet Oncol 2012; 13(12): 1234-41. [http://dx.doi.org/10.1016/S1470-2045(12)70476-X] [PMID: 23153506]

[4] Stylianopoulos T, Jain RK. Combining two strategies to improve perfusion and drug delivery in solid tumors. Proc Natl Acad Sci USA 2013; 110(46): 18632-7. [http://dx.doi.org/10.1073/pnas.1318415110] [PMID: 24167277]

[5] Danielli R, Patuzzo R, Ruffini PA, *et al.* Armed antibodies for cancer treatment: a promising tool in a changing era. Cancer Immunol Immunother 2015; 64(1): 113-21.

[http://dx.doi.org/10.1007/s00262-014-1621-0] [PMID: 25314912]

[6] Tang P, Shen T, Wang H, *et al.* Challenges and opportunities for improving the druggability of natural product: Why need drug delivery system? Biomed Pharmacother 2023; 164114955 [http://dx.doi.org/10.1016/j.biopha.2023.114955] [PMID: 37269810]

[7] Hawe A, Hulse WL, Jiskoot W, Forbes RT. Taylor dispersion analysis compared to dynamic light scattering for the size analysis of therapeutic peptides and proteins and their aggregates. Pharm Res 2011; 28(9): 2302-10. [http://dx.doi.org/10.1007/s11095-011-0460-3] [PMID: 21560019]

[8] Bertrand N, Wu J, Xu X, Kamaly N, Farokhzad OC. Cancer nanotechnology: The impact of passive and active targeting in the era of modern cancer biology. Adv Drug Deliv Rev 2014; 66: 2-25. [http://dx.doi.org/10.1016/j.addr.2013.11.009] [PMID: 24270007]

[9] Anand U, Dey A, Chandel AKS, *et al.* Cancer chemotherapy and beyond: Current status, drug candidates, associated risks and progress in targeted therapeutics. Genes Dis 2023; 10(4): 1367-401. [http://dx.doi.org/10.1016/j.gendis.2022.02.007] [PMID: 37397557]

[10] Liu B, Zhou H, Tan L, Siu KTH, Guan XY. Exploring treatment options in cancer: tumor treatment strategies. Signal Transduct Target Ther 2024; 9(1): 175. [http://dx.doi.org/10.1038/s41392-024-01856-7] [PMID: 39013849]

[11] Kciuk M, Gielecińska A, Mujwar S, *et al.* Doxorubicin—An Agent with Multiple Mechanisms of Anticancer Activity. Cells 2023; 12(4): 659. [http://dx.doi.org/10.3390/cells12040659] [PMID: 36831326]

[12] Szebeni J, Alving CR, Muggia FM. Complement activation by Cremophor EL as a possible contributor to hypersensitivity to paclitaxel: an in vitro study. J Natl Cancer Inst 1998; 90(4): 300-6. [http://dx.doi.org/10.1093/jnci/90.4.300] [PMID: 9486816]

[13] Bhave G, Lewis JB, Chang SS. Association of gadolinium based magnetic resonance imaging contrast agents and nephrogenic systemic fibrosis. J Urol 2008; 180(3): 830-5. [http://dx.doi.org/10.1016/j.juro.2008.05.005] [PMID: 18635232]

[14] Yao Y, Zhou Y, Liu L, *et al.* Nanoparticle-Based Drug Delivery in Cancer Therapy and Its Role in Overcoming Drug Resistance. Front Mol Biosci 2020; 7: 193. [http://dx.doi.org/10.3389/fmolb.2020.00193] [PMID: 32974385]

[15] Ma P, Mumper RJ. Paclitaxel Nano-Delivery Systems: A Comprehensive Review. J Nanomed Nanotechnol 2013; 4(2)1000164 [http://dx.doi.org/10.4172/2157-7439.1000164] [PMID: 24163786]

[16] Navarro G, Sawant RR, Biswas S, Essex S, Tros de Ilarduya C, Torchilin VP. P-glycoprotein silencing with siRNA delivered by DOPE-modified PEI overcomes doxorubicin resistance in breast cancer cells. Nanomedicine (Lond) 2012; 7(1): 65-78. [http://dx.doi.org/10.2217/nnm.11.93] [PMID: 22191778]

[17] Chen N, Brachmann C, Liu X, *et al.* Albumin-bound nanoparticle (nab) paclitaxel exhibits enhanced paclitaxel tissue distribution and tumor penetration. Cancer Chemother Pharmacol 2015; 76(4): 699-712. [http://dx.doi.org/10.1007/s00280-015-2833-5] [PMID: 26231955]

[18] Hoffman RM, Bouvet M. Nanoparticle albumin-bound-paclitaxel: a limited improvement under the current therapeutic paradigm of pancreatic cancer. Expert Opin Pharmacother 2015; 16(7): 943-7. [http://dx.doi.org/10.1517/14656566.2015.1016912] [PMID: 25887245]

[19] Bakhtiary Z, Saei AA, Hajipour MJ, Raoufi M, Vermesh O, Mahmoudi M. Targeted superparamagnetic iron oxide nanoparticles for early detection of cancer: Possibilities and challenges. Nanomedicine 2016; 12(2): 287-307. [http://dx.doi.org/10.1016/j.nano.2015.10.019] [PMID: 26707817]

[20] Barenholz YC. Doxil® — The first FDA-approved nano-drug: Lessons learned. J Control Release

2012; 160(2): 117-34.
[http://dx.doi.org/10.1016/j.jconrel.2012.03.020] [PMID: 22484195]

[21] Matsumura Y, Maeda H. A new concept for macromolecular therapeutics in cancer chemotherapy: mechanism of tumoritropic accumulation of proteins and the antitumor agent smancs. Cancer Res 1986; 46(12 Pt 1): 6387-92.
[PMID: 2946403]

[22] Rizzo JD, Somerfield MR, Hagerty KL, *et al.* Use of epoetin and darbepoetin in patients with cancer: 2007 American Society of Clinical Oncology/American Society of Hematology clinical practice guideline update. J Clin Oncol 2008; 26(1): 132-49.
[http://dx.doi.org/10.1200/JCO.2007.14.3396] [PMID: 17954713]

[23] Awada A, Bondarenko IN, Bonneterre J, *et al.* A randomized controlled phase II trial of a novel composition of paclitaxel embedded into neutral and cationic lipids targeting tumor endothelial cells in advanced triple-negative breast cancer (TNBC). Ann Oncol 2014; 25(4): 824-31.
[http://dx.doi.org/10.1093/annonc/mdu025] [PMID: 24667715]

[24] Burstein HJ, Krilov L, Aragon-Ching JB, *et al.* Clinical cancer advances 2017: annual report on progress against cancer from the American Society of Clinical Oncology. J Clin Oncol 2017; 35(12): 1341-67.
[http://dx.doi.org/10.1200/JCO.2016.71.5292] [PMID: 28148207]

[25] Shen Z, Wu A, Chen X. Iron oxide nanoparticle based contrast agents for magnetic resonance imaging. Mol Pharm 2017; 14(5): 1352-64.
[http://dx.doi.org/10.1021/acs.molpharmaceut.6b00839] [PMID: 27776215]

[26] Mohajeri M, Salehi P, Heidari B, *et al.* PEGylated Pemetrexed and PolyNIPAM decorated gold nanoparticles: A biocompatible and highly stable CT contrast agent for cancer imaging. ACS Appl Bio Mater 2024; 7(9): 5977-91.
[http://dx.doi.org/10.1021/acsabm.4c00563] [PMID: 39120942]

[27] Wong C, Stylianopoulos T, Cui J, *et al.* Multistage nanoparticle delivery system for deep penetration into tumor tissue. Proc Natl Acad Sci USA 2011; 108(6): 2426-31.
[http://dx.doi.org/10.1073/pnas.1018382108] [PMID: 21245339]

[28] Tang L, Fan TM, Borst LB, Cheng J. Synthesis and biological response of size-specific, monodisperse drug-silica nanoconjugates. ACS Nano 2012; 6(5): 3954-66.
[http://dx.doi.org/10.1021/nn300149c] [PMID: 22494403]

[29] Anselmo AC, Zhang M, Kumar S, *et al.* Elasticity of nanoparticles influences their blood circulation, phagocytosis, endocytosis, and targeting. ACS Nano 2015; 9(3): 3169-77.
[http://dx.doi.org/10.1021/acsnano.5b00147] [PMID: 25715979]

[30] Bogart LK, Pourroy G, Murphy CJ, *et al.* Nanoparticles for imaging, sensing, and therapeutic intervention. ACS Nano 2014; 8(4): 3107-22.
[http://dx.doi.org/10.1021/nn500962q] [PMID: 24641589]

[31] Hansen AE, Petersen AL, Henriksen JR, *et al.* Positron emission tomography based elucidation of the enhanced permeability and retention effect in dogs with cancer using copper-64 liposomes. ACS Nano 2015; 9(7): 6985-95.
[http://dx.doi.org/10.1021/acsnano.5b01324] [PMID: 26022907]

[32] McNeil SE. Evaluation of nanomedicines: stick to the basics. Nat Rev Mater 2016; 1(10): 16073.
[http://dx.doi.org/10.1038/natrevmats.2016.73]

[33] Xu R, Zhang G, Mai J, *et al.* An injectable nanoparticle generator enhances delivery of cancer therapeutics. Nat Biotechnol 2016; 34(4): 414-8.
[http://dx.doi.org/10.1038/nbt.3506] [PMID: 26974511]

[34] Kirpotin DB, Drummond DC, Shao Y, *et al.* Antibody targeting of long-circulating lipidic nanoparticles does not increase tumor localization but does increase internalization in animal models.

Cancer Res 2006; 66(13): 6732-40.
[http://dx.doi.org/10.1158/0008-5472.CAN-05-4199] [PMID: 16818648]

[35] Schmidt MM, Wittrup KD. A modeling analysis of the effects of molecular size and binding affinity on tumor targeting. Mol Cancer Ther 2009; 8(10): 2861-71.
[http://dx.doi.org/10.1158/1535-7163.MCT-09-0195] [PMID: 19825804]

[36] Sahay G, Querbes W, Alabi C, *et al.* Efficiency of siRNA delivery by lipid nanoparticles is limited by endocytic recycling. Nat Biotechnol 2013; 31(7): 653-8.
[http://dx.doi.org/10.1038/nbt.2614] [PMID: 23792629]

[37] Gilleron J, Querbes W, Zeigerer A, *et al.* Image-based analysis of lipid nanoparticle–mediated siRNA delivery, intracellular trafficking and endosomal escape. Nat Biotechnol 2013; 31(7): 638-46.
[http://dx.doi.org/10.1038/nbt.2612] [PMID: 23792630]

[38] Kedmi R, Veiga N, Ramishetti S, *et al.* A modular platform for targeted RNAi therapeutics. Nat Nanotechnol 2018; 13(3): 214-9.
[http://dx.doi.org/10.1038/s41565-017-0043-5] [PMID: 29379205]

[39] Yuan F, Dellian M, Fukumura D, *et al.* Vascular permeability in a human tumor xenograft: molecular size dependence and cutoff size. Cancer Res 1995; 55(17): 3752-6.
[PMID: 7641188]

[40] Bertrand N, Leroux JC. The journey of a drug-carrier in the body: An anatomo-physiological perspective. J Control Release 2012; 161(2): 152-63.
[http://dx.doi.org/10.1016/j.jconrel.2011.09.098] [PMID: 22001607]

[41] Caracciolo G, Farokhzad OC, Mahmoudi M. Biological identity of nanoparticles *in vivo*: clinical implications of the protein corona. Trends Biotechnol 2017; 35(3): 257-64.
[http://dx.doi.org/10.1016/j.tibtech.2016.08.011] [PMID: 27663778]

[42] Kedmi R, Ben-Arie N, Peer D. The systemic toxicity of positively charged lipid nanoparticles and the role of Toll-like receptor 4 in immune activation. Biomaterials 2010; 31(26): 6867-75.
[http://dx.doi.org/10.1016/j.biomaterials.2010.05.027] [PMID: 20541799]

[43] Aradhya SV, Venkataraman L. Single-molecule junctions beyond electronic transport. Nat Nanotechnol 2013; 8(6): 399-410.
[http://dx.doi.org/10.1038/nnano.2013.91] [PMID: 23736215]

[44] Rodriguez PL, Harada T, Christian DA, Pantano DA, Tsai RK, Discher DE. Minimal "Self" peptides that inhibit phagocytic clearance and enhance delivery of nanoparticles. Science 2013; 339(6122): 971-5.
[http://dx.doi.org/10.1126/science.1229568] [PMID: 23430657]

[45] Hu Q, Sun W, Qian C, Wang C, Bomba HN, Gu Z. Anticancer platelet-mimicking nanovehicles. Adv Mater 2015; 27(44): 7043-50.
[http://dx.doi.org/10.1002/adma.201503323] [PMID: 26416431]

[46] Poon Z, Chang D, Zhao X, Hammond PT. Layer-by-layer nanoparticles with a pH-sheddable layer for *in vivo* targeting of tumor hypoxia. ACS Nano 2011; 5(6): 4284-92.
[http://dx.doi.org/10.1021/nn200876f] [PMID: 21513353]

[47] Sahoo P, Kundu S, Roy S, *et al.* Fundamental understanding of the size and surface modification effects on r_1, the relaxivity of Prussian blue nanocube@ *m* -SiO_2 : a novel targeted chemo-photodynamic theranostic agent to treat colon cancer. RSC Advances 2022; 12(38): 24555-70. [http://dx.doi.org/10.1039/D2RA03995H] [PMID: 36128364]

[48] Yameen B, Choi WI, Vilos C, Swami A, Shi J, Farokhzad OC. Insight into nanoparticle cellular uptake and intracellular targeting. J Control Release 2014; 190: 485-99.
[http://dx.doi.org/10.1016/j.jconrel.2014.06.038] [PMID: 24984011]

[49] Colombo M, Fiandra L, Alessio G, *et al.* Tumour homing and therapeutic effect of colloidal nanoparticles depend on the number of attached antibodies. Nat Commun 2016; 7(1): 13818.

[http://dx.doi.org/10.1038/ncomms13818] [PMID: 27991503]

[50] Yatvin MB, Weinstein JN, Dennis WH, Blumenthal R. Design of liposomes for enhanced local release of drugs by hyperthermia. Science 1978; 202(4374): 1290-3. [http://dx.doi.org/10.1126/science.364652] [PMID: 364652]

[51] Li J, Mater NA, Mura S, *et al.* Couvreur. Nat Mater 2013; 12: 991-1003.

[52] Liu C, Liu F, Feng L, Li M, Zhang J, Zhang N. The targeted co-delivery of DNA and doxorubicin to tumor cells via multifunctional PEI-PEG based nanoparticles. Biomaterials 2013; 34(10): 2547-64. [http://dx.doi.org/10.1016/j.biomaterials.2012.12.038] [PMID: 23332321]

[53] Ahmed F, Pakunlu RI, Brannan A, Bates F, Minko T, Discher DE. Biodegradable polymersomes loaded with both paclitaxel and doxorubicin permeate and shrink tumors, inducing apoptosis in proportion to accumulated drug. J Control Release 2006; 116(2): 150-8. [http://dx.doi.org/10.1016/j.jconrel.2006.07.012] [PMID: 16942814]

[54] Patel NR, Rathi A, Mongayt D, Torchilin VP. Reversal of multidrug resistance by co-delivery of tariquidar (XR9576) and paclitaxel using long-circulating liposomes. Int J Pharm 2011; 416(1): 296-9. [http://dx.doi.org/10.1016/j.ijpharm.2011.05.082] [PMID: 21703341]

[55] Guo X, Shi C, Wang J, Di S, Zhou S. pH-triggered intracellular release from actively targeting polymer micelles. Biomaterials 2013; 34(18): 4544-54. [http://dx.doi.org/10.1016/j.biomaterials.2013.02.071] [PMID: 23510854]

[56] Sahoo P, Nandi SK, Das M, *et al.* GSH-pH dual-responsive engineered codoped Prussian blue multimodal theranostic nanoplatform induces TP53 deregulated apoptotic death of MDA-MB-231 with enhanced T_1 - T_2 W MRI. ACS Appl Nano Mater 2024; 7(23): 26617-28. [https://doi.org/10.1021/acsanm.4c05556]. [http://dx.doi.org/10.1021/acsanm.4c05556]

[57] Kato T, Hatakeyama R. Site- and alignment-controlled growth of graphene nanoribbons from nickel nanobars. Nat Nanotechnol 2012; 7(10): 651-6. [http://dx.doi.org/10.1038/nnano.2012.145] [PMID: 22961304]

[58] Sekhon BS, Kamboj SR. Inorganic nanomedicine—Part 1. Nanomedicine 2010; 6(4): 516-22. [http://dx.doi.org/10.1016/j.nano.2010.04.004] [PMID: 20417313]

[59] Wolfram J, Ferrari M. Clinical cancer nanomedicine. Nano Today 2019; 25: 85-98. [http://dx.doi.org/10.1016/j.nantod.2019.02.005] [PMID: 31360214]

[60] Wang R, Billone PS, Mullett WM. Nanomedicine in action: an overview of cancer nanomedicine on the market and in clinical trials. J Nanomater 2013; 2013(1)629681 [http://dx.doi.org/10.1155/2013/629681]

[61] Chen G, Qiu H, Prasad PN, Chen X. Upconversion nanoparticles: design, nanochemistry, and applications in theranostics. Chem Rev 2014; 114(10): 5161-214. [http://dx.doi.org/10.1021/cr400425h] [PMID: 24605868]

[62] Kim H, Chung K, Lee S, Kim DH, Lee H. Near□infrared light□responsive nanomaterials for cancer theranostics. Wiley Interdiscip Rev Nanomed Nanobiotechnol 2016; 8(1): 23-45. [http://dx.doi.org/10.1002/wnan.1347] [PMID: 25903643]

[63] Wang Y, Song S, Zhang S, Zhang H. Stimuli-responsive nanotheranostics based on lanthanide-doped upconversion nanoparticles for cancer imaging and therapy: current advances and future challenges. Nano Today 2019; 25: 38-67. [http://dx.doi.org/10.1016/j.nantod.2019.02.007]

[64] Loo JFC, Chien YH, Yin F, Kong S-K, Ho H-P, Yong K-T. Upconversion and downconversion nanoparticles for biophotonics and nanomedicine. Coord Chem Rev 2019; 400213042 [http://dx.doi.org/10.1016/j.ccr.2019.213042]

[65] Wang H, Lu W, Zeng T, *et al.* Multi-functional $NaErF_4$:Yb nanorods: enhanced red upconversion

emission, in vitro cell, in vivo X-ray, and T_2-weighted magnetic resonance imaging. Nanoscale 2014; 6(5): 2855-60.
[http://dx.doi.org/10.1039/C3NR05782H] [PMID: 24469246]

[66] Liu J, Bu W, Pan L, Shi J. NIR-triggered anticancer drug delivery by upconverting nanoparticles with integrated azobenzene-modified mesoporous silica. Angew Chem Int Ed 2013; 52(16): 4375-9.
[http://dx.doi.org/10.1002/anie.201300183] [PMID: 23495013]

[67] Lu H, He S, Zhang Q, *et al.* Dual-sensitive dual-prodrug nanoparticles with light-controlled endo/lysosomal escape for synergistic photoactivated chemotherapy. Biomater Sci 2021; 9(21): 7115-23.
[http://dx.doi.org/10.1039/D1BM01154E] [PMID: 34569561]

[68] Ding B, Sheng J, Zheng P, *et al.* Biodegradable upconversion nanoparticles induce pyroptosis for cancer immunotherapy. Nano Lett 2021; 21(19): 8281-9.
[http://dx.doi.org/10.1021/acs.nanolett.1c02790] [PMID: 34591494]

[69] Zhao J, Zhang X, Fang L, Gao C, Xu C, Gou S. Iridium (III) complex–derived polymeric micelles with low dark toxicity and strong NIR excitation for phototherapy and chemotherapy. Small 2020; 16(14)2000363
[http://dx.doi.org/10.1002/smll.202000363] [PMID: 32174002]

[70] Jin J, Xu Z, Zhang Y, Gu YJ, Lam MHW, Wong WT. Upconversion nanoparticles conjugated with Gd(3+) -DOTA and RGD for targeted dual-modality imaging of brain tumor xenografts. Adv Healthc Mater 2013; 2(11): 1501-12.
[http://dx.doi.org/10.1002/adhm.201300102] [PMID: 23630101]

[71] Liu Q, Sun Y, Li C, *et al.* 18F-Labeled magnetic-upconversion nanophosphors via rare-Earth cation-assisted ligand assembly. ACS Nano 2011; 5(4): 3146-57.
[http://dx.doi.org/10.1021/nn200298y] [PMID: 21384900]

[72] Yang Y, Sun Y, Cao T, *et al.* Hydrothermal synthesis of $NaLuF_4$:153Sm,Yb,Tm nanoparticles and their application in dual-modality upconversion luminescence and SPECT bioimaging. Biomaterials 2013; 34(3): 774-83.
[http://dx.doi.org/10.1016/j.biomaterials.2012.10.022] [PMID: 23117216]

[73] Indhu AR, Keerthana L, Dharmalingam G. Plasmonic nanotechnology for photothermal applications – an evaluation. Beilstein J Nanotechnol 2023; 14: 380-419.
[http://dx.doi.org/10.3762/bjnano.14.33] [PMID: 37025366]

[74] Sharifi M, Attar F, Saboury AA, *et al.* Plasmonic gold nanoparticles: Optical manipulation, imaging, drug delivery and therapy. J Control Release 2019; 311-312: 170-89.
[http://dx.doi.org/10.1016/j.jconrel.2019.08.032] [PMID: 31472191]

[75] Sahoo P, Mukherjee A, Ghosh CK. Gold nanoparticles for photothermal and photodynamic therapy. 2025.
[http://dx.doi.org/10.1016/B978-0-443-15897-1.00002-9]

[76] Fang J, Chen YC. Nanomaterials for photohyperthermia: a review. Curr Pharm Des 2013; 19(37): 6622-34.
[http://dx.doi.org/10.2174/1381612811319370006] [PMID: 23621537]

[77] Hwang J, An EK, Kim SJ, Zhang W, Jin JO. Escherichia coli mimetic gold nanorod-mediated photo- and immunotherapy for treating cancer and its metastasis. ACS Nano 2022; 16(5): 8472-83.
[http://dx.doi.org/10.1021/acsnano.2c03379] [PMID: 35466668]

[78] Gowsalya K, Rithisa B, Shyamsivappan S, *et al.* Immune-theranostic gold nanorod-based NIR-responsive nanomedicine for the delivery of TLR7/8 adjuvant-induced effective anticancer therapy. RSC Pharmaceutic 2024.
[http://dx.doi.org/10.1039/D4PM00033A]

[79] Khoobchandani M, Katti KK, Karikachery AR, *et al.* Targeted phytochemical-conjugated gold

nanoparticles in cancer treatment. Biotechnology Products in Everyday Life 2019; pp. 37-52. [http://dx.doi.org/10.1007/978-3-319-92399-4_3]

[80] Lee CS, Kim TW, Kang Y, *et al.* Targeted drug delivery nanocarriers based on hyaluronic acid-decorated dendrimer encapsulating gold nanoparticles for ovarian cancer therapy. Mater Today Chem 2022; 26101083 [http://dx.doi.org/10.1016/j.mtchem.2022.101083]

[81] Tunç CÜ, Aydin O. Co-delivery of Bcl-2 siRNA and doxorubicin through gold nanoparticle-based delivery system for a combined cancer therapy approach. J Drug Deliv Sci Technol 2022; 74103603 [http://dx.doi.org/10.1016/j.jddst.2022.103603]

[82] Chen C, Ma Y, Du S, *et al.* Controlled CRISPR□Cas9 ribonucleoprotein delivery for sensitized photothermal therapy. Small 2021; 17(33)2101155 [http://dx.doi.org/10.1002/smll.202101155] [PMID: 34269521]

[83] Na HB, Song IC, Hyeon T. Inorganic nanoparticles for MRI contrast agents. Adv Mater 2009; 21(21): 2133-48. [http://dx.doi.org/10.1002/adma.200802366]

[84] Yu J, Huang DY, Yousaf MZ, Hou Y-L, Gao S. Magnetic nanoparticle-based cancer therapy. Chin Phys B 2013; 22(2)027506 [http://dx.doi.org/10.1088/1674-1056/22/2/027506]

[85] Sahoo P, Choudhury D, Kundu S, *et al.* Nanoparticles in Biomedical Applications: MRI Contrast Agents.Advanced Nanomaterials and Their Applications 139-188.

[86] Ren X, Chen H, Yang V, Sun D. Iron oxide nanoparticle-based theranostics for cancer imaging and therapy. Front Chem Sci Eng 2014; 8(3): 253-64. [http://dx.doi.org/10.1007/s11705-014-1425-y]

[87] Liu HL, Hua MY, Yang HW, *et al.* Magnetic resonance monitoring of focused ultrasound/magnetic nanoparticle targeting delivery of therapeutic agents to the brain. Proc Natl Acad Sci USA 2010; 107(34): 15205-10. [http://dx.doi.org/10.1073/pnas.1003388107] [PMID: 20696897]

[88] Li J, Zheng L, Cai H, *et al.* Polyethyleneimine-mediated synthesis of folic acid-targeted iron oxide nanoparticles for *in vivo* tumor MR imaging. Biomaterials 2013; 34(33): 8382-92. [http://dx.doi.org/10.1016/j.biomaterials.2013.07.070] [PMID: 23932250]

[89] Zhang Y, Shen T, Deng X, *et al.* Design of a versatile nanocomposite for 'seeing' drug release and action behavior. J Mater Chem B Mater Biol Med 2015; 3(43): 8449-58. [http://dx.doi.org/10.1039/C5TB01367D] [PMID: 32262684]

[90] Yuan Y, Ding Z, Qian J, *et al.* Casp3/7-instructed intracellular aggregation of Fe_3O_4 nanoparticles enhances T_2 MR imaging of tumor apoptosis. Nano Lett 2016; 16(4): 2686-91. [http://dx.doi.org/10.1021/acs.nanolett.6b00331] [PMID: 27031226]

[91] Ryu C, Lee H, Kim H, *et al.* Highly optimized iron oxide embedded poly (lactic acid) nanocomposites for effective magnetic hyperthermia and biosecurity. Int J Nanomedicine 2022; 17: 31-44. [http://dx.doi.org/10.2147/IJN.S344257] [PMID: 35023918]

[92] Hajikarimi Z, Khoei S, Khoee S, Mahdavi SR. Evaluation of the cytotoxic effects of PLGA coated iron oxide nanoparticles as a carrier of 5- fluorouracil and mega-voltage X-ray radiation in DU145 prostate cancer cell line. IEEE Trans Nanobiosci 2014; 13(4): 403-8. [http://dx.doi.org/10.1109/TNB.2014.2328868] [PMID: 25051558]

[93] Javid A, Ahmadian S, Saboury AA, Kalantar SM, Rezaei-Zarchi S. Chitosan-coated superparamagnetic iron oxide nanoparticles for doxorubicin delivery: synthesis and anticancer effect against human ovarian cancer cells. Chem Biol Drug Des 2013; 82(3): 296-306. [http://dx.doi.org/10.1111/cbdd.12145] [PMID: 23594157]

[94] Shirangi A, Mottaghitalab F, Dinarvand S, Atyabi F. Theranostic silk sericin/SPION nanoparticles for

targeted delivery of ROR1 siRNA: Synthesis, characterization, diagnosis and anticancer effect on triple-negative breast cancer. Int J Biol Macromol 2022; 221: 604-12.
[http://dx.doi.org/10.1016/j.ijbiomac.2022.09.020] [PMID: 36084874]

[95] Tang F, Li L, Chen D. Mesoporous silica nanoparticles: synthesis, biocompatibility and drug delivery. Adv Mater 2012; 24(12): 1504-34.
[http://dx.doi.org/10.1002/adma.201104763] [PMID: 22378538]

[96] Zhang Z, Wang L, Wang J, *et al.* Mesoporous silica-coated gold nanorods as a light-mediated multifunctional theranostic platform for cancer treatment. Adv Mater 2012; 24(11): 1418-23.
[http://dx.doi.org/10.1002/adma.201104714] [PMID: 22318874]

[97] Xie W, Deng WW, Zan M, *et al.* Cancer cell membrane camouflaged nanoparticles to realize starvation therapy together with checkpoint blockades for enhancing cancer therapy. ACS Nano 2019; 13(3): 2849-57.
[http://dx.doi.org/10.1021/acsnano.8b03788] [PMID: 30803232]

[98] Fu LH, Hu YR, Qi C, *et al.* Biodegradable manganese-doped calcium phosphate nanotheranostics for traceable cascade reaction-enhanced anti-tumor therapy. ACS Nano 2019; 13(12): 13985-94.
[http://dx.doi.org/10.1021/acsnano.9b05836] [PMID: 31833366]

[99] Lee D, Shin J, Son H, *et al.* Organic and inorganic nanomedicine for combination cancer therapies. Nanoscale Adv 2023; 5(6): 1600-10.
[http://dx.doi.org/10.1039/D3NA00043E] [PMID: 36926565]

[100] Zhou J, Yang Y, Zhang C. Toward biocompatible semiconductor quantum dots: from biosynthesis and bioconjugation to biomedical application. Chem Rev 2015; 115(21): 11669-717.
[http://dx.doi.org/10.1021/acs.chemrev.5b00049] [PMID: 26446443]

[101] Guo W, chen N, Tu Y, *et al.* Synthesis of Zn-Cu-In-S/ZnS core/shell quantum dots with inhibited blue-shift photoluminescence and applications for tumor targeted bioimaging. Theranostics 2013; 3(2): 99-108.
[http://dx.doi.org/10.7150/thno.5361] [PMID: 23422883]

[102] Sasaki A, Tsukasaki Y, Komatsuzaki A, Sakata T, Yasuda H, Jin T. Recombinant protein (EGFP-Protein G)-coated PbS quantum dots for *in vitro* and *in vivo* dual fluorescence (visible and second-NIR) imaging of breast tumors. Nanoscale 2015; 7(12): 5115-9.
[http://dx.doi.org/10.1039/C4NR06480A] [PMID: 25564367]

[103] del Rosal B, Carrasco E, Ren F, *et al.* Infrared□emitting QDs for Thermal therapy with real□time subcutaneous temperature feedback. Adv Funct Mater 2016; 26(33): 6060-8.
[http://dx.doi.org/10.1002/adfm.201601953]

[104] Lian HY, Hu M, Liu CH, Yamauchi Y, Wu KCW. Highly biocompatible, hollow coordination polymer nanoparticles as cisplatin carriers for efficient intracellular drug delivery. Chem Commun (Camb) 2012; 48(42): 5151-3.
[http://dx.doi.org/10.1039/c2cc31708g] [PMID: 22514015]

[105] Cheng L, Gong H, Zhu W, *et al.* PEGylated Prussian blue nanocubes as a theranostic agent for simultaneous cancer imaging and photothermal therapy. Biomaterials 2014; 35(37): 9844-52.
[http://dx.doi.org/10.1016/j.biomaterials.2014.09.004] [PMID: 25239041]

[106] Li ZH, Chen Y, Sun Y, Zhang XZ. Platinum-doped prussian blue nanozymes for multiwavelength bioimaging guided photothermal therapy of tumor and anti-inflammation. ACS Nano 2021; 15(3): 5189-200.
[http://dx.doi.org/10.1021/acsnano.0c10388] [PMID: 33703878]

[107] Sahoo P, Jana P, Kundu S, *et al.* Quercetin@Gd $^{3+}$ doped Prussian blue nanocubes induce the pyroptotic death of MDA-MB-231 cells: combinational targeted multimodal therapy, dual modal MRI, intuitive modelling of $r_1 - r_2$ relaxivities.r1-r2 J Mater Chem B Mater Biol Med 2023; 11(28): 6646-63.
[http://dx.doi.org/10.1039/D3TB00316G] [PMID: 37366114]

[108] Zhou B, Jiang BP, Sun W, *et al.* Water-dispersible Prussian blue hyaluronic acid nanocubes with near-infrared photoinduced singlet oxygen production and photothermal activities for cancer theranostics. ACS Appl Mater Interfaces 2018; 10(21): 18036-49.
[http://dx.doi.org/10.1021/acsami.8b01387] [PMID: 29745229]

[109] Zhang W, Hu S, Yin JJ, *et al.* Prussian blue nanoparticles as multienzyme mimetics and reactive oxygen species scavengers. J Am Chem Soc 2016; 138(18): 5860-5.
[http://dx.doi.org/10.1021/jacs.5b12070] [PMID: 26918394]

[110] Chen H, Ma Y, Wang X, Zha Z. Multifunctional phase-change hollow mesoporous Prussian blue nanoparticles as a NIR light responsive drug co-delivery system to overcome cancer therapeutic resistance. J Mater Chem B Mater Biol Med 2017; 5(34): 7051-8.
[http://dx.doi.org/10.1039/C7TB01712J] [PMID: 32263896]

[111] Xue P, Cheong KKY, Wu Y, Kang Y. An in-vitro study of enzyme-responsive Prussian blue nanoparticles for combined tumor chemotherapy and photothermal therapy. Colloids Surf B Biointerfaces 2015; 125: 277-83.
[http://dx.doi.org/10.1016/j.colsurfb.2014.10.059] [PMID: 25465756]

[112] Wang C, Jia X, Zhen W, Zhang M, Jiang X. Small-sized MOF-constructed multifunctional diagnosis and therapy platform for tumor. ACS Biomater Sci Eng 2019; 5(9): 4435-41.
[http://dx.doi.org/10.1021/acsbiomaterials.9b00813] [PMID: 33438409]

[113] Kim T, Lemaster JE, Chen F, Li J, Jokerst JV. Photoacoustic imaging of human mesenchymal stem cells labeled with Prussian blue–poly (l-lysine) nanocomplexes. ACS Nano 2017; 11(9): 9022-32.
[http://dx.doi.org/10.1021/acsnano.7b03519] [PMID: 28759195]

[114] Shukla M, Verma NV, Mohanta Z, Tripathi S, Pandya A. A review on tunable multi-functional Prussian blue nanoparticles; their promising biological applications & future directions. Coord Chem Rev 2023; 496215414 [https://doi.org/10.1016/j.ccr.2023.215414].
[http://dx.doi.org/10.1016/j.ccr.2023.215414]

[115] Tian W, Su Y, Tian Y, *et al.* Periodic Mesoporous Organosilica Coated Prussian Blue for MR/PA Dual□Modal Imaging□Guided Photothermal□Chemotherapy of Triple Negative Breast Cancer. Adv Sci (Weinh) 2017; 4(3)1600356
[http://dx.doi.org/10.1002/advs.201600356] [PMID: 28331788]

[116] U S, Basu U, Paira P. Current context of designing phototheranostic cyclometalated iridium (III) complexes to open a new avenue in cancer therapy. ChemMedChem 2025; 20(5)e202400649
[http://dx.doi.org/10.1002/cmdc.202400649] [PMID: 39495110]

[117] Wu C, Cui M, Cai L, *et al.* NIR-responsive photodynamic nanosystem combined with antitumor immune optogenetics bacteria for precise synergetic therapy. ACS Appl Mater Interfaces 2022; 14(11): 13094-106.
[http://dx.doi.org/10.1021/acsami.2c01138] [PMID: 35262323]

[118] Emami F, Banstola A, Vatanara A, *et al.* Doxorubicine and anti-PD-L1 antibody conjugated gold nanoparticles for colorectal cancer phototherapy. Mol Pharm 2019; 16(3): 1184-99.
[http://dx.doi.org/10.1021/acs.molpharmaceut.8b01157] [PMID: 30698975]

[119] Gowsalya K, Rithisa B, Shyamsivappan S, *et al.* Immune-theranostic gold nanorod-based NIR-responsive nanomedicine for the delivery of TLR7/8 adjuvant-induced effective anticancer therapy. RSC Pharmaceutics 2024.
[http://dx.doi.org/10.1039/D4PM00033A]

[120] Libutti SK, Paciotti GF, Byrnes AA, *et al.* Phase I and pharmacokinetic studies of CYT-6091, a novel PEGylated colloidal gold-rhTNF nanomedicine. Clin Cancer Res 2010; 16(24): 6139-49.
[http://dx.doi.org/10.1158/1078-0432.CCR-10-0978] [PMID: 20876255]

[121] Zhang Z, Zhang L, Huang C, *et al.* Gas-generating mesoporous silica nanoparticles with rapid localized drug release for enhanced chemophotothermal tumor therapy. Biomater Sci 2020; 8(23):

6754-63.
[http://dx.doi.org/10.1039/D0BM01502D] [PMID: 33140761]

[122] Huang C, Zhang L, Guo Q, *et al.* Robust nanovaccine based on polydopamine□coated mesoporous silica nanoparticles for effective photothermal□immunotherapy against melanoma. Adv Funct Mater 2021; 31(18)2010637
[http://dx.doi.org/10.1002/adfm.202010637]

[123] Benezra M, Penate-Medina O, Zanzonico PB, *et al.* Multimodal silica nanoparticles are effective cancer-targeted probes in a model of human melanoma. J Clin Invest 2011; 121(7): 2768-80.
[http://dx.doi.org/10.1172/JCI45600] [PMID: 21670497]

[124] Chen Z, Yu T, Zhou B, *et al.* Mg(II)-Catechin nanoparticles delivering siRNA targeting EIF5A2 inhibit bladder cancer cell growth in vitro and *in vivo.* Biomaterials 2016; 81: 125-34.
[http://dx.doi.org/10.1016/j.biomaterials.2015.11.022] [PMID: 26731576]

[125] Vimala K, Soundarapandian K. 129P Inhibition of breast cancer cell explosion rate by irinotecan loaded zinc oxide nanoparticles through E2F3/Akt signaling circuits: A milestone in cancer gene therapy. Ann Oncol 2016; 27: ix38-9.
[http://dx.doi.org/10.1016/S0923-7534(21)00288-X]

[126] Sharma H, Kumar K, Choudhary C, Mishra PK, Vaidya B. Development and characterization of metal oxide nanoparticles for the delivery of anticancer drug. Artif Cells Nanomed Biotechnol 2016; 44(2): 672-9.
[http://dx.doi.org/10.3109/21691401.2014.978980] [PMID: 25406734]

[127] Sudhagar S, Sathya S, Pandian K, Lakshmi BS. Targeting and sensing cancer cells with ZnO nanoprobes in vitro. Biotechnol Lett 2011; 33(9): 1891-6.
[http://dx.doi.org/10.1007/s10529-011-0641-5] [PMID: 21553287]

[128] Zhao W, Wei JS, Zhang P, *et al.* Self-assembled ZnO nanoparticle capsules for carrying and delivering isotretinoin to cancer cells. ACS Appl Mater Interfaces 2017; 9(22): 18474-81.
[http://dx.doi.org/10.1021/acsami.7b02542] [PMID: 28541041]

[129] Sun C, Fang C, Stephen Z, *et al.* Tumor-targeted drug delivery and MRI contrast enhancement by chlorotoxin-conjugated iron oxide nanoparticles. Nanomedicine (Lond) 2008; 3(4): 495-505.
[http://dx.doi.org/10.2217/17435889.3.4.495] [PMID: 18694312]

[130] Shahbazi-Gahrouei D, Abdolahi M. Detection of MUC1-expressing ovarian cancer by C595 monoclonal antibody-conjugated SPIONs using MR imaging. ScientificWorldJournal 2013; 2013(1)609151
[http://dx.doi.org/10.1155/2013/609151] [PMID: 24194685]

[131] Birkhäuser FD, Studer UE, Thoeny HC. Ferumoxtran-10 Ultrasmall Superparamagnetic Iron Oxide–Enhanced Diffusion-weighted Imaging Magnetic Resonance Imaging for Detection of Metastases in Normal-sized Lymph Nodes in Patients with Bladder and Prostate Cancer: Do We Enter the Era After Extended Pelvic Lymph Node Dissection? Eur Urol 2013; 64: 961–3. Eur Urol 2013; 6(64): 963-4.

[132] Hedgire S, Mino- Kenudson M, Elmi A, Thayer S, Fernandez-del Castillo C, Harisinghani M. Enhanced primary tumor delineation in pancreatic adenocarcinoma using ultrasmall super paramagnetic iron oxide nanoparticle-ferumoxytol: an initial experience with histopathologic correlation. Int J Nanomedicine 2014; 9: 1891-6.
[http://dx.doi.org/10.2147/IJN.S59788] [PMID: 24790431]

[133] Liu T, Wang C, Gu X, *et al.* Drug delivery with PEGylated MoS_2 nano-sheets for combined photothermal and chemotherapy of cancer. Adv Mater 2014; 26(21): 3433-40.
[http://dx.doi.org/10.1002/adma.201305256] [PMID: 24677423]

[134] Maggiorella L, Barouch G, Devaux C, *et al.* Nanoscale radiotherapy with hafnium oxide nanoparticles. Future Oncol 2012; 8(9): 1167-81.
[http://dx.doi.org/10.2217/fon.12.96] [PMID: 23030491]

[135] Monti A, de Groot HJM, Buda F. In-silico design of a donor–antenna–acceptor supramolecular complex for photoinduced charge separation. J Phys Chem C 2014; 118(29): 15600-9. [http://dx.doi.org/10.1021/jp505105a]

[136] Ng KK, Zheng G. Molecular interactions in organic nanoparticles for phototheranostic applications. Chem Rev 2015; 115(19): 11012-42. [http://dx.doi.org/10.1021/acs.chemrev.5b00140] [PMID: 26244706]

[137] Layek B, Gidwani B, Tiwari S, Joshi V, Jain V, Vyas A. Recent advances in lipid-based nanodrug delivery systems in cancer therapy. Curr Pharm Des 2020; 26(27): 3218-33. [http://dx.doi.org/10.2174/1381612826666200622133407] [PMID: 32568015]

[138] Trivedi R, Arora S, Lamptey RN, *et al.* A summarized view of lipid, polyplex, inorganic, and carbon-based nanotherapeutics for hepatocellular carcinoma treatment. Nanotherapeutics for the Treatment of Hepatocellular Carcinoma 2022; p. 248. [http://dx.doi.org/10.2174/9789815039740122010008]

[139] Sercombe L, Veerati T, Moheimani F, Wu SY, Sood AK, Hua S. Advances and challenges of liposome assisted drug delivery. Front Pharmacol 2015; 6: 286. [http://dx.doi.org/10.3389/fphar.2015.00286] [PMID: 26648870]

[140] Liu P, Chen G, Zhang J. A review of liposomes as a drug delivery system: current status of approved products, regulatory environments, and future perspectives. Molecules 2022; 27(4): 1372. [http://dx.doi.org/10.3390/molecules27041372] [PMID: 35209162]

[141] Taléns-Visconti R, Díez-Sales O, de Julián-Ortiz JV, Nácher A. Nanoliposomes in cancer therapy: marketed products and current clinical trials. Int J Mol Sci 2022; 23(8): 4249. [http://dx.doi.org/10.3390/ijms23084249] [PMID: 35457065]

[142] Immordino ML, Dosio F, Cattel L. Stealth liposomes: review of the basic science, rationale, and clinical applications, existing and potential. Int J Nanomedicine 2006; 1(3): 297-315. [PMID: 17717971]

[143] Suk JS, Xu Q, Kim N, Hanes J, Ensign LM. PEGylation as a strategy for improving nanoparticle-based drug and gene delivery. Adv Drug Deliv Rev 2016; 99(Pt A): 28-51. [http://dx.doi.org/10.1016/j.addr.2015.09.012] [PMID: 26456916]

[144] Gabizon A, Catane R, Uziely B, *et al.* Prolonged circulation time and enhanced accumulation in malignant exudates of doxorubicin encapsulated in polyethylene-glycol coated liposomes. Cancer Res 1994; 54(4): 987-92. [PMID: 8313389]

[145] Dai Y, Su J, Wu K, *et al.* Multifunctional thermosensitive liposomes based on natural phase-change material: near-infrared light-triggered drug release and multimodal imaging-guided cancer combination therapy. ACS Appl Mater Interfaces 2019; 11(11): 10540-53. [http://dx.doi.org/10.1021/acsami.8b22748] [PMID: 30807086]

[146] Naseri N, Valizadeh H, Zakeri-Milani P. Solid lipid nanoparticles and nanostructured lipid carriers: structure, preparation and application. Adv Pharm Bull 2015; 5(3): 305-13. [http://dx.doi.org/10.15171/apb.2015.043] [PMID: 26504751]

[147] Mehnert W, Mäder K. Solid lipid nanoparticles. Adv Drug Deliv Rev 2012; 64: 83-101. [http://dx.doi.org/10.1016/j.addr.2012.09.021] [PMID: 11311991]

[148] Bayón-Cordero L, Alkorta I, Arana L. Application of solid lipid nanoparticles to improve the efficiency of anticancer drugs. Nanomaterials (Basel) 2019; 9(3): 474. [http://dx.doi.org/10.3390/nano9030474] [PMID: 30909401]

[149] Rodenak-Kladniew B, Islan GA, de Bravo MG, Durán N, Castro GR. Design, characterization and in vitro evaluation of linalool-loaded solid lipid nanoparticles as potent tool in cancer therapy. Colloids Surf B Biointerfaces 2017; 154: 123-32. [http://dx.doi.org/10.1016/j.colsurfb.2017.03.021] [PMID: 28334689]

[150] Wang W, Chen T, Xu H, *et al.* Curcumin-loaded solid lipid nanoparticles enhanced anticancer efficiency in breast cancer. Molecules 2018; 23(7): 1578.
[http://dx.doi.org/10.3390/molecules23071578] [PMID: 29966245]

[151] Zheng G, Zheng M, Yang B, Fu H, Li Y. Improving breast cancer therapy using doxorubicin loaded solid lipid nanoparticles: Synthesis of a novel arginine-glycine-aspartic tripeptide conjugated, pH sensitive lipid and evaluation of the nanomedicine in vitro and *in vivo.* Biomed Pharmacother 2019; 116109006
[http://dx.doi.org/10.1016/j.biopha.2019.109006] [PMID: 31152925]

[152] Guimarães KL, Ré MI. 2011.

[153] Jain P, Rahi P, Pandey V, *et al.* Nanostructure lipid carriers: a modish contrivance to overcome the ultraviolet effects 2017.
[http://dx.doi.org/10.1016/j.ejbas.2017.02.001]

[154] Karn-orachai K, Smith SM, Phunpee S, *et al.* The effect of surfactant composition on the chemical and structural properties of nanostructured lipid carriers. J Microencapsul 2014; 31(6): 609-18.
[http://dx.doi.org/10.3109/02652048.2014.911374] [PMID: 24861323]

[155] Fernandes RS, Silva JO, Monteiro LOF, *et al.* Doxorubicin-loaded nanocarriers: A comparative study of liposome and nanostructured lipid carrier as alternatives for cancer therapy. Biomed Pharmacother 2016; 84: 252-7.
[http://dx.doi.org/10.1016/j.biopha.2016.09.032] [PMID: 27664949]

[156] Rizwanullah M, Ahmad MZ, Garg A, Ahmad J. Advancement in design of nanostructured lipid carriers for cancer targeting and theranostic application. Biochim Biophys Acta, Gen Subj 2021; 1865(9)129936
[http://dx.doi.org/10.1016/j.bbagen.2021.129936] [PMID: 34058266]

[157] González-Vallinas M, González-Castejón M, Rodríguez-Casado A, Ramírez de Molina A. Dietary phytochemicals in cancer prevention and therapy: a complementary approach with promising perspectives. Nutr Rev 2013; 71(9): 585-99.
[http://dx.doi.org/10.1111/nure.12051] [PMID: 24032363]

[158] Poonia N, Kaur Narang J, Lather V, *et al.* Resveratrol loaded functionalized nanostructured lipid carriers for breast cancer targeting: Systematic development, characterization and pharmacokinetic evaluation. Colloids Surf B Biointerfaces 2019; 181: 756-66.
[http://dx.doi.org/10.1016/j.colsurfb.2019.06.004] [PMID: 31234063]

[159] Gagliardi A, Giuliano E, Venkateswararao E, *et al.* Biodegradable polymeric nanoparticles for drug delivery to solid tumors. Front Pharmacol 2021; 12601626
[http://dx.doi.org/10.3389/fphar.2021.601626] [PMID: 33613290]

[160] Layek B, Mandal S. Natural polysaccharides for controlled delivery of oral therapeutics: a recent update. Carbohydr Polym 2020; 230115617
[http://dx.doi.org/10.1016/j.carbpol.2019.115617] [PMID: 31887888]

[161] Liyanage PY, Hettiarachchi SD, Zhou Y, *et al.* Nanoparticle-mediated targeted drug delivery for breast cancer treatment. Biochim Biophys Acta Rev Cancer 2019; 1871(2): 419-33.
[http://dx.doi.org/10.1016/j.bbcan.2019.04.006] [PMID: 31034927]

[162] Masood F. Polymeric nanoparticles for targeted drug delivery system for cancer therapy. Mater Sci Eng C 2016; 60: 569-78.
[http://dx.doi.org/10.1016/j.msec.2015.11.067] [PMID: 26706565]

[163] Hasnain MS, Ahmad SA, Chaudhary N, *et al.* Biodegradable polymer matrix nanocomposites for bone tissue engineering.Applications of nanocomposite materials in orthopedics. Woodhead Publishing 2019; pp. 1-37.
[http://dx.doi.org/10.1016/B978-0-12-813740-6.00001-6]

[164] Rehman U, Parveen N, Sheikh A, Abourehab MAS, Sahebkar A, Kesharwani P. Polymeric

nanoparticles-siRNA as an emerging nano-polyplexes against ovarian cancer. Colloids Surf B Biointerfaces 2022; 218112766
[http://dx.doi.org/10.1016/j.colsurfb.2022.112766] [PMID: 35994990]

[165] Cai J, Qian K, Zuo X, *et al.* PLGA nanoparticle-based docetaxel/LY294002 drug delivery system enhances antitumor activities against gastric cancer. J Biomater Appl 2019; 33(10): 1394-406.
[http://dx.doi.org/10.1177/0885328219837683] [PMID: 30952195]

[166] Yadav B, Chauhan M, Shekhar S, *et al.* RGD-decorated PLGA nanoparticles improved effectiveness and safety of cisplatin for lung cancer therapy. Int J Pharm 2023; 633122587
[http://dx.doi.org/10.1016/j.ijpharm.2023.122587] [PMID: 36623741]

[167] Al-Nemrawi NK, Altawabeyeh RM, Darweesh RS. Preparation and characterization of docetaxel-PLGA nanoparticles coated with folic acid-chitosan conjugate for cancer treatment. J Pharm Sci 2022; 111(2): 485-94.
[http://dx.doi.org/10.1016/j.xphs.2021.10.034] [PMID: 34728172]

[168] Layek B, Haldar MK, Sharma G, Lipp L, Mallik S, Singh J. Hexanoic acid and polyethylene glycol double grafted amphiphilic chitosan for enhanced gene delivery: influence of hydrophobic and hydrophilic substitution degree. Mol Pharm 2014; 11(3): 982-94.
[http://dx.doi.org/10.1021/mp400633r] [PMID: 24499512]

[169] Kumar GA, Salar RK. Chitosan nanoparticle delivery systems: an effective approach to enhancing efficacy and safety of anticancer drugs. Nano TransMed 2024; p. 100040.

[170] Qu J, Tian M, Wang Q, *et al.* Photo-thermal properties of MWCNT-H_2O nanofluid. CIESC Joournal 2016; 67: 113-9.

[171] Liang C, Diao S, Wang C, *et al.* Tumor metastasis inhibition by imaging-guided photothermal therapy with single-walled carbon nanotubes 2014.
[http://dx.doi.org/10.1002/adma.201401825]

[172] Liu J, Wang C, Wang X, *et al.* Mesoporous silica coated single□walled carbon nanotubes as a multifunctional light□responsive platform for cancer combination therapy. Adv Funct Mater 2015; 25(3): 384-92.
[http://dx.doi.org/10.1002/adfm.201403079]

[173] Gaillard PJ, Appeldoorn CCM, Dorland R, *et al.* Pharmacokinetics, brain delivery, and efficacy in brain tumor-bearing mice of glutathione pegylated liposomal doxorubicin (2B3-101). PLoS One 2014; 9(1)e82331
[http://dx.doi.org/10.1371/journal.pone.0082331] [PMID: 24416140]

[174] Tardi PG, Dos Santos N, Harasym TO, *et al.* Drug ratio–dependent antitumor activity of irinotecan and cisplatin combinations *in vitro* and *in vivo*. Mol Cancer Ther 2009; 8(8): 2266-75.
[http://dx.doi.org/10.1158/1535-7163.MCT-09-0243] [PMID: 19671743]

[175] Xu Z, Zhang Z, Chen Y, Chen L, Lin L, Li Y. The characteristics and performance of a multifunctional nanoassembly system for the co-delivery of docetaxel and iSur-pDNA in a mouse hepatocellular carcinoma model. Biomaterials 2010; 31(5): 916-22.
[http://dx.doi.org/10.1016/j.biomaterials.2009.09.103] [PMID: 19846217]

[176] Batist G, Gelmon KA, Chi KN, *et al.* Safety, pharmacokinetics, and efficacy of CPX-1 liposome injection in patients with advanced solid tumors. Clin Cancer Res 2009; 15(2): 692-700.
[http://dx.doi.org/10.1158/1078-0432.CCR-08-0515] [PMID: 19147776]

[177] Landen CN Jr, Chavez-Reyes A, Bucana C, *et al.* Therapeutic EphA2 gene targeting *in vivo* using neutral liposomal small interfering RNA delivery. Cancer Res 2005; 65(15): 6910-8.
[http://dx.doi.org/10.1158/0008-5472.CAN-05-0530] [PMID: 16061675]

[178] Suzuki R, Takizawa T, Kuwata Y, *et al.* Effective anti-tumor activity of oxaliplatin encapsulated in transferrin–PEG-liposome. Int J Pharm 2008; 346(1-2): 143-50.
[http://dx.doi.org/10.1016/j.ijpharm.2007.06.010] [PMID: 17640835]

[179] Matsumura Y, Gotoh M, Muro K, *et al.* Phase I and pharmacokinetic study of MCC-465, a doxorubicin (DXR) encapsulated in PEG immunoliposome, in patients with metastatic stomach cancer. Ann Oncol 2004; 15(3): 517-25. [http://dx.doi.org/10.1093/annonc/mdh092] [PMID: 14998859]

[180] Senzer N, Nemunaitis J, Nemunaitis D, *et al.* Phase I study of a systemically delivered p53 nanoparticle in advanced solid tumors. Mol Ther 2013; 21(5): 1096-103. [http://dx.doi.org/10.1038/mt.2013.32] [PMID: 23609015]

[181] Ko AH, Tempero MA, Shan Y-S, *et al.* A multinational phase 2 study of nanoliposomal irinotecan sucrosofate (PEP02, MM-398) for patients with gemcitabine-refractory metastatic pancreatic cancer. Br J Cancer 2013; 109(4): 920-5. [http://dx.doi.org/10.1038/bjc.2013.408] [PMID: 23880820]

[182] Zhang Y, Wang J, Bian D, Zhang X, Zhang Q. Targeted delivery of RGD-modified liposomes encapsulating both combretastatin A-4 and doxorubicin for tumor therapy: In vitro and *in vivo* studies. Eur J Pharm Biopharm 2010; 74(3): 467-73. [http://dx.doi.org/10.1016/j.ejpb.2010.01.002] [PMID: 20064608]

[183] Shim G, Han SE, Yu YH, *et al.* Trilysinoyl oleylamide-based cationic liposomes for systemic co-delivery of siRNA and an anticancer drug. J Control Release 2011; 155(1): 60-6. [http://dx.doi.org/10.1016/j.jconrel.2010.10.017] [PMID: 20971142]

[184] Kroemer G, Zitvogel L, Galluzzi L. Victories and deceptions in tumor immunology. OncoImmunology 2013; 2(1)e23687 [http://dx.doi.org/10.4161/onci.23687] [PMID: 23483762]

[185] Beutel G, Glen H, Schöffski P, *et al.* Phase I study of OSI-7904L, a novel liposomal thymidylate synthase inhibitor in patients with refractory solid tumors. Clin Cancer Res 2005; 11(15): 5487-95. [http://dx.doi.org/10.1158/1078-0432.CCR-05-0104] [PMID: 16061865]

[186] Izbicka E, Diaz A, Campos D, *et al.* Evaluation of antitumor activity and biomarkers for MBP-42 in human pancreatic cancer xenograft models in vivo. Cancer Res 2007; 67(9) (Suppl.): 5586-6.

[187] Yang SH, Lin CC, Lin ZZ, Tseng YL, Hong RL. A phase I and pharmacokinetic study of liposomal vinorelbine in patients with advanced solid tumor. Invest New Drugs 2012; 30(1): 282-9. [http://dx.doi.org/10.1007/s10637-010-9522-3] [PMID: 20809205]

[188] Prados MD, Yung WKA, Jaeckle KA, *et al.* Phase 1 trial of irinotecan (CPT-11) in patients with recurrent malignant glioma: A North American Brain Tumor Consortium study. Neuro-oncol 2004; 6(1): 44-54. [http://dx.doi.org/10.1215/S1152851703000292] [PMID: 14769140]

[189] Sarris AH, Hagemeister F, Romaguera J, *et al.* Liposomal vincristine in relapsed non-Hodgkin's lymphomas: Early results of an ongoing phase II trial. Ann Oncol 2000; 11(1): 69-72. [http://dx.doi.org/10.1023/A:1008348010437] [PMID: 10690390]

[190] Duffaud F, Borner M, Chollet P, *et al.* Phase II study of OSI-211 (liposomal lurtotecan) in patients with metastatic or loco-regional recurrent squamous cell carcinoma of the head and neck. Eur J Cancer 2004; 40(18): 2748-52. [http://dx.doi.org/10.1016/j.ejca.2004.08.024] [PMID: 15571957]

[191] Gabizon AA, Tzemach D, Horowitz AT, Shmeeda H, Yeh J, Zalipsky S. Reduced toxicity and superior therapeutic activity of a mitomycin C lipid-based prodrug incorporated in pegylated liposomes. Clin Cancer Res 2006; 12(6): 1913-20. [http://dx.doi.org/10.1158/1078-0432.CCR-05-1547] [PMID: 16551877]

[192] Tang S, Yin Q, Su J, *et al.* Inhibition of metastasis and growth of breast cancer by pH-sensitive poly (β-amino ester) nanoparticles co-delivering two siRNA and paclitaxel. Biomaterials 2015; 48: 1-15. [http://dx.doi.org/10.1016/j.biomaterials.2015.01.049] [PMID: 25701027]

[193] Zhou Q, Sun X, Zeng L, Liu J, Zhang Z. A randomized multicenter phase II clinical trial of

mitoxantrone-loaded nanoparticles in the treatment of 108 patients with unresected hepatocellular carcinoma. Nanomedicine 2009; 5(4): 419-23.
[http://dx.doi.org/10.1016/j.nano.2009.01.009] [PMID: 19523421]

[194] Madaan A, Singh P, Awasthi A, *et al.* Efficiency and mechanism of intracellular paclitaxel delivery by novel nanopolymer-based tumor-targeted delivery system, NanoxelTM. Clin Transl Oncol 2013; 15(1): 26-32.
[http://dx.doi.org/10.1007/s12094-012-0883-2] [PMID: 22855169]

[195] Hamaguchi T, Doi T, Eguchi-Nakajima T, *et al.* Phase I study of NK012, a novel SN-38-incorporating micellar nanoparticle, in adult patients with solid tumors. Clin Cancer Res 2010; 16(20): 5058-66.
[http://dx.doi.org/10.1158/1078-0432.CCR-10-0387] [PMID: 20943763]

[196] Harada M, Bobe I, Saito H, *et al.* Improved anti□tumor activity of stabilized anthracycline polymeric micelle formulation, NC□6300. Cancer Sci 2011; 102(1): 192-9.
[http://dx.doi.org/10.1111/j.1349-7006.2010.01745.x] [PMID: 21040218]

[197] Devulapally R, Sekar NM, Sekar TV, *et al.* Polymer nanoparticles mediated codelivery of antimiR-10b and antimiR-21 for achieving triple negative breast cancer therapy. ACS Nano 2015; 9(3): 2290-302.
[http://dx.doi.org/10.1021/nn507465d] [PMID: 25652012]

[198] Wang Y, Gao S, Ye WH, Yoon HS, Yang YY. Co-delivery of drugs and DNA from cationic core–shell nanoparticles self-assembled from a biodegradable copolymer. Nat Mater 2006; 5(10): 791-6.
[http://dx.doi.org/10.1038/nmat1737] [PMID: 16998471]

[199] Jiang T, Mo R, Bellotti A, Zhou J, Gu Z. Gel–liposome□mediated co□delivery of anticancer membrane□associated proteins and small□molecule drugs for enhanced therapeutic efficacy. Adv Funct Mater 2014; 24(16): 2295-304.
[http://dx.doi.org/10.1002/adfm.201303222]

[200] Zheng M, Yue C, Ma Y, *et al.* Single-step assembly of DOX/ICG loaded lipid--polymer nanoparticles for highly effective chemo-photothermal combination therapy. ACS Nano 2013; 7(3): 2056-67.
[http://dx.doi.org/10.1021/nn400334y] [PMID: 23413798]

[201] Hawkins MJ, Soon-Shiong P, Desai N. Protein nanoparticles as drug carriers in clinical medicine. Adv Drug Deliv Rev 2008; 60(8): 876-85.
[http://dx.doi.org/10.1016/j.addr.2007.08.044] [PMID: 18423779]

[202] Wang L, Shi J, Zhang H, *et al.* RETRACTED: Synergistic anticancer effect of RNAi and photothermal therapy mediated by functionalized single-walled carbon nanotubes. Biomaterials 2013; 34(1): 262-74.
[http://dx.doi.org/10.1016/j.biomaterials.2012.09.037] [PMID: 23046752]

[203] Wang P, Kankala RK, Chen B, *et al.* Cancer cytomembrane-cloaked prussian blue nanoparticles enhance the efficacy of mild-temperature photothermal therapy by disrupting mitochondrial functions of cancer cells. ACS Appl Mater Interfaces 2021; 13(31): 37563-77.
[http://dx.doi.org/10.1021/acsami.1c11138] [PMID: 34338525]

[204] Fu G, Liu W, Li Y, *et al.* Magnetic Prussian blue nanoparticles for targeted photothermal therapy under magnetic resonance imaging guidance. Bioconjug Chem 2014; 25(9): 1655-63.
[http://dx.doi.org/10.1021/bc500279w] [PMID: 25109612]

[205] Sahoo P, Nandi SK, Das M, *et al.* GSH-pH dual-responsive engineered codoped Prussian blue multimodal theranostic nanoplatform induces TP53 deregulated apoptotic death of MDA-MB-231 with enhanced T_1 - T_2 W MRI. ACS Appl Nano Mater 2024; 7(23): 26617-28.
[http://dx.doi.org/10.1021/acsanm.4c05556]

[206] Kundu S, Jana P, Sahoo P, *et al.* Curcumin-based Nanoformulation for the Pyroptotic Death of MDA-MB-231 Cells. ACS Appl Nano Mater 2024; 7(5): 4895-912.
[http://dx.doi.org/10.1021/acsanm.3c05662]

[207] Chen G, Roy I, Yang C, Prasad PN. Nanochemistry and nanomedicine for nanoparticle-based diagnostics and therapy. Chem Rev 2016; 116(5): 2826-85.
[http://dx.doi.org/10.1021/acs.chemrev.5b00148] [PMID: 26799741]

[208] Li H, Jin H, Wan W, Wu C, Wei L. Cancer nanomedicine: mechanisms, obstacles and strategies. Nanomedicine (Lond) 2018; 13(13): 1639-56.
[http://dx.doi.org/10.2217/nnm-2018-0007] [PMID: 30035660]

[209] Ravi Kiran AVVV, Kusuma Kumari G, Krishnamurthy PT, Khaydarov RR. Tumor microenvironment and nanotherapeutics: intruding the tumor fort. Biomater Sci 2021; 9(23): 7667-704.
[http://dx.doi.org/10.1039/D1BM01127H] [PMID: 34673853]

[210] Sia CS, Lim HP, Tey BT, Goh BH, Low LE. Stimuli-responsive nanoassemblies for targeted delivery against tumor and its microenvironment. Biochim Biophys Acta Rev Cancer 2022; 1877(5)188779
[http://dx.doi.org/10.1016/j.bbcan.2022.188779] [PMID: 35977690]

[211] Carneiro BA, El-Deiry WS. Targeting apoptosis in cancer therapy. Nat Rev Clin Oncol 2020; 17(7): 395-417.
[http://dx.doi.org/10.1038/s41571-020-0341-y] [PMID: 32203277]

[212] Jiang Y, Jiang Z, Wang M, Ma L. Current understandings and clinical translation of nanomedicines for breast cancer therapy. Adv Drug Deliv Rev 2022; 180114034
[http://dx.doi.org/10.1016/j.addr.2021.114034] [PMID: 34736986]

[213] Sharifi S, Behzadi S, Laurent S, Laird Forrest M, Stroeve P, Mahmoudi M. Toxicity of nanomaterials. Chem Soc Rev 2012; 41(6): 2323-43.
[http://dx.doi.org/10.1039/C1CS15188F] [PMID: 22170510]

[214] Li J, Chang X, Chen X, *et al.* Toxicity of inorganic nanomaterials in biomedical imaging. Biotechnol Adv 2014; 32(4): 727-43.
[http://dx.doi.org/10.1016/j.biotechadv.2013.12.009] [PMID: 24389087]

[215] Yang RSH, Chang LW, Wu JP, *et al.* Persistent tissue kinetics and redistribution of nanoparticles, quantum dot 705, in mice: ICP-MS quantitative assessment. Environ Health Perspect 2007; 115(9): 1339-43.
[http://dx.doi.org/10.1289/ehp.10290] [PMID: 17805425]

[216] Yang J, Wang X, Wang B, Park K, Wooley K, Zhang S. Challenging the fundamental conjectures in nanoparticle drug delivery for chemotherapy treatment of solid cancers. Adv Drug Deliv Rev 2022; 190114525
[http://dx.doi.org/10.1016/j.addr.2022.114525] [PMID: 36100142]

[217] Younis MA, Tawfeek HM, Abdellatif AAH, Abdel-Aleem JA, Harashima H. Clinical translation of nanomedicines: Challenges, opportunities, and keys. Adv Drug Deliv Rev 2022; 181114083
[http://dx.doi.org/10.1016/j.addr.2021.114083] [PMID: 34929251]

CHAPTER 6

An Efficient Machine Learning-based Approach to Detect the Alzheimer's Disease

Suparna Biswas[1,*], **Moloy Dhar**[1], **Soumik Podder**[2] and **Suparna Karmakar**[1]

[1] *Guru Nanak Institute of Technology, Panihati, West Bengal, India*

[2] *Department of Basic Science & Humanities, Institute of Engineering and Management, New Town, University of Engineering & Management, Kolkata, India*

Abstract: The primary reason behind dementia, which is distinguished by a decrease in cognition, freedom within everyday tasks, is Alzheimer's Disease (AD), a disorder that causes brain cells to deteriorate. AD is addressed as a complex illness, with the cholinergic and amyloid hypotheses proposed as two primary theories underlying its pathology.. Additionally, a number of risk factors, such as aging, genetics, head trauma, vascular disease, pollution, as well as environmental elements, all participate in the illness. In this chapter, we have presented machine learning-based automatic identification of Alzheimer's Disease (AD). As features, Socioeconomic Status, Mini-Mental State Examination, Estimated total intracranial volume, Normalized whole-brain volume, and the Clinical Dementia Rating have been used. For classification, the KNN classifier has been used with different distance metrics and by varying the number of K-values. Here are mainly three types of distance metrics: Euclidean distance, Manhattan distance, and Minkowski distance, among others, to compute the performance measures of Accuracy, Recall, Precision, and F1-values.

Keywords: Alzheimer's disease, Accuracy, F1-values, Euclidean distance, KNN classifier, Machine learning, Manhattan distance,minkowski distance, Precision, Recall.

INTRODUCTION

A considerable reduction in cognitive function that affects an individual's capacity to carry out daily tasks is referred to as dementia. More than two-thirds of dementia cases in those 65 years of age and older are caused by AD, a neurological illness that gradually impairs both mental and behavioral abilities. Recall, understanding, language, focus, logic, and verdict are some of these abilities. Although AA does not directly cause mortality, it does significantly

[*] **Corresponding author Suparna Biswas:** Guru Nanak Institute of Technology, Panihati, West Bengal, India; E-mail: suparna.biswas@gnit.ac.in

Soumik Podder & Amalesh Samanta (Eds.)

increase a person's susceptibility to additional issues that may ultimately result in death. Information from the Centers for Disease Control and Prevention shows that in 2022, AD will rank as the seventh most frequent cause of death in the US, with COVID-19 coming in at number one. After a stroke, AD was the sixth most common cause of death prior to the COVID-19 pandemic. AD is dementia's most prevalent type, and it is defined as developing neurodegenerative illness that is triggered by an accumulation of amyloid-beta peptide (Aβ) in the damaged areas of the brain, medial temporal lobe and neocortical frameworks. This form of dementia is characterized by the presence of neuritic plaques and neurofibrillary tangles [1]. Late-onset Alzheimer's Disease (LOAD) is the term used to describe AD, which usually appears after the age of 65. About 5% of AD patients have Early-onset Alzheimer's disease (EOAD), which is less prevalent and occurs before the age of 65. The symptoms of EOAD are frequently unusual, and the condition is typically diagnosed later, which causes the illness to progress more quickly [2]. Over the last decade, substantial developments have been made in creating biomarkers for the specific and early identification of AD. Cerebrospinal Fluid (CSF), plasma markers including phospho-tau, tau, and amyloid levels, and neuroimaging markers from amyloid and tau PET scans are examples of these biomarkers [3]. While there is no known remedy for AD, there are helpful therapies for control and lessening some of its symptoms. With the identification of novel disease biomarkers, the development of drugs intended to slow the disease's course has advanced significantly in recent years [3].

The manifestation of AD can differ according to the illness's stage. Depending on how much cognitive impairment there is and disability that each person experiences, AD is divided into several phases. The progression of Alzheimer's disease includes the preclinical (or presymptomatic) stage, moderate cognitive impairment, and dementia [4]. Dementia itself is further classified into three stages: mild, moderate, and severe.

The diagnostic standards contained in the Diagnostic and Statistical Manual of Mental Disorders, Fifth Edition (DSM-5) for AD differ from this staging method [5].

Following these initial indicators of cognitive decline are visuospatial impairment and linguistic disorders. In the intermediate to advanced phases, neuropsychiatric symptoms like disinhibition, agitation, wandering, psychosis, and apathy are also common. Late-stage symptoms include dyspraxia, difficulties with learning motor tasks, olfactory dysfunction, sleep difficulties, and extrapyramidal motor indications like dystonia, akathisia, and Parkinsonian symptoms. This is followed by incontinence, primitive reflexes, and complete reliance on caregivers [6 - 8].

A common AD patient's first and most frequently presenting symptom is episodic short-term memory loss. People might find it challenging to remember new information while still recalling long-term memories. Short-term memory loss may give rise to deficits in judgment, problem-solving abilities, executive functioning, and organizational skills. Tasks requiring abstract thought and multitasking may be difficult for them. Executive functioning deficits can range from mild to severe in the initial phases of the disease. Relatively early in their dementia, essential daily activities such as operating a vehicle, managing money, cooking, and meticulously organizing tasks are impacted [4].

When Alois Alzheimer looked into the brain of his first patient, who had memory loss and a personality shift before expiration, he observed amyloid plaques and an enormous neuronal loss. He described the state of the patient as an awful illness affecting the brain cortex. In his psychiatric manual, the 8th version, Emil Kraepelin 1st referred to this neurological clutter as AD. Cerebral problems such as AD or additional illnesses such as infections, intoxications, anomalies within the circulatory and pulmonary systems, which lower the oxygen content reaching the brain, malnutrition, low vitamin B12, tumors, and additionally more can all lead to an increasing cognitive decline [5]. Currently, there are roughly 50 million AD patients worldwide. By 2050, the total number is anticipated to have doubled every 5 years to 152 million. The burden of AD affects people, the economy, and their families; the annual worldwide expenses are estimated to be $1 trillion. AD, as of right, has no known treatment; nevertheless, there exist treatments that can aid in symptom relief [7]. This evaluation aims to provide a concise summary of AD pathology, investigation, causes, and current treatments. It additionally emphasizes the discovery of novel compounds that target numerous pathogenic mechanisms, such as tau and Aβ aggregation, inflammation, oxidative damage, misfolding, and others, and may be used to treat or prevent AD.

In addition to a medical and family history review, a patient suspected of having AA should undergo various examinations, including a neurological test, Magnetic Resonance Imaging (MRI) of the brain, laboratory testing for vitamin B12, and other diagnostic tests [8]. Due to specific research, vitamin B12 deficiency has been associated with neurologic problems as well as increased chances of AD. High levels of homocysteine are a distinctive sign of vitamin B12 deficiency and can lead to brain injury *via* oxidative damage, enhanced calcium influx, and cell death. Serum vitamin B12 levels, whole blood counts, additionally serum homocysteine levels can all be evaluated to identify inadequate vitamin B12 [9 - 11]. The AD, Related Disorders Association (ADRDA), and the National Institute of Neurological and Communicative Disorders and Stroke (NINCDS) created the study group NIDCS-ADRD in 1984 to develop clinical diagnostic standards for AD. Criteria for diagnosing AD comprise the following: (1) dementia, that is supported by neuropsychological testing, increasing loss of memory that gets worse every day, and additional symptoms such as aphasia (a language deficiency), apraxia (a problem due to motor skills), and agnosia (a decline in perception). When no systemic or neurological conditions are present, any among these signs and symptoms can emerge in the age range of 40 and 90, (2) feasible AD able to diagnosed in the following situations: (1) no neurologic or psychiatric chaos, (2) another illness, such as a brain or systemic illness, nevertheless, these conditions are not considered the main reason behind dementia, and (3) a diagnosis of AD that is validated by histopathology verification from an autopsy or biopsy [12].

The chapter is organized as follows: Section 2 provides a brief review of AD detection techniques, Section 3 presents the proposed method, and Section 4 presents the simulation results and discussions. At last, Section 5 concludes the paper with important notifications and a discussion of future scope.

LITERATURE REVIEW

Neuronal cell death resulting in progressive and slow neurodegeneration is the distinguishing feature of AD. The brain's entorhinal cortex hippocampal region is where the neurodegenerative process usually starts. It has been determined that genetic factors have a role in both late-onset and early-onset AD. For instance, trisomy 21 is a risk factor linked to dementia with early onset. AD is a complex illness with numerous risk variables. The most crucial factor is age, and aging is the primary cause. Beginning at age 65, the prevalence of AD increases by double every five years [9].Cardiovascular Disorders (CVD) are recognized as significant risk factors for Alzheimer’s Disease (AD). They also increase the likelihood of developing other forms of dementia, including vascular dementia caused by strokes or impaired blood flow. The prevalence of CVD is continuing to rise.

Diabetes and obesity are two more significant modifiable risk factors for AD. Obesity brings up the risk of type II diabetes and can impede glucose tolerance. Prolonged hyperglycemia can lead to the buildup of beta-amyloid (A-beta) and neuroinflammation, which can impair cognitive function. By encouraging insulin resistance and inducing the release of pro-inflammatory cytokines, obesity further increases the risk [10].

Depression, traumatic brain damage, heart disease, strokes, smoking, higher paternal age at birth, a high homocysteine level, a family history of dementia, and the APOE e4 allele are additional possible risk factors for AD. AD raises one's chance of getting the disease by 10% to 30% if they have a first-degree relative who has it. A person's chance of developing AD with two or more late-onset siblings is three times greater compared to the whole population [11 - 13].

It has been demonstrated that certain elements may potentially reduce the risk of developing AD. A balanced diet, regular cardiovascular exercise, reading and music-making as hobbies, the use of estrogen in women, higher education, and anti-inflammatory drugs are a few of these. AD is most commonly seen in older people. In 1990, there were 20.3 million cases of dementia worldwide. By 2016, that number had risen to 43.8 million, a stunning 116% growth. The prevalence and incidence of AD and the prevalence of other dementias rose by 160.84% and 147.95%, respectively, between 1990 and 2019. According to projections, there will be four times as many people living with dementia by 2050—150 million people [14].

Following the age of 65, the likelihood of developing AD increases by approximately 5 years. Age-specific incidence rates rise sharply, from less than 1% a year to 6% annually after the age of 85. After the age of 65, prevalence rates increase from 10% to 40% by the age of 85. Women have a somewhat higher incidence of AD than men do, in particular after the age of 85 [15].

The 1984 NINCDS-ADRDA criteria were revised in 2011 by the National Institute on Aging and the Alzheimer's Association to improve the specificity and sensitivity of AD's prognosis. The recently proposed criteria include clinical biomarkers and likely or conceivable AD brain disease with pathophysiological proof for scientific investigations, besides likely or feasible AD brain disease for application in therapeutic settings. Alzheimer disease biomarkers can be divided into two categories: (a) brain amyloid markers, as positron emission tomography and Cerebrospinal Fluid (CSF); and (b) neuronal injury markers, as tau in the CSF, Fluorodeoxyglucose (FDG) for metabolic activity, and Magnetic Resonance Imaging (MRI) for measuring atrophy [14, 15].

Two distinct kinds of neuropathological alterations in AD have been identified, offering insight into the course and manifestation of the disease. These are: (1) positive lesions (because of accumulation), which are distinguished by the build-up of deposits like amyloid plaques, dystrophic neurites, neuropil threads, and neurofibrillary tangles in the brains of AD patients. Furthermore, there are (2) adverse lesions (caused by losses) that exhibit significant atrophy due to neuron loss, neuropils, and synapses. Additionally, oxidative stress, neuroinflammation, and harm to cholinergic neurons can all contribute to neurodegeneration [16 - 19].

Beta-amyloid protein (Aβ) extracellular deposits, referred to as senile plaques, can take on several morphological forms, including diffuse, neuritic, classic, dense-cored, or condensed type plaques. The transmembrane Amyloid Precursor Protein (APP) is the origin of Aβ deposits, which are produced by proteolytic cleavage enzymes such as β- and γ-secretase [20, 21].

Those enzymes break down APP into fragments of amino acids that combine to generate the completed forms of Aβ40 and Aβ42. Aβ monomers come in many forms: soluble oligomers, which can proliferate through the brain, and enormous, insoluble amyloid fibrils that may build up to form amyloid plaques. Because Aβ is involved in neurotoxicity and neural function, the formation of denser plaques in the amygdala, cerebral cortex, and hippocampus can result in cognitive disabilities in addition to harm to dendrites, axons, and dying synapses, as well as stimulation of astrocytes and microglia [21 - 23].

PROPOSED METHOD

The flow diagram of the proposed technique is depicted in Fig. (**1**). It consists of three main modules: dataset reading, Preprocessing, and classification. In this proposed technique, socioeconomic status, mini-mental state examination, estimated total intracranial volume, and normalized whole-brain volumes are used as input features. This dataset is available online [24]. All are explained below:

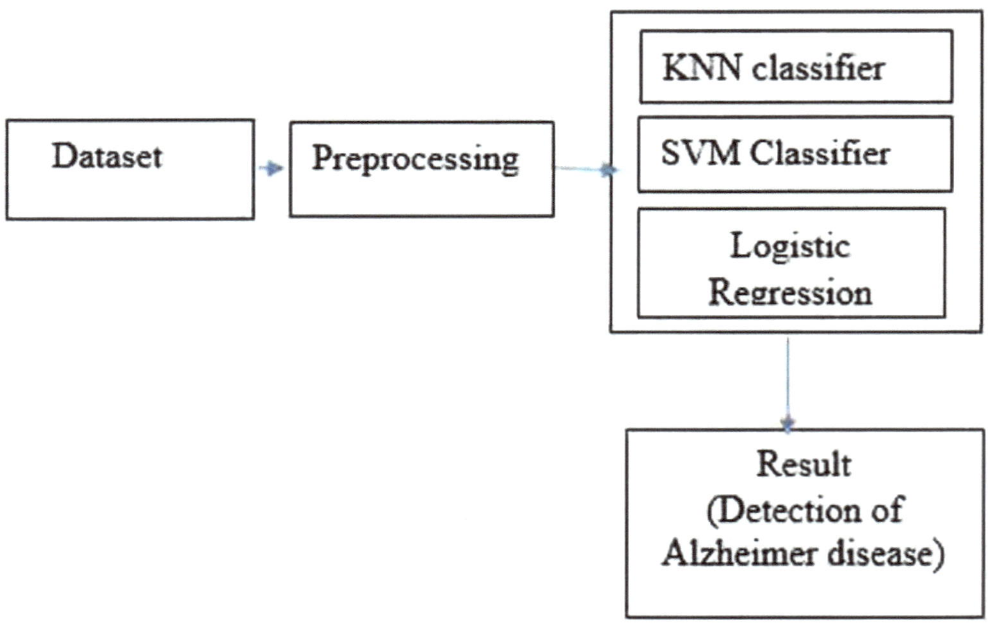

Fig. (1). Flow diagram of the proposed method.

SES - Socioeconomic Status: According to the Hollingshead Index of Social Position (lowest = 5, highest = 1), it is a reflection of a person's social and economic factors, such as their work experience, financial access to resources, and social position. SES is commonly measured by educational level, income level, and occupation. Low SES is associated with an increased risk of dementia and dementia-related death.

MMSE - Mini-Mental State Examination: Score (min = 0, max = 30) is a screening tool that doctors and other healthcare professionals use to assess cognitive impairment. It is the most well-known and commonly used tool for this purpose.

eTIV - Estimated Total Intracranial Volume (cm3) is a clinical variable that is used in studies of Alzheimer's disease.

nWBV - Normalized Whole-Brain Volume refers to the proportion of the brain's volume relative to the Total Intracranial Volume (TIV).

CDR - The **Clinical Dementia Rating** is a scale (0 = no dementia, 0.5 = questionable, 1 = mild, 2 = moderate, 3 = severe [13]) that evaluates the severity of dementia. It is a commonly used tool for staging dementia severity.

In the preprocessing step, all features are standardized using the StandardScaler function in Python.The StandardScaler function, which is used to standardize features by scaling them to unit variance and deleting the mean. In order to guarantee that every feature contributes equally to the outcome, this preprocessing step is often employed in machine learning. After preprocessing, the features are passed to the classifier to detect the classification performance. Here, the KNN classifier has been used to compute the performance for 3-different distance metrics: Euclidean distance, Manhattan distance, and Minkowski distance.

EXPERIMENTAL RESULTS AND DISCUSSION

The proposed method is simulated on the Python platform, and we have varied the value of K up to 10. Among the entire dataset, 80% has been used for training, and the remaining 20% has been used as test data. Tables **1**, **2** and **3** present the simulation results for various distance metrics. Table **1** shows that Euclidean distance metrics yield the best results for K=3, whereas Table **2** shows that Manhattan distance yields the best results for K=8. Performance measures for Minkowski distance are mentioned in Table **3**. From Table **3**, it is observed that Minkowski distance provides the best result for K=3.For all cases, Precision, Recall, and F1-values are also computed, as shown in Tables **1**, **2**, and **3**. Comparing Tables **1**, **2** and **3**, it is observed that the proposed technique provides the best result for the Manhattan distance at K-3.

Table 1. Accuracy, precision, recall, and F1 values for Euclidean distance.

K	Accuracy	Precision	Recall	F1 values
2	0.76	0.75	0.73	0.72
3	0.78	0.74	0.76	0.74
4	0.76	0.73	0.72	0.70
5	0.77	0.72	0.72	0.71
6	0.78	0.75	0.73	0.73
7	0.78	0.75	0.73	0.73
8	0.74	0.71	0.66	0.66
9	0.73	0.69	0.65	0.65
10	0.74	0.68	0.62	0.64

Table 2. Accuracy, precision, recall, and F1 values for Manhattan distance.

K	Accuracy	Precision	Recall	F1-Score
2	0.76	0.71	0.69	0.69
3	0.76	0.71	0.73	0.71
4	0.76	0.72	0.70	0.69
5	0.76	0.69	0.68	0.67
6	0.77	0.73	0.69	0.69
7	0.74	0.70	0.69	0.68
8	0.8	0.81	0.74	0.76
9	0.76	0.74	0.71	0.71
10	0.76	0.73	0.70	0.70

Table 3. Accuracy, precision, recall, and F1 values for Minkowski distance.

K	Accuracy	Precision	Recall	F1
2	0.76	0.75	0.73	0.72
3	0.78	0.74	0.76	0.74
4	0.76	0.73	0.72	0.70
5	0.77	0.72	0.72	0.71
6	0.78	0.75	0.73	0.73
7	0.78	0.75	0.73	0.73
8	0.74	0.71	0.66	0.66
9	0.73	0.69	0.65	0.65
10	0.74	0.68	0.62	0.64

CONCLUSION

In this chapter, we present a machine learning-based Alzheimer's Disease detection technique. Here, only four different features, such as Socioeconomic Status, Mini-Mental State Examination, Estimated total intracranial volume, and normalized whole-brain volume, have been used for the identification of AD. For the classification, K-NN classifier has been used by varying the distance metrics and different K-values. With an accuracy of 80%, a precision of 0.81, a recall of 0.74, and an F1-Score of 0.76 at K=8, the suggested method yields the best results for the Manhattan distance.

As we know, K-NN does not create a model during training because it is a lazy learner. Rather, it performs the costly processing during prediction by memorizing the training data. The more features that are irrelevant or only marginally important, the worse the performance gets. It consumes a significant amount of memory, particularly for large datasets, to store all the training data. In our future work, we will try other classifiers to improve accuracy.

In our future work, we plan to utilize additional features to enhance the recognition rate. Another objective of our future work is to achieve high accuracy with low-dimensional features by applying feature selection techniques. Explainable AI can be utilized in our future work to determine the significance of each feature.

REFERENCES

[1] De-Paula VJ, Radanovic M, Diniz BS, Forlenza OV. Alzheimer’s Disease. Subcell Biochem 2012; 65: 329-52.
[http://dx.doi.org/10.1007/978-94-007-5416-4_14] [PMID: 23225010]

[2] Cipriani G, Dolciotti C, Picchi L, Bonuccelli U. Alzheimer and his disease: a brief history. Neurol Sci 2011; 32(2): 275-9.
[http://dx.doi.org/10.1007/s10072-010-0454-7] [PMID: 21153601]

[3] Blass JP Alzheimer's disease. Dis Mon 1985; 31(4): 1-69.
[http://dx.doi.org/10.1016/0011-5029(85)90025-2]

[4] Terry RD, Davies P. Dementia of the Alzheimer type. Annu Rev Neurosci 1980; 3(1): 77-95.
[http://dx.doi.org/10.1146/annurev.ne.03.030180.000453] [PMID: 6251745]

[5] Rathmann KL, Conner CS. Alzheimer’s disease: clinical features, pathogenesis, and treatment. Drug Intell Clin Pharm 1984; 18(9): 684-91.
[http://dx.doi.org/10.1177/106002808401800902] [PMID: 6383752]

[6] Yiannopoulou KG, Papageorgiou SG. Current and future treatments in alzheimer ailment: An update. J Cent Nerv Syst Dis 2020; 12
[http://dx.doi.org/10.1177/1179573520907397] [PMID: 32165850]

[7] Livingston G, Huntley J, Sommerlad A, *et al.* Dementia prevention, intervention, and care: 2020 report of the Lancet Commission. Lancet 2020; 396(10248): 413-46.
[http://dx.doi.org/10.1016/S0140-6736(20)30367-6] [PMID: 32738937]

[8] Schachter AS, Davis KL. Alzheimer's disease. Dialogues Clin Neurosci 2000; 2(2): 91-100. [http://dx.doi.org/10.31887/DCNS.2000.2.2/asschachter] [PMID: 22034442]

[9] Jatoi S, Hafeez DRA, Riaz SU, Ali A, Ghauri MI, Zehra M. Low Vitamin B12 levels: An underestimated cause of minimal cognitive impairment and dementia. Cureus 2020; 12(2): e6976. [http://dx.doi.org/10.7759/cureus.6976] [PMID: 32206454]

[10] Cho HS, Huang LK, Lee YT, Chan L, Hong CT. Suboptimal baseline serum Vitamin B12 is associated with cognitive decline in people with Alzheimer's ailment undergoing cholinesterase inhibitor treatment. Front Neurol 2018; 9: 325. [http://dx.doi.org/10.3389/fneur.2018.00325] [PMID: 29867734]

[11] McKhann G, Drachman D, Folstein M, Katzman R, Price D, Stadlan EM. Clinical diagnosis of Alzheimer's disease. Neurology 1984; 34(7): 939-44. [http://dx.doi.org/10.1212/WNL.34.7.939] [PMID: 6610841]

[12] Neugroschl J, Wang S. Alzheimer's disease: diagnosis and treatment across the spectrum of disease severity. Mt Sinai J Med 2011; 78(4): 596-612. [http://dx.doi.org/10.1002/msj.20279] [PMID: 21748748]

[13] McKhann GM, Knopman DS, Chertkow H, *et al.* The diagnosis of dementia due to Alzheimer's disease: Recommendations from the National Institute on Aging-Alzheimer's Association workgroups on diagnostic guidelines for Alzheimer's disease. Alzheimers Dement 2011; 7(3): 263-9. [http://dx.doi.org/10.1016/j.jalz.2011.03.005] [PMID: 21514250]

[14] Mayeux R, Stern Y. Epidemiology of Alzheimer disease. Cold Spring Harb Perspect Med 2012; 2(8): a006239. [http://dx.doi.org/10.1101/cshperspect.a006239] [PMID: 22908189]

[15] Yaari R, Fleisher AS, Tariot PN. Updates to diagnostic guidelines for Alzheimer's disease. Prim Care Companion CNS Disord 2011; 13(5): PCC.11f01262. [http://dx.doi.org/10.4088/PCC.11f01262] [PMID: 22295259]

[16] Serrano-Pozo A, Frosch MP, Masliah E, Hyman BT. Neuropathological alterations in Alzheimer disease. Cold Spring Harb Perspect Med 2011; 1(1): a006189. [http://dx.doi.org/10.1101/cshperspect.a006189] [PMID: 22229116]

[17] Spires-Jones TL, Hyman BT. The intersection of amyloid beta and tau at synapses in Alzheimer's disease. Neuron 2014; 82(4): 756-71. [http://dx.doi.org/10.1016/j.neuron.2014.05.004] [PMID: 24853936]

[18] Singh SK, Srivastav S, Yadav AK, Srikrishna S, Perry G. Overview of Alzheimer's ailment and some therapeutic approaches targeting abeta by using several synthetic and herbal compounds. Oxid Med Cell Longev 2016; 2016(1): 7361613. [http://dx.doi.org/10.1155/2016/7361613] [PMID: 27034741]

[19] Cras P, Kawai M, Lowery D, Gonzalez-DeWhitt P, Greenberg B, Perry G. Senile plaque neurites in Alzheimer disease accumulate amyloid precursor protein. Proc Natl Acad Sci USA 1991; 88(17): 7552-6. [http://dx.doi.org/10.1073/pnas.88.17.7552] [PMID: 1652752]

[20] Perl DP. Neuropathology of Alzheimer's disease. Mt Sinai J Med 2010; 77(1): 32-42. [http://dx.doi.org/10.1002/msj.20157] [PMID: 20101720]

[21] Armstrong RA. The molecular biology of senile plaques and neurofibrillary tangles in Alzheimer's disease. Folia Neuropathol 2009; 47(4): 289-99. [PMID: 20054780]

[22] Chen G, Xu T, Yan Y, *et al.* Amyloid beta: structure, biology and structure-based therapeutic development. Acta Pharmacol Sin 2017; 38(9): 1205-35. [http://dx.doi.org/10.1038/aps.2017.28] [PMID: 28713158]

[23] Tabaton M, Piccini A. Role of water-soluble amyloid-β in the pathogenesis of Alzheimer's disease. Int J Exp Pathol 2005; 86(3): 139-45.
[http://dx.doi.org/10.1111/j.0959-9673.2005.00428.x] [PMID: 15910548]

[24] Available from: https://www.kaggle.com/datasets/brsdincer/alzheimer-features

CHAPTER 7

Artificial Intelligence in Drug Delivery: An Alternative Approach to Traditional Nano-Theranostic Systems

Shreeja Sinha[1], **Sucharita Bhattacharyya**[1,*], **Sayani Konar**[1] and **Soumik Podder**[2]

[1] *Guru Nanak Institute of Technology, Panihati, West Bengal, India*

[2] *Department of Basic Science & Humanities, Institute of Engineering and Management, New Town, University of Engineering & Management, Kolkata, India*

Abstract: Nanomaterials have been extensively investigated to be used in clinical and pharmaceutical applications due to their unique features, such as shape, size, surface properties, reactive oxygen species (ROS) scavenging, targeted drug delivery, improved cell imaging due to excellent fluorescence property, precise personalized diagnosis, reduced side effects, and excellent sensing property. Despite all advantages, nanomaterials are signified as a potential generator of ROS, a symbol of toxicity. Although some clinical practices utilize ROS to prevent cancer, bacterial infection, *etc*., non-customized morphology can yield excessive ROS that may cause harm to normal cells. Another disadvantage is the infant research stages; more modulation in design is needed, and evaluation, as well as validation in nanotoxicity, is required. Although there exist a few stories of nano-medicine-mediated theranostic applications, the emerging challenges are increasingly prompting researchers to explore the optimal use of artificial intelligence (AI) in designing personalized drug delivery systems, potentially offering a more effective alternative to traditional nano-theranostic approaches. Accordingly, an elaborate governance framework is needed to develop and implement innovative AI systems successfully in the healthcare sector. The present work provides a comprehensive overview of the role of AI technologies in drug delivery, along with its ethical and regulatory concerns. Additionally, it illuminates the numerous challenges met in the employment of AI systems in clinical practice.

Keywords: Artificial intelligence in drug delivery, AI bot, Drug discovery, Drug delivery, NLP, Toxicity profile.

* **Corresponding author Sucharita Bhattacharyya:** Guru Nanak Institute of Technology, Panihati, West Bengal, India; E-mail: sucharita.gnit@gmail.com

Soumik Podder & Amalesh Samanta (Eds.)

INTRODUCTION

Drug

The word 'drug' is derived from the French word 'drogue', meaning 'dry herb'. The use of medicines dates back to ancient civilizations, making it nearly impossible to identify the very first person responsible for drug discovery. Early written records of medicinal drugs are known to have existed in a range of cultures, including Greek, Egyptian, Chinese, and Indian civilizations. This strongly suggests that ancient people treated diseases with conventional methods, most of them involving plants, while others involving animal products and minerals. Chinese medicine, Ayurveda, and the traditional Greek approaches are also proof of plant-based treatment. The positive fact is that those medicines have minimal or negligible side effects [1].

Both Arabic and European countries studied drugs in the medieval era. No sooner than the renaissance in the 19th century, the pharmaceutical approach made its appearance in the pre-modern era. Chemicals were discovered and tested actively in clinical research. It started as an attempt to reduce the load on rare medicinal herbs [1].

With the advancement of technology and the discovery of various viruses, bacteria, and disease-causing microbes, pharmaceutics played an important role in combating them and saving human lives as much as possible [2]. Antiseptics, vaccines, and anesthetics were slowly and steadily brought into existence. More elements were explored by mixtures and mutations to create recreational drugs. At present, both medicinal as well as recreational drugs have become major worldwide industries [3].

Thus, modern drugs are a combination of various chemical components. Any edible substance other than food, which causes changes in mood, hormones, behavior, thoughts, or feelings, can be referred to as a drug [4]. They are essentially used to prevent or suppress existing diseases, infections, abnormal behavior, or other symptoms. Other than treatment and diagnosis, these doses play an instrumental role in the functioning of the brain, glands, and various organs. Such pharmaceutical amalgams also play a significant role in reducing stress, anxiety, pressure levels, and many more physical and mental conditions. However, drugs, such as opioids, are highly addictive and harmful to human health [3].

Traditional methods of designing medicines have recently been replaced by CADD (computer-aided drug design). It refurbishes design techniques and also helps normalize the time taken in drug discovery. AI-based technology can be highly utilized in every process of drug formulation, thus aiding in reducing health hazards and fatalities associated with pre-clinical trials. AI, recognized as an efficient tool for data mining, can easily deal with the bulky pharmacological data and machine learning (ML) processes in every formulation step. AI possesses the ability to optimize all the operations associated with each step, such as improving quality control (QC) and the critical parameters, as well as increasing production by many folds without any hassle, hence upgrading the pharmaceutical industry.

Drugs are segregated into different types and forms, which are listed below.

On the Basis of Administration [5]

- **Oral route:** It is the safest and most common way of drug administration. The drugs are ingested directly as and flow into the human stomach before the action commences.
    - Liquids
    - Capsules
    - Tablets
    - Chewable tablets
    - Suspensions
- **Injection route:** These drugs are administered directly into the skin through any of the following approaches, *via* a needle and syringe, depending upon the affected area (Fig. **1**).
    - Subcutaneous layer (skin)
    - Intramuscular layer (in muscles)
    - Intravenous layer (in veins)
    - Intrathecal layer (around the spinal cord)

- **Sublingually and buccally:** Some doses are placed under the tongue or between teeth and gums for absorption.
- **Vaginal route:** The drugs are administered vaginally to women to combat infections and relieve symptoms during menopause in the form of
    - Cream
    - Solution
    - Tablet
    - Gel
    - Suppository
- **Ocular way:** This way of drug administration is used to treat optical diseases by applying the drugs in or around the eyes. The drugs are in the form of
    - Liquid (drops)
    - Gel

  - Ointment
- **Nasal route:** These drugs are inhaled as prescribed. They are breathed in and absorbed by the thin mucous layer within the nose.

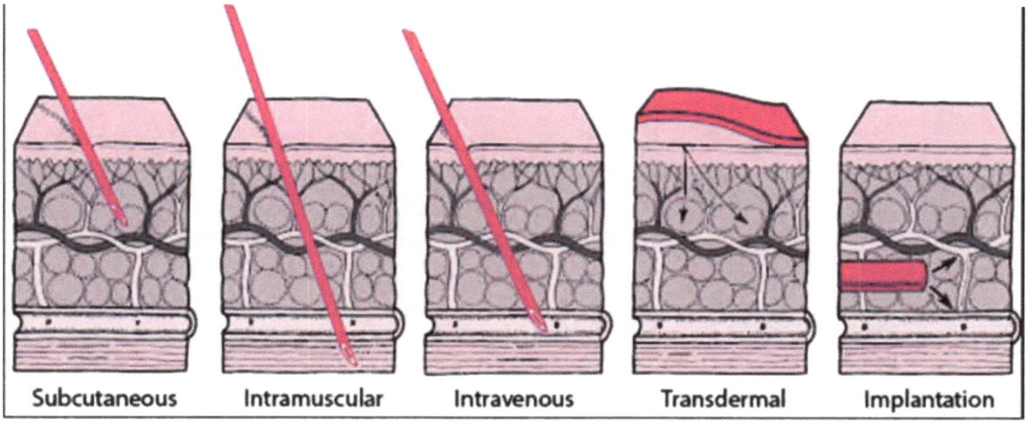

Fig. (1). Drug administration by injection [5].

On the Basis of Function [6]

- **CNS (central nervous system) depressants:** These drugs slow down the operation of the brain and the body.
- **CNS stimulants:** These drugs increase the heart rate, leading to high blood pressure levels, or excessively stimulate the body.
- **Hallucinogens:** These drugs enable the recipient to perceive differently.
- **Anesthetics:** These drugs inhibit the brain's perception of pain.
- **Analgesics:** These drugs are responsible for reducing inflammation or the way of pain reception in the brain.
- **Inhalants:** These are volatile substances producing chemical vapours that induce psychoactive effects.

With the help of different AI methods, drugs can be administered effectively to only the affected cells, not disturbing the surrounding cells. This precise activity is possible with the help of image-sensing technologies along with deep learning and computer vision. It also addresses side effects and prevents malignancy in healthy cells.

Drug Delivery

Depending on foreign substances causing diseases, various chemical components are combined in a highly measured and controlled environment to form a drug. Here, pharmaceutical elements are mixed in specific proportions depending upon the effects of multiple properties of the infectious microbe, such as DNA sequence, RNA molecule, protein, or metabolite. This entire process of creating a medicine and its administration in the body is termed drug delivery. Medicines created are effective for particular diseases and their symptoms.

Drug delivery for patient consumption includes the following five phases [7]:

- **Discovery and Development**

Chemical amalgamation is done on the basis of microbe properties. This is done by continuous tests on a sample virus or microbe. Experiments are also conducted by researchers to check the viability and performance of the drug synthesized. Factors, such as absorption, administration, and side effects, are analyzed here in detail.

- **Pre-clinical Research**

Drugs created are tested either *in vitro* (in a test tube) or *in vivo* (in an animal) before use on a human. Additionally, the candidates undergo testing for pharmacodynamics and pharmacokinetics, examining the effects of the drugs on the body and vice versa. Preclinical research also plays a crucial role in determining pharmaceutical formulation development, including factors, such as stability, bioavailability, and administration methods.

- **Clinical Research**

Clinical research is typically divided into four phases: phase I, phase II, phase III, and phase IV. According to the Food and Drug Administration (FDA), phase I involves 20 to 100 healthy volunteers or individuals with the disease or condition, phase II involves up to several hundred affected people, phase III involves 300 to 3,000 people with the disease or condition, and phase IV involves several thousand of the affected people. If a drug compound successfully demonstrates safety and efficacy during clinical trials, it can advance to the FDA review.

- **FDA Review**

A panel of doctors, microbiologists, chemists, pharmacologists, and statisticians reviews the safety of components of a drug and findings from its clinical trials. When a biotechnological or pharmaceutical organization seeks FDA review, they are required to submit a new drug application (NDA) for drugs or a biologics license application (BLA) for biologics. If accepted, the panel efficiently reviews clinical research comprising patient outcomes, potential adverse effects, and the drug's risk-benefit analysis.

- **FDA Post-market Safety Manufacturing**

The FDA has multiple programs in place to help with public-use safety monitoring, such as MedWatch and Med Sun. MedWatch assists healthcare professionals and consumers in reporting serious problems with medical products. Med Sun collaboratively works with clinical professionals to identify, understand, and provide solutions to problems specifically related to the use of medical devices. Additionally, the FDA conducts regular compliance checks on a drug product's manufacturing environment and facilities to ensure they are in line with regulatory standards. They also monitor medicine advertisements and labelling to ensure pharmaceutical companies' vigilance in case of the spread of any false or misleading claims.

Toxicity Profile of a Drug [8]

Another important phase before drug delivery includes toxicity profiling. 'Drug toxicity' can be defined as a diverse array of adverse effects that are encountered while using the drug at either therapeutic or non-therapeutic doses. The toxic effects and therapeutic doses are usually predictable from the pharmacological properties of the drug, which are prone to affect most patients [9]. Toxicity tasks are essential to predict the potential poisonousness of drugs in humans. Toxicity is one of the essential and most primitive causes of compound attrition, and this is estimated from the pharmaceutical components and reactions caused by a dose. This is an essential step strictly followed to ensure the safety of patients and minimize physical or internal harm [10]. The toxicity predictions are categorised as follows:

- Acute toxicity prediction: Acute toxicity assessments focus on immediate, short-term drug reactions. The assessment is conducted on mice or rats. It is evaluated through the lethal dose half (LD50) value. It is the foundational metric of determining acute toxicity. The LD50 value employs the classification and regression task for determining toxicity.
- Clinical toxicity prediction: Clinical toxicity refers to the damage caused to human organs or tissues. The experiment is conducted at the human level. *In vitro* testing is most fine-grained and captures the chemical's ability to block biological pathways at the cellular level, *i.e.*, experiments done outside a living organism in the laboratory environment. However, *in vivo* testing is coarse-grained and captures the chemical interactions at multiple levels in the human

body, *i.e.*, experiments conducted inside a living organism. Morgan fingerprints and pre-trained simplified molecular input line entry system (SMILES) embeddings are used as input.

- Carcinogenicity prediction: The development of cancer caused by a drug, anticancer agents, or analgesics is called carcinogenicity. Metabokiller ensemble learning model has been created by combining six biochemical models with GBM-based predictions. The local interpretable model-agnostic explanations (LIME) algorithm is used to identify key biochemical features.
- Hepatotoxicity prediction: The damage to the liver by the drug or its metabolite is known as drug hepatotoxicity. ResNet18DNN, a DNN model, has been developed to improve hepatotoxicity prediction.
- Cardiotoxicity prediction: The effect of a drug on the myocardium is called cardiotoxicity. The RF model achieves good performance in predicting the cardiotoxicity [11].

Artificial Intelligence in Drug Delivery

The integration of machine learning (ML) alongside artificial intelligence (AI) in drug delivery showcases a paradigm shift in the biotechnology and pharmaceutical industries. These technologies have the ability to identify patterns, predict outcomes, and optimize processes, being highly adaptable and scalable. Designing of drugs, which is a critical commencing phase in drug delivery, has essentially relied on brute force methods, which are time-consuming and overpriced. AI algorithms, especially deep learning models, can successfully predict the binding affinities, molecular behaviour, and unrealized toxicity of compounds with high accuracy. Upon analysing vast biological and chemical databases, AI can rapidly single out promising drug elements, noticeably condensing the drug discovery phase. These models, trained on historical data, can predict which molecular structures are most likely to interact effectively with specific biological targets, streamlining the onset of drug development [12].

One of the most widespread connotations of AI in drug delivery is the approach to personalized medicine. AI can customize drug formulations and dosages for an individual by integrating specific data, such as proteomics, genomics, and metabolomics of the patient. ML models analyse these datasets to predict differences in patients' behaviour and their response to a given drug, considering countless factors, such as lifestyle, genetic variations, and other health conditions. This approach minimizes unfavourable effects and maximizes effectiveness, leading to a more accurate and reliable treatment plan. AI-driven drug delivery systems are becoming increasingly advanced by utilizing nanotechnology. They can optimize the design of nanoparticles that meticulously target drugs to tissues or cells, reducing vast exposure and side effects. These nanoparticles can be trained to release their payload when vulnerable to specific environmental conditions, such as the presence of certain enzymes and pH changes, to ensure accurate and effective drug delivery [13]. AI models can be used to create dose delivery appliances that release therapeutic agents in a systematic and administered manner over time by examining pharmacodynamic and pharmacokinetic data. AI effectively optimizes the drug release profile, ensuring that reparative levels are maintained in the bloodstream of an individual for favourable periods. This not only enhances the drug's efficacy, but also improves patients' health and side effect ratio by reducing dosing frequency [14].

Artificial intelligence also optimizes the cost and resources and provides medicinal solutions to patients in a customized manner.

This is done in different stages/steps (Fig. **2**). These are as follows:

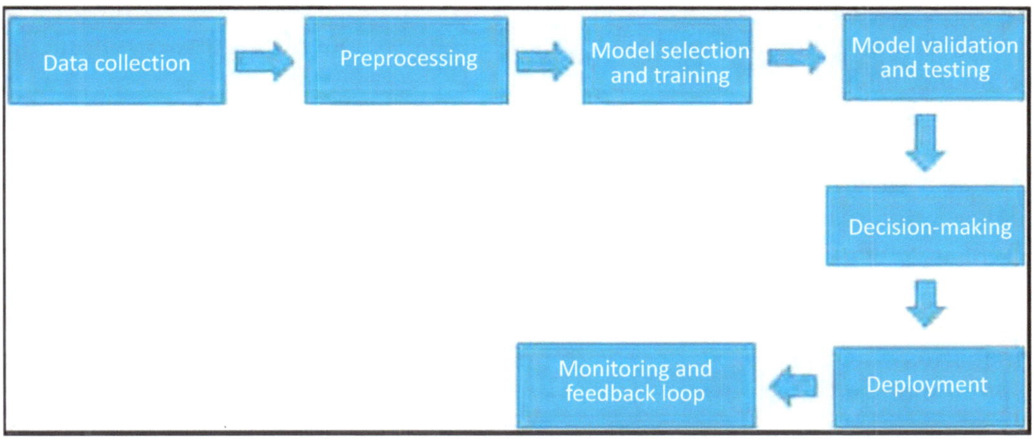

Fig. (2). Steps involved in creating an ML model [14].

- Data collection: Raw data is gathered from various sources (sensors, databases, surveys, *etc.*). This data forms the foundation of the model.
- Preprocessing: The data is cleaned, normalized, and transformed. Missing values and outliers are handled, and data is converted into a suitable format for modelling.
- Model selection and training: The appropriate machine learning algorithm is chosen. The model is trained on a portion of the dataset (training set) to learn patterns.
- Model validation and testing: The model's performance is evaluated on unseen data (validation/test set). Metrics like accuracy, precision, recall, *etc.*, are assessed.

- Decision-making: The validated model is used to make predictions or decisions. The results are ensured to be interpretable and actionable.
- Deployment: The trained model is integrated into a real-world application or system. The model is then made available for use (*e.g.*, *via* API or software tool).
- Monitoring and feedback loop: The model's performance is continuously monitored. The feedback is collected, and the model is retrained/updated if needed to maintain accuracy over time.

Data collection is done on the basis of the type of ML (machine learning).

There are three different types of machine learning [15], which are described as follows:

- Supervised learning: A model is trained by a labelled dataset, whereby every input data is compared and paired with its corresponding correct output, for example, image classification.
- Unsupervised learning: The model is trained with raw and unstructured/unlabelled data without instructions on how to interpret it. Instead, the system needs to identify structures and patterns autonomously from the dataset, for example, clustering.
- Reinforcement learning: This method involves training the model with either labelled or unlabelled data. A feedback segment is added for continuous improvement in the training dataset for further predictions. It is often used in scenarios where the model needs to make a series of decisions, for example, in autonomous vehicles.

Once data is successfully collected in a proper format, such as csv, jpg, time-series, graphs, *etc*., it is pre-processed. Data cleaning is done at this stage. It is the process where unwanted values, null values, and other missing information are handled carefully. It is one of the most important stages in training the AI model to prevent bias and other anomalies. The dataset is then split into training and testing data.

Following the data pre-processing, a suitable AI model is selected for training purposes. This selection is made depending on the function to be carried out. Data is then fed to the model and trained thoroughly.

Testing data then comes into the picture, whereby accuracy is checked. This can be done using F1 score, confusion matrix, or other prediction checkers. These can be directly coded into the environment or accessed from open-source tools.

After achieving the desired accuracy, the model is deployed for public use. The collected feedbacks are then utilized to continuously train the AI model for further enhancement of the use and accuracy, giving a real-time feel.

AI Technologies for Customized Access [16]

AI models, to provide customized treatment plans with real-time data, use much advanced algorithms than machine learning (Fig. **3**).

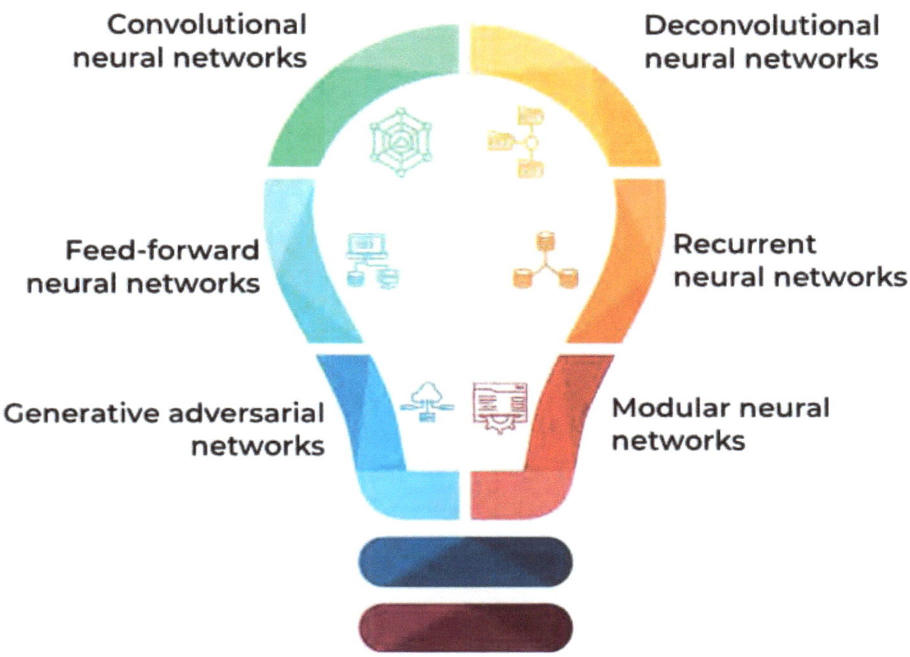

Fig. (3). Types of neural networks [16].

Deep learning models are used for this purpose. They include the application of neural networks. Neural networks are designed to resemble the functioning of neurons in a human brain. They consist of the input layer, multiple hidden layers, and the output layer. The input layer takes input from the user in the form of a questionnaire or image. The hidden layer consists of the logic, activation functions, and optimization algorithms. The output layer is responsible for predicting outcomes, providing insights along with the solutions, bringing about a real-time customized feedback.

The artificial intelligence (AI) policies are best illustrated by natural language processing (NLP), which is utilized widely to enhance usage by multi-lingual patients. It boosts healthcare opportunities by leveraging its immense power to process the available unstructured data from the language of humans to extract patterns for enhancing clinical decision-making. It thus helps to improve operational efficiency [17]. It also facilitates the healthcare industry by cost optimization and managerial job automation, and hence, the optimal quality of care is ensured, enriching the patient's experience using real-time data. NLP thus reflects one of the most significant shifts of the century towards AI-driven healthcare solutions.

NLP in healthcare is applied across various domains. These include computer-assisted coding (CAC), speech recognition, clinical documentation, clinical trial matching, clinical decision support, data mining research, AI chatbots and virtual scribe, computational phenotyping, risk adjustment and hierarchical condition categories, review management and sentiment analysis, root cause analysis, *etc* [17].

In real life, NLP is being utilized by renowned healthcare providers and hospitals in the USA to automate administrative tasks, improve clinical documentation, and streamline patient flow management. Major tech companies, like Google, Amazon, and Microsoft, are integrating NLP into their healthcare solutions. For instance, patient-doctor interactions are summarized, and accordingly automated for processing the insurance claims by the MedLM of Google, while the doctor-patient conversations are analysed by Amazon's HealthScribe to create clinical notes [17]. In the pharmaceutical sector, AstraZeneca employs NLP for research on drug discovery and its clinical trial tests. Here, it may be mentioned that NLP is used to analyse clinical trial protocols in this sector, where a specific pharmaceutical NLP model has been developed for helping Boehringer Ingelheim, the German pharma company, to process their clinical trial protocols [18]. Also, companies, like Genentech, utilize AI tools for efficient analysis of their huge datasets. The U.S. Food and Drug Administration (FDA) has also collaborated with John Snow Labs to leverage NLP for understanding the medicinal effects on mass populations [17].

CNNs (convolutional neural networks) can also be explored for drug analysis and delivery. They can analyse 2D or 3D structures of complex molecules, making them easier to comprehend. A multilayer CNN structure enables large-scale targeted drug detection, which can be highly helpful in monitoring drug toxicity and profiling.

CV (computer vision) is a necessary tool to visualize image data, such as blood test reports, prescriptions, *etc*.

In the case of drug delivery, multiple AI models are in use, especially in remote and rural areas with few medical resources. These models are trained by numerous datasets consisting of diseases, medicines, chemical components, side effects, allergens, and so on.

Datasets

The following are some of the datasets currently used all over the tech domain in terms of healthcare.

- The dataset presented in Table **1** consists of various drugs used for medical conditions, like acne, HIV, Alzheimer's disease, *etc*. The side effects and other details of the drugs can be found in previous works [19].

Table 1. Sample data of various drugs and their side effects.

Drug namename	Medical condition	Medical condition description	Activity	Rx-OTC	Pregnancy category	CSA (Controlled Substances Act)
Doxycycline	Acne	Acne (*Acne vulgaris*, blackheads, breakouts, cystic acne, pimples, whiteheads, *etc.*)	87%	Rx	D	N
Spironolactone	Acne	Acne (*Acne vulgaris*, blackheads, breakouts, cystic acne, pimples, whiteheads, *etc.*)	82%	Rx	C	N
Minocycline	Acne	Acne (*Acne vulgaris*, blackheads, breakouts, cystic acne, pimples, whiteheads, *etc.*)	48%	Rx	D	N
Vyvanse	ADHD	ADHD (attention deficit hyperactivity disorder), ADD (attention deficit disorder)	100%	Rx	C	2
Adderall	ADHD	ADHD (attention deficit hyperactivity disorder), ADD (attention deficit disorder)	95%	Rx	C	2
Truvada	AIDS/HIV	HIV infection (acquired immune deficiency syndrome)	97%	Rx	B	N

(Table 1) cont.....

Drug namename	Medical condition	Medical condition description	Activity	Rx-OTC	Pregnancy category	CSA (Controlled Substances Act)
Biktarvy	AIDS/HIV	HIV infection (acquired immune deficiency syndrome)	805	Rx	-	N
Doxylamine	Allergies	Allergies (dust mite allergies are an overreaction by the patients' immune systems)	9%	Rx/OTC	B	N
Aricept	Alzheimer's disease	Alzheimer's disease [presenile dementia, SDAT (senile dementia of Alzheimer's type)]	98%	Rx	C	N
Gabapentin	Anxiety	Anxiety (anxiety states, nervousness; anxiety is an emotion characterized by feel)	26%	Rx	C	N

OTC (over-the-counter): Medication that can be purchased without a medical prescription Rx: Prescription needed

Rx/OTC = Prescription or over-the-counter

Pregnancy Category

B: Animal reproduction studies have failed to demonstrate a risk to the foetus, and no adequate and well-controlled studies have been conducted on pregnant women. C: Animal reproduction studies have shown an adverse effect on the foetus, and no adequate and well-controlled studies are available in humans. D: There is positive evidence of human foetal risk based on adverse reaction data from investigational or marketing experience or studies involving humans.

CSA

N: Is not subject to the Controlled Substances Act. 2: Has a high potential for abuse.

- Table **2** entails all the medicines identified during our research, including details, such as their compositions, types, market availability, pricing, and other relevant information. The data consist of medicines from various pharmaceutical companies [20].

Table 2. Sample data of various medicines, including their price, manufacturer's name, *etc*.

Name	Augmentin 625 duo tablet	Azithral 500 tablet	Ascoril LS syrup	Allegra 120mg tablet	Avil 25 tablet	Glucosa 500mg tablet	Montelor 5mg/10mg tablet	Nervilead NT 75mg/10mg tablet	Rabicare 20mg tablet	Scabsafe-plus oral suspension
Price/pack	223.42	132.36	118	218.81	10.96	58.5	126	150	55	36
Pack size label	Strip of 10 tablets	Strip of 5 tablets	Bottle of 100 ml syrup	Strip of 10 tablets	Strip of 15 tablets	Strip of 10 tablets	Strip of 10 tablets	Strip of 10 tablets	Strip of 10 tablets	Bottle of 10 ml oral suspension
Is discontinued	False	False	False	False	False	False	False	False	False	False
Manufacturer	GlaxoSmithKline Pharmaceuticals Ltd.	Alembic Pharmaceuticals Ltd.	Glenmark Pharmaceuticals Ltd.	Sanofi India Ltd.	Sanofi India Ltd.	Redvia Pharmaceutical	Meethi Pharmaceuticals	Vilead Healthcare	Medico Healthcare	Rowlinges Life sciences
Short composition 1	Amoxycillin (500mg)	Azithromycin (500mg)	Ambroxol (30mg/5ml)	Fexofenadine (120mg)	Pheniramine (25mg)	Glucosamine (500mg)	Desloratadine (5mg)	Pregabalin (75mg)	Rabeprazole (20mg)	Ivermectin (6mg)
Short composition 2	Clavulanic acid (125mg)	-	Levosalbutamol (1mg/5ml)	-	-	-	Montelukast (10mg)	Nortriptyline (10mg)	-	Albendazole (400mg)

Table **3** contains a list of FDA, CPIC-A, and GPS medications with available germline pharmacogenomic information [21].

Table 3. Sample data of FDA, CPIC-A, and GPS medicines.

FDA drugs		CPIC A drugs	GPS drugs
Abacavir	Metroclopramide	Abacavir	Amlodipine
Atomoxetine	Modafinil	Azathioprine	Atorvastatin
Capecitabine	Nalidixic acid	Capecitabine	Benazepril
Chloroquine	Paroxetine	Escitalopram	Doxorubicin
Clomipramine	Perphenazine	Ivacaftor	Fluorouracil
Diazepam	Pyrazinamide	Ribavirin	Mercaptopurine
Flurbiprofen	Sodium nitrite	Warfarin	Pegylated interferon
Galantamine	Sulfamethoxazole	-	Pravastatin
Imipramine	Ticagrelor	-	Sunitinib

Table **4** consists of an available CSV (computer system validation) dataset containing details of all medicines, components, carcinogen content, and the effects on human health validated by the European Medicines Agency [22].

Table 4. Sample data of medicines, components, carcinogens, and their effects.

Category	Human	Veterinary	Veterinary
Name of medicine	Baiama	Biobhyo	Bravecto CombiUNO
EMA product number	EMEA/H/C/005980	EMEA/V/C/006336	EMEA/V/C/006358
Medicine status	Authorised	Opinion	Opinion
Opinion status	-	Positive	Positive

(Table 4) cont.....

Category	Human	Veterinary	Veterinary
Latest procedure affecting product information	VR/0000266291	-	-
International non-proprietary name (INN)/common name	Aflibercept	Swine dysentery vaccine (inactivated)	Fluralaner; Milbemycin oxime
Active substance	Aflibercept	*Brachyspira hyodysenteriae*, strain AqDys057, inactivated	Fluralaner; Milbemycin oxime
Therapeutic area (MeSH)	Wet macular degeneration, macular edema, retinal vein occlusion, choroidal neovascularization, diabetes complications	-	-
Species (veterinary)	-	Pigs	Dogs
Patient safety	No	No	No
ATC code (human)	S01LA05	-	-
ATCvet code (veterinary)	-	QI09AV	QP54AB51
Pharmacotherapeutic group (human)	Antineovascularisation agents, ocular vascular disorder agents	-	-
Pharmacotherapeutic group (veterinary)	-	Immunologicals for suidae	Endectocides
Therapeutic indication	Baiama is indicated for adults for the treatment of neovascular (wet) age-related macular degeneration (AMD), visual impairment due to macular oedema, diabetic macular oedema (DME), *etc.*	For the active immunisation of pigs against infections caused by *Brachyspira hyodysenteriae*, reducing the occurrence of dysenteric diarrhoea and minimising the widespread use of antibiotics.	It is a monthly treatment for dogs used to protect against a wide range of internal and external parasites. It provides fast and lasting protection against fleas and ticks for one month, helping to prevent flea infestations and flea allergy dermatitis (FAD).

(Table 4) cont.....

Category	Human	Veterinary	Veterinary
			The product also reduces the risk of infection with *Babesia canis* by killing the transmitting tick and lowers the risk of *Dipylidium caninum* by killing the transmitting flea. Bravecto CombiUNO also treats and controls several types of intestinal worms, including roundworms and whipworms.
Accelerated assessment	No	No	No
Additional monitoring	Yes	No	No
Advanced therapy	No	No	No
Biosimilar	Yes	No	No
Conditional approval	No	No	No

Once the AI model is successfully trained on the data, it is tested with common diseases and remedies. When accuracy is achieved, the model is used publicly.

However, not all reports are 100% accurate. Hence, in times of critical urgency, it is advised to consult a doctor. Nevertheless, these types of AI tools and bots are capable of providing primary treatment and first aid.

Design of an AI Bot Providing Enhanced Medications

Training

Different datasets are fed using Pandas (a Python package to read and manipulate data). Some examples of datasets are given above. These essentially consist of diseases, their symptoms, and the medicine with the corresponding chemical components. The dataset containing allergen information (Table **5**) and its chemical components is also fed into the system. Image datasets are also available for certain diseases, such as autism, cancer, *etc*., and for X-rays, MRIs, and all other types of scanned images. These image datasets are read *via* OpenCV (a tool used to visualize data in computer vision). Different prescriptions are also fed into the AI model for it to understand all types of hand-written data easily.

Table 5. Sample dataset containing allergen information.

Medicine name	Active ingredient	Allergenic chemicals	Disease treated	Potential allergic effects/side effects
Amoxicillin	Amoxicillin	Penicillin	Bacterial infections (*e.g.*, pneumonia, bronchitis)	Rash, anaphylaxis, difficulty breathing, swelling (angioedema)
Aspirin	Acetylsalicylic acid	Salicylates	Pain, inflammation, fever, arthritis	Rashes, gastrointestinal bleeding, asthma (aspirin sensitivity)
Penicillin V	Penicillin V potassium	Penicillin	Bacterial infections (*e.g.*, strep throat, pneumonia)	Rash, anaphylaxis, difficulty breathing, swelling (angioedema)
Ibuprofen	Ibuprofen	None (except for rare allergic reactions)	Pain, inflammation, fever, arthritis	Rash, gastrointestinal upset, kidney damage
Cetirizine	Cetirizine	None (antihistamine)	Allergies (*e.g.*, hay fever, allergic rhinitis)	Drowsiness, dry mouth, dizziness
Ciprofloxacin	Ciprofloxacin	None (may cause rare reactions)	Bacterial infections (*e.g.*, UTI, respiratory infection)	Rash, photosensitivity, tendonitis, nausea
Clindamycin	Clindamycin	Lincomycin, clindamycin-related allergens	Bacterial infections (*e.g.*, skin infections)	Rash, diarrhoea, anaphylaxis
Fexofenadine	Fexofenadine	None (antihistamine)	Allergies (*e.g.*, hay fever, allergic rhinitis)	Headache, drowsiness, dry mouth (rare)

Deep Learning Model

Different large language models (LLMs), transformers, and gen AI models are tools used to manage such huge data and provide customized outputs. These are based on distinct neural networks, such as CNN, RNN, and ANN. They consist of three main layers (Fig. **4**).

The input layer is responsible for accepting data, either labelled or unlabelled. The hidden layer contains all conditions, samples, comparisons, and other factors required for prediction. The output layer provides output based on training data. This output is again used as feedback to update the database in the input layer.

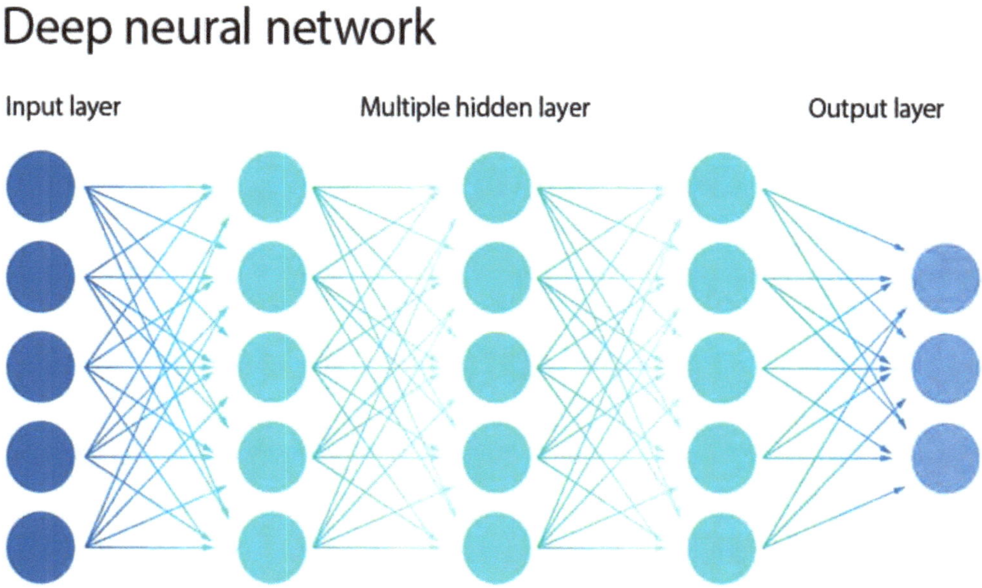

Fig. (4). Layers in deep learning [23].

Output

In a healthcare chatbot, the input layer collects symptoms and details of patients in the form of a questionnaire. It also collects test reports if necessary. The hidden layer processes the input data and finally suggests medications as required or further tests if necessary. AI chatbot also has the capability to provide customized medications depending on the allergen information of patients.

Advancement in Usage Worldwide [24]

Key statistics from the past few years strongly flaunt the use of chatbot tools at a much higher rate. Human intervention has drastically reduced in recent years.

The global use of AI in healthcare grew from $1.1 billion in 2016 to $22.4 billion in 2023. By 2030, the global AI healthcare market is projected to soar to $188 billion, driven by a 37% CAGR from 2022 to 2030. AI has also been expected to reduce healthcare costs by $13 billion by 2025 (Fig. **5**).

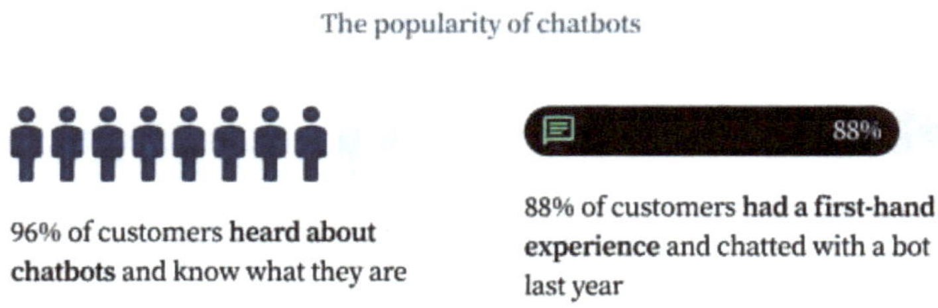

Fig. (5). The increase in use of chatbots globally [24].

Especially in remote areas with poor medical facilities, AI tools and bots have become a boon to ensure health quality on a regular basis. The AI nursing assistant market is forecast to reduce 20% of nurses' maintenance tasks [25].

AI plays a huge role in following up with critical treatments, such as cancer, cardiac diseases, and other organ ailments. Presently, in 2025, 90% of hospitals are expected to utilize AI-powered technology for early diagnosis and remote patient monitoring.

Currently, most countries' healthcare systems have successfully infused the use of robots in various ways. Robotic surgeries are pretty common in many countries. Remote patient monitoring systems are also widely used (Fig. **6** and Table **6**).

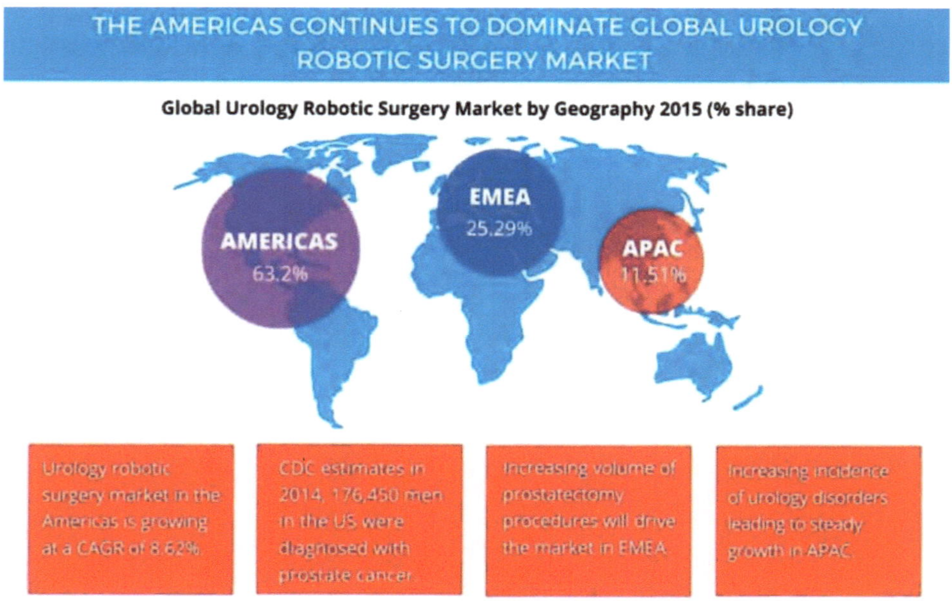

Fig. (6). The advancement of robotic surgery in urological sector [26].

Table 6. Statistics showing research and development of AI in healthcare country-wise [27].

No.	Country	Total papers	% papers	Cite rate	Total downloads	Total institutes	Total country	% papers with international collaboration
1	United States	10,623	30.8	3.4	25,384	6.8	1.5	33.6%
2	China	2617	7.6	2.9	15,995	7.3	1.7	44.8%
3	Italy	1834	5.3	2.8	3343	8.4	2.1	55.2%
4	Germany	1553	4.5	3.3	3415	8.9	2.1	53.1%
5	Canada	1312	3.8	2.9	3343	8.0	1.8	48.5%
6	France	1308	3.8	3.1	2623	9.0	2.2	63.7%
7	India	1264	3.7	2.1	3350	4.9	1.6	31.6%
8	Spain	1029	3.0	2.6	2852	7.7	2.0	49.3%
9	Australia	910	2.6	3.5	3337	7.5	2.0	50.5%
10	Japan	841	2.4	2.2	2107	7.5	1.7	35.7%
11	Turkey	787	2.3	1.8	1121	4.4	1.4	20.3%
12	Iran	713	2.1	2.2	1599	4.6	1.4	30.2%
13	Brazil	489	1.4	2.6	1380	8.1	1.9	44.6%
14	Israel	384	1.1	3.4	950	9.8	2.4	69.8%

Hence, artificial intelligence is experiencing rapid growth across multiple sectors in the healthcare industry. These include robotic surgery, remote medical prescribers, AI bots to suggest medications, remote patient monitoring, and even critical health care.

Artificial Intelligence: The Ethics and the Regulations

The introduction of AI in clinical workflows to assist in diagnostics and drug delivery for enabling personalized patient care has led to the emergence of various tools and applications that often lack regulatory approvals, hence posing serious challenges in ethical and legal matters.

The exponential growth of medical data raises significant concerns regarding the security and safe handling of vast data storage, which is critical for reshaping privacy and security frameworks in the healthcare landscape. Thus, plans should be established to address any breaches that may occur.

The ethical guidelines should categorize all AI products with precision based on their potential risk to fundamental rights, including health and safety, dignity and equality, democracy and the right of no discrimination, and data protection. Accordingly, on April 21, 2021, the European Regulation was enacted [28].

In the literature, six fundamental ethical principles and guidelines have been identified to address various operational parameters of decision-making algorithms of AI techniques used in the service of society. Some of them are fundamental, and others are drawn considering moral and legal standards. They include the following:

- ensuring inconclusivity and equity
- ensuring transparency and explainability
- autonomy protection
- promoting welfare and safety
- promoting responsiveness and sustainability
- promoting accountability and responsibility

They play a major role for all stakeholders, the physicians, system developers, health authority policymakers, healthcare system administrators, and the government, responsible for the advancement, deployment, and assessment of AI technologies in healthcare [28].

The Challenges Posed by AI and the Limitations of AI Models

Naturally, many challenges emerge in the healthcare sector with the growing application of AI in diagnosis and healthcare systems, suggesting reassessment of the conventional doctor-patient relationship. Physicians and healthcare professionals may become susceptible to numerous cognitive biases with the use of AI, which may lead to errors in diagnosis. They can arise from biased training data or algorithmic biases, so proper evaluation should be carried out to eliminate these biases and provide impartial results [28].

Deep learning in AI systems operates as a black box. It takes inputs and generates outputs, but does not reveal the reasoning or underlying calculations, as the learning outcomes are reflected in node weights that cannot be directly interpreted by humans. Here, reasons for the results of the discrimination and anomaly detection are not always explicable, which creates serious concerns, particularly in industrial applications, as people's lives and health are their main considerations. So, in AI development guidelines, transparency as well as accountability are the two most important requirements, which are not met with the black box machine learning presently [29]. To tackle such issues and prevent healthcare practitioners from being questionable for AI errors, standardized policies' implementation and measures at the government level should be introduced.

Another point must be considered in deep learning, which uses deep neural networks (DNNs). DNN works with multilayers and a large number of parameters related to complex structures, and thus is prone to overfitting. Here, generalization is impossible, and so with unknown data, an accurate output is not expected. A large amount of training data is required to handle these challenges. Data sharing among the researchers can help in overcoming this problem. Again, a large-scale DNN takes a long time to input such datasets for executing the learning process [29]. Also, complex algorithms make it difficult to understand the reasoning behind the prediction.

AI integration in the healthcare sector thus faces notable limitations in managing health record data, including patients' complete medical history, physical examination details, the investigation, and treatment records, which are stored in electronic forms. Electronic health records raise ethical concerns related to autonomy, fidelity, and justice, especially when patients' health data are shared without their knowledge or when healthcare organizations fail to implement adequate safeguards.

So, the idea that AI, due to its ability to analyze data rapidly, can perform increasingly complex tasks to replace physicians in clinical decision-making is practically far from reality. Here, it must be noted that AI applications are relatively new to be applied regularly in all clinical cases with precision.

CONCLUSION

AI algorithms can process variables, like age, socioeconomic factors, income, ethnicity, and geographic location, to find disparities in healthcare coverage. ML models have identified disparities in the treatment of chronic diseases, like diabetes and hypertension. AI can thus be used to reduce disparities by developing personalized treatment plans.

At present, there exist numerous AI bots all over the world, helping in prescribing medicines based on symptoms. Such virtual consultations are provided to patients of rural and underserved regions where they can access healthcare professionals without any travel. Here, telemedicine acts as immediate first aid in remote locations. Another application includes providing medications to patients from low-income backgrounds. AI chatbots and drug delivery robots are also used in many countries to enhance treatments in areas with poor facilities. They are trained using vast datasets to predict output. However, these bots are incapable of providing new medicines as they have no human intelligence.

Although AI-driven drug discovery is beginning to yield promising results, its efficiency needs to be enhanced, particularly in identifying lead compounds with larger and more complex molecular structures, such as biopharmaceuticals. So, AI is indeed a developing platform that may promote a data-driven drug discovery target search approach in combination with genomes.

Further research and development are in demand, particularly in addressing allergen issues. Existing AI bots may be upgraded to provide prescriptions based on the patient's allergen details. This can be highly helpful in reducing side effects and other health issues. In upcoming years, robotic surgeries may also be used on a larger scale, ranging from minor to major critical operations. Critical diseases, such as cancer, organ failure, long Covid, neurotic issues, *etc*., are also significant sectors where AI can be highly infused.

REFERENCES

[1] Wadud A, Prasad PVV, Rao MM, Narayana A. Evolution of drug: a historical perspective. Bull Indian Inst Hist Med Hyderabad 2007; 37(1): 69-80.
[PMID: 19569453]

[2] Anand SS, Philip BK, Mehendale HM. Interactive Toxicity. Encyclopedia of Toxicology (Third Edition) 2014; 1061-1064.
[http://dx.doi.org/10.1016/B978-0-12-386454-3.00323-7]

[3] Pearce JL. EDCs impacts on human populations Addressing multiple chemicals in human exposure and epidemiological studies. Environmental Contaminants and Endocrine Health 2023; pp. 63-70.
[http://dx.doi.org/10.1016/B978-0-12-824464-7.00019-2]

[4] Afrin S, Gupta V. Pharmaceutical Formulation. StatPearls Publishing 2023.

[5] Le J. Drug Administration [homepage on the internet]. Administration and Kinetics of Drugs [revised: Nov 2024]. Available from: https://www.msdmanuals.com/home/drugs/administration-and-kineti-s-of-drugs/drug-administration

[6] The International Association of Chiefs of Police (IACP) [homepage on the Internet]. Available from: https://www.theiacp.org/7-drug-categories

[7] Exploring the five phases of drug development [homepage on the Internet]. Patheon pharma services [Oct 2023]. Available from: https://www.patheon.com/us/en/insights-resources/blog/dru--development-phases.html

[8] Egan WJ, Zlokarnik G, Grootenhuis PDJ. In silico prediction of drug safety: despite progress there is abundant room for improvement. Drug Discov Today Technol 2004; 1(4): 381-7.
[http://dx.doi.org/10.1016/j.ddtec.2004.11.002] [PMID: 24981618]

[9] Silakari O, Singh PK. ADMET tools: Prediction and assessment of chemical ADMET properties of NCEs. Concepts and Experimental Protocols of Modelling and Informatics in Drug Design 2021; pp. 299-320.
[http://dx.doi.org/10.1016/B978-0-12-820546-4.00014-3]

[10] Benigni R. Computational prediction of drug toxicity: the case of mutagenicity and carcinogenicity. Drug Discov Today Technol 2004; 1(4): 457-63.
[http://dx.doi.org/10.1016/j.ddtec.2004.09.003] [PMID: 24981627]

[11] Bai C, Wu L, Li R, Cao Y, He S, Bo X. Machine Learning□Enabled Drug□Induced Toxicity Prediction. Adv Sci (Weinh) 2025; 12(16): 2413405.
[http://dx.doi.org/10.1002/advs.202413405] [PMID: 39899688]

[12] Lim S, Lee S, Piao Y, *et al.* On modeling and utilizing chemical compound information with deep learning technologies: A task-oriented approach. Comput Struct Biotechnol J 2022; 20: 4288-304.

[http://dx.doi.org/10.1016/j.csbj.2022.07.049] [PMID: 36051875]

[13] A guide to pharmaceutical mixing [homepage on the Internet]. Available from: https://www.pharmahygieneproducts.com/2023/05/22/a-guide-to-pharmaceutical-mixing/

[14] Jena GK, Patra CN, Jammula S, Rana R, Chand S. Artificial Intelligence and Machine Learning Implemented Drug Delivery Systems: A Paradigm Shift in the Pharmaceutical Industry [Review]. Journal of Bio-X Research 2024. [http://dx.doi.org/10.34133/jbioxresearch.0016]

[15] Accuracy in AI: Artificial Intelligence Explained [homepage on the Internet]. Available from: https://www.netguru.com/glossary/accuracy-in-ai

[16] Ashtari H. What is a Neural Network? Definition, Working, Types, and Applications in 2022 [homepage on the Internet]. Available from: https://www.spiceworks.com/tech/artificial-intelligence/articles/what-is-a-neural-network/ https://doi.org/10.3390/biomedinformatics2040039

[17] Ariwala P. NLP in Healthcare: Top 14 Use Cases [homepage on the internet]. Available from: https://marutitech.com/use-cases-of-natural-language-processing-in-healthcare/

[18] NLP in pharma: NLP clinical trial analysis [homepage on the internet]. Available from: https://fastdatascience.com/ai-in-pharma/clinical-trials-analysis/

[19] Varghese J. Drugs Related to Medical Conditions [homepage on the Internet]. Available from: https://www.kaggle.com/datasets/jithinanievarghese/drugs-related-to-common-treatments

[20] Singh S. A-Z Medicine of India [homepage on the Internet]. Available from: https://www.kaggle.com/datasets/shudhanshusingh/az-medicine-dataset-of-india

[21] Hussain S, Kenigsberg BB, Danahey K, *et al.* Disease–drug database for pharmacogenomic□based prescribing. Clin Pharmacol Ther 2016; 100(2): 179-90. [http://dx.doi.org/10.1002/cpt.364] [PMID: 26940584]

[22] European Medicines agency 2024 [homepage on the Internet]. Available from: https://www.ema.europa.eu/en/medicines/download-medicine-data

[23] Shaik S. The Deep Learning Ecosystem-Inspired by the human brain [homepage on the Internet] Available from: https://medium.com/@saleema2002shaik/the-deep-learning-ecosystem-inspir-d-by-the-human-brain-ea780126d88e

[24] Fakina M. The future of Chatbots: 80+ Chatbot statistics for 2025 [homepage on the Internet] [updated Oct 2024].Available from: https://www.tidio.com/blog/chatbot-statistics/

[25] Roy S. AI in Healthcare Statistics: Comprehensive List for 2025 [homepage on the Internet]. Available from: https://www.dialoghealth.com/post/ai-healthcare-statistics

[26] Andreas H, Noveriansyah S. Identifying GNSS market in Indonesia before and the future. E3S Web of Conferences 94 2019. [http://dx.doi.org/10.1051/e3sconf/20199403010]

[27] Tran BX, Vu GT, Ha GH, *et al.* Global Evolution of Research in Artificial Intelligence in Health and Medicine: A Bibliometric Study. J Clin Med 2019; 8(3): 360. [http://dx.doi.org/10.3390/jcm8030360] [PMID: 30875745]

[28] Mennella C, Maniscalco U, Pietro GD, Esposito M. Ethical and regulatory challenges of AI technologies in healthcare: A narrative review 2024; 10(4). [http://dx.doi.org/10.1016/j.heliyon.2024.e26297]

[29] Matsuzaka Y, Yashiro R. Applications of Deep Learning for Drug Discovery Systems with BigData. BioMedInformatics 2022; 2(4): 603-24. [http://dx.doi.org/10.3390/biomedinformatics2040039]

CHAPTER 8

Artificial Intelligence in Nanomedicine Formulation and Applications

Shouvik Sarkar[1,2,*] and **Debaprasad Das**[2]

[1] *Department of Computer Science and Engineering-AI, Brainware University, Barasat, Kolkata, West Bengal, India*

[2] *Department of Electronics and Communication Engineering, Assam University, Silchar, Assam, India*

Abstract: Artificial intelligence is emerging as a transformative factor in the development of nanomedicine—the integration of nanotechnology and biomedical science to solve complex health problems. This paper reports on the synergistic integration of AI and nanomedicine, with a focus on the contributions it makes towards creating nanoscale materials, upgrading nanomaterials, and applications in diagnostics, drug delivery, and regenerative therapy. AI-driven approaches rapidly identify the ideal properties of nanomaterials, enhance the interaction between drugs and nanoparticles, and improve the accuracy of their mechanism for targeting diseases. Here, predictive modeling using machine learning algorithms accelerates progress in nanocarriers, nanosensors, and imaging technologies, while providing an opportunity to detect diseases at early stages and customize targeted therapeutic strategies [1].

The article highlights revolutionary breakthroughs enabled by AI in addressing the aforementioned limitations of nanomedicine, specifically in terms of production scales, regulatory burdens, and nano-material toxicity. Case studies illustrating AI-driven breakthroughs in treatments for cancer, cardiovascular diseases, and neurological disorders describe improved clinical results through targeted and advanced diagnostics and treatments. However, the convergence of AI and nanomedicine also raises ethical, regulatory, and data-related issues that require interdisciplinary collaboration and robust frameworks for responsible implementation. This study highlights the potential of AI in transforming nanomedicine, paving the way for next-generation medical solutions that are more secure, efficient, and tailored to meet the unique needs of patients. By connecting computational technologies with biomedical applications, the research envisions a future in which AI-driven nanomedicine revolutionizes healthcare delivery worldwide [2].

* **Corresponding author Shouvik Sarkar:** Department of Computer Science and Engineering-AI, Brainware University, Barasat, Kolkata, West Bengal, India; E-mail: shouviksarkar08@gmail.com

Soumik Podder & Amalesh Samanta (Eds.)

Keywords: Artificial intelligence, Drug delivery systems, Deep learning, Machine learning, Nanosensors, Nanomedicine, Nanotechnology, Personalized medicine, Predictive modeling, Targeted therapy.

INTRODUCTION

Overview of Nanomedicine

Nanomedicine is a rapidly emerging field that combines nanotechnology with healthcare to identify and prevent diseases at the molecular level. Nanomedicine provides unique opportunities to enhance therapeutic effectiveness and facilitate precision medicine. Nanoparticles, nanosensors, and drug delivery systems are essential elements that have transformed fields such as oncology, infectious diseases, and regenerative medicine [3]. Nanomedicine utilizes physical and chemical characteristics that develop at the nanometer scale, ranging from 1 to 100 nanometers in diameter. Nanotechnology advancements have enabled the development of biocompatible nanoparticles, including liposomes, dendrimers, and polymeric micelles, which can be tailored for targeted drug delivery and focused therapies. Nanomedicine has experienced significant advancements in creating nanosensors that can detect biomarkers at extremely low levels, thereby facilitating the early detection and monitoring of diseases. A major obstacle to nanomedicine is the scalability of production, regulatory issues, and the potential toxicity of nanomaterials. These issues necessitate a multidisciplinary strategy that incorporates material science, biology, and computational methods. Artificial Intelligence stands out as a vital facilitator in addressing these problems, promoting innovation, and accelerating the progress of nanomedical solutions [3].

The Function of Artificial Intelligence in Contemporary Healthcare

Artificial Intelligence has emerged as a revolutionary influence in the modern healthcare system. It enhances the system by leveraging machine learning, deep learning, and data analysis to improve patient outcomes. AI enhances diagnostic precision, predicts treatment responses, and streamlines complex workflows. It is applied from medical imaging and tailored healthcare to predictive analytics and robotic surgery. AI offers solutions for complex issues, including molecular modeling, nanomaterial production, and precision medicine, such as precision drug delivery. AI is transforming the healthcare sector by enabling informed decisions through data analysis. Machine learning algorithms examine large volumes of clinical data, revealing patterns and insights that may be missed by human analysis. AI-based diagnostic systems have enhanced medical imaging, demonstrating higher accuracy in identifying conditions such as cancer, heart disease, and neurological disorders [4]. These systems minimize diagnostic errors and help healthcare providers make informed decisions. In nanomedicine, AI aids in the development and enhancement of nanomaterials by anticipating their physicochemical characteristics and interactions with biological systems. For example, AI models can replicate the behavior of nanoparticles within the human body, enabling the optimization of their size, shape, and surface characteristics for improved therapeutic outcomes. Additionally, AI-powered platforms facilitate the high-throughput evaluation of nanomaterials, thereby accelerating the discovery of candidates with ideal characteristics for drug delivery and various applications [4].

Significance of AI in Nanomedicine Development and Uses

The development of AI and nanomedicine has created new opportunities for innovation. AI-based methods facilitate the creation and enhancement of nanocarriers, predictive modeling of drug-nanoparticle interactions, and effective examination of extensive datasets from clinical trials. AI accelerates the identification of new nanomaterials and enhances the accuracy of treatment methods. This section focuses on the capability of AI to address current challenges in nanomedicine and facilitate its transition from laboratory to clinical application. The capability of AI to analyze and process intricate datasets is especially beneficial in nanomedicine. Conventional experimental methods for designing and testing nanoparticles can be laborious and costly [5]. AI algorithms can easily analyze data from high-throughput experiments, recognizing patterns and correlations that guide the development of more efficient nanocarriers. AI can forecast the optimal arrangement of nanoparticles for precise drug delivery, thereby minimizing the need for extensive trial-and-error testing. Predictive modeling is another field in which AI performs exceptionally good. Machine learning models are capable of predicting how nanomaterials interact with biological systems, taking into account aspects such as biodistribution, cellular uptake, and toxicity. These forecasts enable scientists to develop nanomaterials with enhanced safety and effectiveness characteristics, thereby reducing potential risks to patients. Moreover, AI-based evaluation of clinical trial data helps pinpoint elements that affect treatment outcomes, guiding the development of tailored nanomedicine approaches. AI plays a crucial role in enhancing diagnostics in nanomedicine. Researchers have created systems that can detect diseases early with high sensitivity and specificity by combining AI with nanosensors and imaging technologies. For example, nanosensors augmented with AI can instantly evaluate biomarker information, facilitating quick diagnosis and tracking of conditions such as cancer, Alzheimer's, and infectious diseases [5].

FUNDAMENTALS OF NANOMEDICINE

Essential Ideas in Nanomedicine

Nanomedicine relies on nanotechnology, utilizing materials and devices that function at the nanoscale to fulfill specific biomedical goals. Nanoparticles play a significant role in this area and consist of various structures, such as liposomes, polymeric nanoparticles, and metallic nanoparticles. Table **1** illustrates the application areas of key functional nanomaterials in their active structural forms. Liposomes, polymeric nanoparticles, and metallic nanoparticles are designed to carry out tasks such as targeted drug delivery, transporting therapeutic agents directly to disease sites, and improving treatment effectiveness. Nanocarriers are a type of nanoparticles that are uniquely designed for use in drug delivery. It includes sophisticated characteristics like stimuli-responsive release mechanisms that trigger in response to pH, temperature, and enzymatic activity. This accuracy enables regulated drug delivery that minimizes overall toxicity and enhances patient outcomes. Nanosensors capable of identifying biological and chemical signals with remarkable sensitivity [6]. These sensors are often combined with AI algorithms to evaluate data instantly. It offers diagnostic insights that can inform treatment choices. Functional Characteristics of Nanomaterials: Nanomaterials exhibit distinct properties, including high surface-to-volume ratios, adjustable optical and electronic characteristics, and enhanced reactivity. These characteristics allow for applications like imaging, where nanoparticles improve contrast in medical scans, and therapy, where their surfaces can be modified with drugs or targeting agents.

Table 1. Key functional nanomaterials and their biomedical applications.

Nanomaterial Type	Structure/Form	Application
Liposomes	Phospholipid bilayer	Drug delivery
Polymeric nanoparticles	Biodegradable polymers	Controlled drug release
Metallic nanoparticles	Gold/silver particles	Imaging, photothermal therapy
Dendrimers	Branched polymers	Gene delivery
Quantum Dots	Semiconductor crystals	Fluorescent imaging

Applications in Healthcare

Drug Delivery Systems - Nanomedicine alters drug delivery by enabling the development of systems that can overcome biological barriers, such as the blood-brain barrier. Nanocarriers, such as liposomes and polymeric nanoparticles, protect therapeutic agents from degradation and enhance their bioavailability [7].

Innovations in this area include multifunctional carriers capable of simultaneous imaging and therapy, known as theragnostic. The various drug administration routes are illustrated in Fig. (**1**).

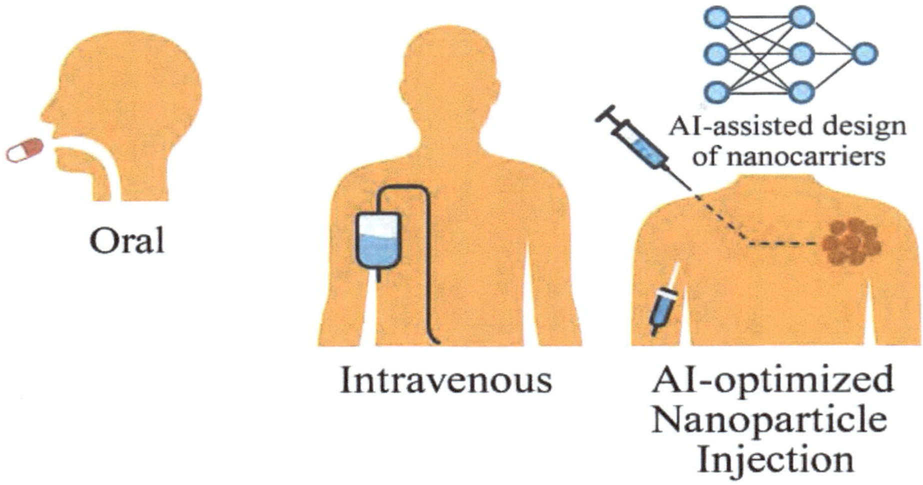

Fig. (1). Drug administration routes.

Diagnostics and Imaging: Nanoparticles enhance the capabilities of diagnostic imaging modalities, such as MRI and CT scans. Quantum dots offer superior fluorescence properties for optical imaging, while superparamagnetic nanoparticles enhance the sensitivity of MRI. Combined with AI, these technologies offer real-time analysis and improved diagnostic accuracy [8].

Regenerative Medicine- Nanotechnology contributes to regenerative medicine by supporting tissue engineering and the development of biomimetic scaffolds. Nanomaterials such as hydrogels and nanofibers promote cell adhesion, growth, and differentiation. Additionally, nanoparticles can deliver growth factors or genetic material to specific tissues, facilitating repair and regeneration [9].

Challenges in Nanomedicine Development

Nanomedicine faces significant challenges that hinder its widespread adoption. Manufacturing scalability remains a critical issue, as producing nanoparticles with consistent quality and functionality is a complex process. Regulatory pathways for nanomedicine products are also underdeveloped, creating uncertainty for researchers and manufacturers. In addition, the potential toxicity and long-term effects of nanomaterials require thorough investigation. These challenges necessitate collaborative efforts across disciplines as well as the integration of AI tools to streamline development and ensure safety and efficacy. Through ongoing research and innovation, the field of nanomedicine continues to evolve, offering new solutions to some of healthcare's most pressing challenges [10].

ARTIFICIAL INTELLIGENCE IN HEALTHCARE

AI leverages algorithms and computational models to interpret data, make predictions, and assist in decision-making. Machine learning techniques, including supervised learning, unsupervised learning, and reinforcement learning, as well as deep learning methods, are foundational components of this technology.

Supervised, Unsupervised, and Reinforcement Learning

Supervised learning involves training algorithms on labeled datasets, where inputs are paired with corresponding outputs. Annotated datasets guide artificial intelligence in identifying patterns and making accurate diagnoses in tasks like medical image analysis. Popular supervised learning algorithms include decision trees, support vector machines, and ensemble methods such as random forests and gradient boosting [11].

Unsupervised learning: It works with unlabeled data, focusing on uncovering hidden structures or relationships. This approach is priceless in exploratory biomedical research, such as clustering patient data to identify subgroups with similar disease characteristics or using dimensionality reduction techniques like principal component analysis (PCA) to simplify complex datasets [11].

Reinforcement learning- RL stands apart by emphasizing sequential decision-making. Agents learn to achieve specific goals by interacting with their environment and receiving feedback in the form of rewards or penalties. RL is used in optimizing treatment protocols where the agent learns the most effective sequence of interventions for a given patient profile [11]. RL has shown promise in personalized medicine, enabling dynamic treatment strategies for chronic diseases such as diabetes and cancer.

Deep Learning and Neural Networks: Deep learning is a subset of machine learning that utilizes artificial neural networks (ANNs) with multiple layers to model complex patterns and relationships in data. Convolutional neural networks are widely employed in medical imaging tasks such as tumor detection in MRI scans or identifying diabetic retinopathy in retinal images. CNNs surpass in processing grid-like data structures that making them ideal for visual tasks. Recurrent neural networks (RNNs) and their advanced variants, such as long short-term memory (LSTM) networks, are particularly well-suited for analyzing sequential data. These models analyze time-series data such as patient vital signs to predict health outcomes or detect early signs of deterioration. Generative adversarial networks are also playing a growing role, specifically in data augmentation for biomedical research. GANs generate synthetic datasets that mimic real-world data, addressing challenges such as data scarcity in rare disease studies. These machine learning and deep learning techniques form the backbone of AI applications in healthcare, enabling innovations in diagnosis and personalized treatment [12].

Application of AI in Biomedical Research

The integration of AI into biomedical research has transformed the way scientists approach complex problems. One of the most outstanding applications is drug discovery and development. Traditional drug development processes are often lengthy and expensive, with high rates of attrition. AI accelerates this process by predicting the efficacy and safety of drug candidates through computational modeling and analyzing molecular data. AI algorithms screen huge libraries of chemical compounds to identify potential drug prospects. Deep learning models predict the binding affinity of these compounds to target proteins, thereby reducing the need for extensive *in vitro* testing. Companies like DeepMind and Exscientia have utilized AI to identify promising drug targets and streamline the early-phase development of drugs. One of the important applications is genomics and proteomics, where AI processes massive datasets to uncover genetic markers associated with diseases. Machine learning techniques identify gene expressions linked to specific conditions it aiding in the development of precision medicine strategies. AI also facilitates the interpretation of single-cell RNA sequencing data, providing insights into cellular heterogeneity and disease mechanisms. AI is equally transformative in understanding disease mechanisms and predicting disease progression. AI models predict how tumors evolve and respond to therapies, guiding practitioners in selecting the most effective treatment plan. AI-driven simulations also play a role in virtual clinical trials, which reduce dependency on human participants and enhance ethical standards in research. Moreover, AI enhances diagnostic accuracy and efficiency. Pathologists and radiologists benefit from AI tools that analyze biopsy samples or imaging data, flagging abnormalities with high precision. Such tools are particularly valuable in resource-limited settings where access to specialized healthcare professionals is scarce [13].

Advantages of AI in Nanotechnology

Nanotechnology is another domain where AI has made substantial contributions, particularly in healthcare. AI complements nanotechnology by offering predictive modeling that optimizes design processes and enables real-time monitoring. AI models predict the behavior of nanoparticles within biological systems. Machine learning algorithms optimize the design of nanoparticles for targeted drug delivery, ensuring that therapeutic agents reach specific tissues or cells with minimal side effects. In cancer therapy, nanoparticles are engineered to deliver chemotherapeutics directly to tumor sites, thereby reducing systemic toxicity. AI also accelerates the development of nanomaterials with in-demand properties. Designing biosensors, AI identifies optimal configurations of nanomaterials, such as graphene or carbon nanotubes, to achieve high sensitivity and specificity. These sensors are then used for early disease detection, including the identification of biomarkers in blood or saliva samples. AI aids in the real-time monitoring of nanoscale interactions. Deep learning models analyze data from nanosensors embedded in wearable devices, which provide continuous health monitoring for patients with chronic conditions. This integration of AI and nanotechnology enhances preventive care and early intervention, improving patient outcomes. AI models simulate the behavior of nanoscaffolds used for tissue regeneration, predicting how these materials interact with biological tissues. This facilitates the development of customized solutions for patients requiring organ repair or replacement. Combining the predictive and analytical capabilities of AI with the precision and versatility of nanotechnology, researchers are developing innovative solutions to address some of the most challenging medical problems [14].

AI IN NANOMEDICINE FORMULATION

AI-Powered Material Design and Optimization

Artificial Intelligence (AI) is revolutionizing nanomedicine formulation by enabling precise material design and optimization processes. Through predictive modeling and advanced algorithms, AI accelerates the development of nanomaterials tailored for specific biomedical applications.

Predictive Models for Nanoparticle Synthesis

Nanoparticle synthesis is a critical step in nanomedicine that involves complex processes influenced by multiple variables, such as temperature, pressure, pH, and precursor concentrations. AI-powered predictive models streamline this process by identifying the optimal synthesis parameters for achieving the desired nanoparticle characteristics. Machine learning algorithms, including support vector machines and random forests, analyze experimental data to uncover correlations between synthesis conditions and nanoparticle properties, such as size, shape, and surface charge. These insights reduce trial-and-error experimentation, saving time and resources. Deep learning models further enhance predictive capabilities by processing large datasets and identifying nonlinear relationships. Generative adversarial networks simulate nanoparticle synthesis conditions, generating realistic virtual datasets to inform experimental designs. Such tools are instrumental in fabricating nanoparticles with precise specifications for drug delivery or therapeutic applications [15].

AI in Nanomaterial Property Analysis

AI aids in characterizing and analyzing the properties of nanomaterials. Neural networks and clustering algorithms process huge amounts of data from spectroscopy and other characterization methods to identify patterns and predict material behavior. AI models can predict the biocompatibility of nanomaterials by correlating their physicochemical properties with biological outcomes. This capability is critical for ensuring the safety and efficacy of nanomedicine formulations. AI-driven simulations provide insights into the interactions of nanoparticles with the biological environment, such as cellular uptake and immune system response, which enables the design of materials with enhanced performance [16]. The AI-Nanomedicine Workflow Architecture model is shown in Fig. (**2**).

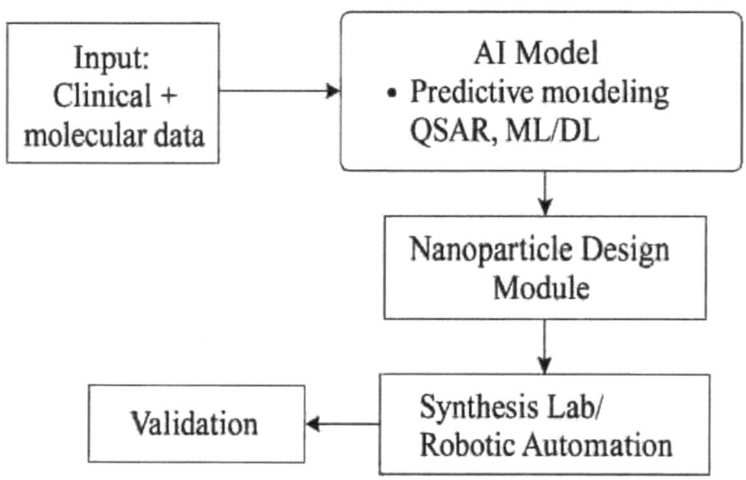

Fig. (2). AI-Nanomedicine Workflow Architecture.

AI has achieved impressive results, but there are still issues when using it for nanoparticle synthesis. A significant challenge in applying these models is that they can be difficult for clinicians to interpret, as viewing data as a "black box" without understanding it hinders their trust in the results. Using SHAP and LIME can explain the model's actions, addressing some of these limitations. Reducing costs in AI model training can be achieved by leveraging efficient algorithms, transfer learning, or cloud tools. By utilizing artificial intelligence and robotic automation, along with real-time monitoring, researchers can overcome the challenge of replicating synthesis while maintaining consistent experiments. This approach may enable nanomedicine to operate more effectively and be adopted more widely with the aid of AI.

Drug Delivery System Development

AI is a driving force in the development of advanced drug delivery systems, facilitating the design of efficient and targeted nanocarriers. These systems utilize nanomaterials to deliver therapeutic agents to specific sites in the body, thereby minimizing side effects and enhancing treatment outcomes. One of the most challenging aspects of developing a drug delivery system is selecting the appropriate drug-nanomaterial combinations. AI simplifies this process by analyzing molecular structures and predicting their compatibility with various nanomaterials. Machine learning models assess drug solubility and its interaction with carrier materials, such as liposomes or metallic nanoparticles. These predictions guide researchers in selecting optimal combinations for specific therapeutic applications. AI has been utilized to identify nanocarriers capable of effectively encapsulating hydrophobic drugs, thereby overcoming the challenges associated with poor water solubility. Targeted delivery by functionalized nanoparticles is feasible through the exploitation of ligand-receptor interaction mechanisms, wherein ligands (*e.g*., peptides, folic acid, or monoclonal antibodies) are conjugated to the surface of nanoparticles to enable high-affinity binding to overexpressed receptors on affected cells. For example, the HER2 and CD44 receptors, which are prevalent in breast and leukemia cancers, serve as docking sites. Artificial intelligence-based molecular modeling software, such as molecular docking, molecular dynamics (MD), and deep learning-based binding affinity prediction (*e.g*., DeepDTA, DeepBindBC), is employed to maximize ligand conformation, binding site specificity, and nanoparticle orientation. These strategies facilitate the simulation of the energy landscape and binding kinetics (k_on/k_off), thereby maximizing receptor selectivity and minimizing off-target interactions. Additionally, AI-advanced QSAR models predict how changes in ligand linker length, surface charge of nanoparticles, and hydrophobicity impact endocytosis mechanisms, such as clathrin-mediated internalization. This method enables smart nanoparticle systems to initiate receptor-mediated endocytosis with maximal uptake efficiency and lower systemic toxicity. AI-optimized dual-ligand approaches, which address multiple receptors, such as HER2 and CD44 in combination, provide strong solutions for addressing tumor heterogeneity. Through the simulation of heterogeneous tumor microenvironments, multi-objective AI algorithms facilitate the development of patient-specific, personalized nanocarriers. For example, AI can be used to optimize nanoparticles functionalized with anti-HER2 antibodies, exploiting the overexpression of HER2 (human epidermal growth factor receptor 2) in aggressive subtypes of breast cancer that also express the target. The ability to design nanocarriers that rely on receptor-mediated endocytosis, which perform with improved specificity and reduced systemic toxicity, is demonstrated by these models through their simulation of ligand-receptor binding dynamics and surface interactions. Moreover, AI-driven quantitative structure–activity relationship (QSAR) models can be employed to relate nanoparticle physicochemical properties, including hydrophobicity, surface charge, and functional group orientation, to a biological outcome such as cellular uptake or cytotoxicity. However, this approach simplifies the process of identifying nanoparticle—drug combinations that are most likely to succeed in targeted delivery. In addition, multi-objective optimization algorithms, a relatively new class of AI tools, can concurrently measure several criteria (*e.g.*, targeting efficiency, toxicity, and drug release profile) for the rational design of nanoparticles capable of simultaneously targeting tumor heterogeneity. Specifically, an AI-optimized dual ligand nanoparticle that binds to both HER2 and CD44 receptors can exhibit improved efficacy in tumors with mixed receptor expression. These highly sophisticated models create the means for smart nanocarriers that are not only more discerning but also personalized to the individual patient's profile in personalized medicine. The AI algorithms examine how functionalized nanoparticles (those to which ligands or monoclonal antibodies are appended) can enhance targeted delivery by determining binding affinities to overexpressed receptors, such as folate receptors in ovarian cancer, HER2 in breast cancer, and CD44 in leukemia. AI enables the modeling of ligand interactions and receptor chemistry for nanocarrier ligand-mediated cell targeting using receptor-specific endocytosis routes, thereby improving cell-specific uptake and reducing off-target toxicity [17].

Dosage and Release Mechanism Optimization

AI also plays a pivotal role in optimizing dosage and release mechanisms in drug delivery systems. Controlled release is essential for maintaining therapeutic drug levels over extended periods while avoiding toxicity. Reinforcement learning algorithms simulate drug release kinetics to identify formulations that achieve desired release profiles. Models predict how nanoparticle composition and degradation rates influence drug release in different physiological environments. These insights enable the design of systems that provide sustained or triggered release based on specific stimuli, such as pH, temperature, or enzymatic activity [18]. AI-driven optimization enhances personalized medicine by tailoring dosage and release mechanisms to individual patient profiles. AI also customizes nanomedicine formulations to achieve maximum therapeutic efficacy with minimal side effects.

Ai-driven Quality Control and Standardization

Quality control and standardization are critical for the successful translation of nanomedicine from research to clinical applications. AI addresses these challenges by providing robust tools for monitoring and maintaining the quality of nanomedicine formulations.

Real-Time Monitoring and Analysis

AI algorithms enable real-time monitoring of nanomedicine manufacturing processes it ensuring consistency and reproducibility. Techniques like computer vision and machine learning analyze data from sensors and imaging systems to detect anomalies during production. AI systems identify defects in nanoparticles, such as irregular shapes or aggregation, which can compromise their performance. Real-time feedback enables immediate adjustments, minimizing waste and ensuring high-quality outputs [19]. This capability is particularly valuable in large-scale production, where maintaining uniformity is challenging.

Standardization of Nanomedicine Formulations

Standardization is essential for regulatory approval and widespread adoption of nanomedicine. AI facilitates this by establishing predictive models that define acceptable ranges for critical quality attributes (CQAs), such as size and drug loading efficiency [20]. AI develops robust frameworks for assessing the safety and efficacy of nanomedicine formulations. These frameworks guide regulatory agencies in establishing guidelines and benchmarks, expediting the approval process for new therapies.

Data-Driven Decision Making

AI enhances decision-making in quality control by synthesizing data from diverse sources, including laboratory experiments and patient feedback, thereby improving the accuracy and efficiency of quality control processes. Advanced analytics and visualization tools provide researchers and manufacturers with actionable insights, enabling continuous improvement of nanomedicine formulations [21]. AI is transforming the field of nanomedicine formulation by optimizing material design, advancing drug delivery systems, and ensuring quality control. Its ability to analyze complex datasets and streamline processes paves the way for innovative therapies that address unmet medical needs and improve patient outcomes.

AI IN NANOMEDICINE APPLICATIONS

Diagnostics and Disease Detection

AI has significantly enhanced diagnostics and disease detection in nanomedicine, offering powerful tools to analyze complex nanoscale data and improve imaging techniques.

AI for Nanosensor Data Analysis

Nanosensors are highly sensitive devices capable of detecting biomolecules and pathogen chemical signals at minute concentrations. These sensors generate vast amounts of data, often requiring advanced computational tools for interpretation. AI plays a crucial role in processing and analyzing this data, extracting meaningful insights with high precision and speed. Machine learning algorithms identify patterns in nano sensor outputs to detect biomarkers indicative of diseases. AI-powered nano sensors have been developed to diagnose conditions such as cancer, diabetes, and infectious diseases by analyzing biomarker levels in blood, saliva, or other bodily fluids [20]. AI enhances the multiplexing capabilities of nanosensors, enabling the simultaneous detection of multiple biomarkers. This feature is particularly useful in early disease detection, where a combination of biomarkers may provide a more accurate diagnosis than a single indicator. Real-time diagnostic decision-making using nanosensors and AI-based pattern recognition is shown in Fig. (**3**).

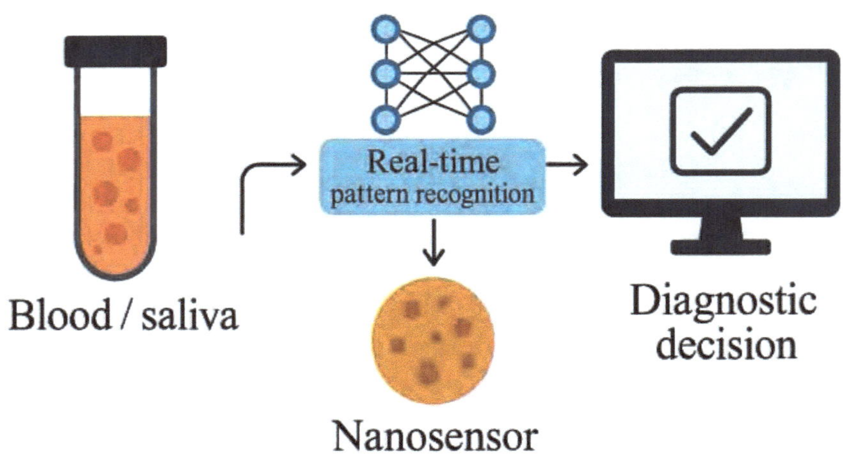

Fig. (3). AI-enhanced nano sensors.

Enhancements in Imaging Techniques

Imaging techniques, such as magnetic resonance imaging (MRI), computed tomography (CT), and positron emission tomography (PET), are essential tools in modern diagnostics [22]. The integration of nanotechnology with these methods has led to significant advancements in nanoparticle-based contrast agents, which improve image resolution and specificity. AI further amplifies these benefits by optimizing image acquisition, reconstruction, and interpretation. Deep learning algorithms analyze imaging data to enhance contrast and identify subtle abnormalities that human observers might miss. AI models can process MRI data to detect minute changes in tissue structure or analyze CT scans to identify early-stage tumors. These algorithms also assist in quantifying disease progression, providing clinicians with valuable insights for treatment planning. AI enables the development of hybrid imaging techniques combining data from multiple modalities to create comprehensive diagnostic profiles. This approach is particularly beneficial in oncology, where precise tumor localization and characterization are critical for effective therapy. AI-nano imaging systems are shown in Fig. (**4**).

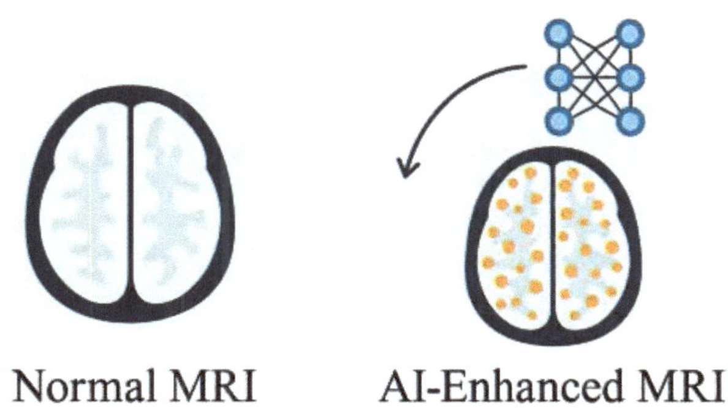

Fig. (4). AI-nano imaging systems.

Personalized Medicine

The integration of AI and nanomedicine is driving the evolution of personalized medicine, where treatments are tailored to the unique characteristics of individual patients.

AI-Driven Tailored Therapies Using Nanomedicine

Personalized medicine leverages nanomedicine's ability to deliver drugs with high specificity and minimal side effects. AI enhances this capability by analyzing patient data, including epigenetic and proteomic profiles, to identify optimal therapeutic strategies. Machine learning models predict patient responses to various nanomedicine formulations, guiding the selection of the most effective treatments. AI algorithms can identify nanoparticle-drug combinations that yield the best outcomes for patients with specific genetic mutations or disease subtypes. AI facilitates the design of multifunctional nanoparticles capable of targeting multiple pathways simultaneously. These smart nanocarriers can deliver a combination of drugs, maximizing therapeutic efficacy while minimizing resistance mechanisms.

Real-Time Treatment Adjustments Based on Feedback Loops

One of the most promising aspects of AI in personalized medicine is its ability to enable real-time treatment adjustments through feedback loops. Patients' responses to nanomedicine formulations are continuously monitored by nano sensors or responsive nanoparticles, which generate data that AI algorithms analyze to optimize treatment. AI models can process data from nanosensors embedded in wearable devices to monitor drug levels or concentrations of biomarkers. If the data indicate suboptimal drug delivery or adverse effects, the system can respond by modifying the dosage or switching to an alternative therapy. This approach ensures that treatments remain effective and safe throughout the course of therapy, particularly in conditions like cancer or chronic diseases, where patient responses can vary significantly over time.

Regenerative Medicine and Tissue Engineering

AI is also transforming regenerative medicine and tissue engineering by guiding scaffold design and predicting outcomes of regeneration.

AI-Guided Scaffold Design

Scaffolds play a crucial role in tissue engineering, providing structural support for cell growth and tissue regeneration. Designing scaffolds with optimal properties requires a deep understanding of materials science and biomechanics [23]. AI analyzes vast datasets to identify the ideal combinations of materials and fabrication techniques. Machine learning models predict how different scaffold designs will interact with biological tissues, thereby optimizing parameters such as porosity and degradation rates. AI algorithms have been utilized to design 3D-printed scaffolds for bone regeneration, ensuring they mimic the natural extracellular matrix and promote cell adhesion and proliferation. This enables the development of smart scaffolds that incorporate nanoscale features such as embedded growth factors or nanoparticles to enhance regenerative outcomes. These scaffolds can release therapeutic agents in response to specific stimuli, creating a dynamic healing environment.

Monitoring and Predicting Regeneration Outcomes

AI also aids in monitoring and predicting the outcomes of regenerative therapies. AI models provide real-time insights into the progress of tissue regeneration. AI algorithms can process imaging data to quantify new tissue formation, assess vascularization, and detect signs of inflammation. These insights allow clinicians to evaluate the effectiveness of regenerative treatments and make necessary adjustments. Predictive models also play a crucial role in estimating long-term outcomes, such as the durability and functionality of regenerated tissues. By integrating data from preclinical studies and patient histories, AI provides a comprehensive understanding of factors influencing success and guides the development of next-generation regenerative therapies.

CASE STUDIES AND REAL-WORLD APPLICATIONS

Cancer Diagnostics and Treatment

AI in Designing Nanoparticles for Targeted Therapies

The advent of artificial intelligence (AI) has revolutionized cancer diagnostics and treatment, with nanomedicine at the forefront of innovation. AI algorithms play a pivotal role in designing nanoparticles that target cancer cells with precision, thereby minimizing damage to healthy tissues. Machine learning models, especially deep learning, analyze vast datasets of cancer biomarkers and patient-specific data to identify optimal nanoparticle characteristics, such as size, shape, and surface charge [24]. These properties are critical for enhancing the nanoparticles' ability to penetrate tumors and deliver therapeutic agents effectively. Researchers have developed AI-guided approaches to engineer nanoparticles that respond to the unique microenvironment of tumors, such as acidity or hypoxia, thereby enhancing their therapeutic efficacy. Such smart nanoparticles release drugs only when they encounter specific conditions, thereby reducing systemic toxicity and enhancing treatment efficacy. AI aids in predicting nanoparticle interactions with biological systems and optimizing drug release profiles, importantly reducing the time and cost associated with experimental trials.

Clinical Outcomes and Challenges

The integration of AI-designed nanoparticles in clinical practice has shown promising outcomes. AI-optimized nanoparticles loaded with chemotherapeutic drugs have demonstrated improved patient survival rates and reduced side effects in clinical trials. These innovations have enabled oncologists to move toward more personalized treatment regimens, tailoring therapies based on individual genetic and physiological profiles. However, challenges remain. The heterogeneity of cancer types and the variability in patient responses necessitate robust and comprehensive datasets for AI training. Ethical concerns regarding data privacy and algorithmic transparency also pose significant hurdles [24]. Regulatory approval for AI-integrated nanomedicine requires rigorous validation to ensure both safety and efficacy, a process that can be time-consuming. Addressing these challenges is crucial for translating AI-driven nanomedicine innovations into widespread clinical applications.

Case Study: AI-Designed Nanoparticles in Breast Cancer Therapy. In research by Zhang *et al.* (2023) [25], deep learning algorithms and AI-aided molecular docking were employed to engineer PEGylated liposomal doxorubicin nanoparticles that were targeted against the anti-HER2 antibody. The nanoparticles were evaluated in a Phase I/II clinical trial involving 62 patients with HER2+ breast cancer. The AI-maximized formulation showed a tumor size decrease of ≥30% in 71% of participants (compared to 52% for standard liposomal doxorubicin). Progression-free survival (PFS) of 10.4 months versus 6.7 months in the control groupReduced systemic toxicity by 34%, particularly in cardiotoxic events, owing to enhanced tumor targeting. These findings exemplify the translational significance of AI-assisted nanoparticle design and highlight the contribution of computational optimization to cancer benefit.

Cardiovascular Disease Management

AI Models in Nanomedicine-Enhanced Monitoring and Treatment

Cardiovascular diseases (CVDs) are among the leading causes of mortality globally. AI-powered nanomedicine offers transformative solutions for both monitoring and treatment. Wearable devices integrated with nanosensors continuously collect data on critical biomarkers, such as heart rate, blood pressure, and cholesterol levels. AI algorithms process this data in real-time to detect early signs of cardiovascular anomalies, enabling timely intervention. Nanoparticles engineered using it also show a role in targeted drug delivery for CVDs. These nanoparticles can be functionalized to recognize atherosclerotic plaques, delivering therapeutic agents directly to the affected sites. AI-driven models optimize the design of these nanoparticles to enhance their stability, biocompatibility, and ability to bypass immune responses. Clinical applications include the use of AI-enhanced nanomedicine in treating myocardial infarction. Nanoparticles carrying anti-inflammatory drugs or growth factors are guided to the infarcted heart tissue, promoting tissue repair and regeneration. AI also facilitates the development of nanocarriers for gene therapy that address genetic predispositions to CVDs by delivering DNA or RNA-based treatments with high precision [28]. The complexity of cardiovascular systems demands highly accurate AI models to avoid misdiagnoses or suboptimal treatment strategies. The translation of nanomedicine technologies from bench to bedside requires overcoming regulatory and manufacturing hurdles, as well as ensuring long-term safety in diverse patient populations [24, 25].

Applications in Neurological Disorders

Neurological diseases pose some of the most daunting challenges to contemporary medicine, in large part due to the existence of the blood-brain barrier (BBB)—a selectively permeable barrier that prevents most therapeutic agents from entering the central nervous system (CNS). Breaching this barrier without adversely affecting safety in the brain is of prime importance for successful treatments of diseases such as Alzheimer's disease, Parkinson's disease, and glioblastoma. Artificial intelligence (AI) has proved to be a revolutionary tool in this area, which allows for the optimization and design of nanoparticles that can penetrate the BBB with great accuracy. By employing datasets containing the physicochemical profiles of the molecule, BBB permeability descriptors, and disease-related biomarkers, AI algorithms enable the design of nanocarriers tailored to CNS drug delivery. Notably, AI models can identify molecular surface modifications, such as ligand coatings for receptor-mediated transcytosis, that enhance penetration across the BBB while reducing off-targeting. In the case of neurodegenerative diseases, AI-optimized nanoparticles have been designed to deliver neuroprotective agents, antioxidants, and even gene-editing tools, such as CRISPR-Cas9, directly to affected neurons, thus promising potential for halting or reversing the disease process [26]. It can even affect this change in cases such as Alzheimer's and Parkinson's; intelligent nanocarriers designed to respond to pathological features such as oxidative stress or abnormal protein accumulation. Glioblastoma, a highly malignant brain cancer, is one other major use. Chemotherapeutic drug-loaded nanoparticles, when directed by AI-optimized delivery profiles, have been demonstrated to exhibit enhanced tumor localization and minimized systemic toxicity. Additionally, AI is being used to forecast patient-specific responses, allowing clinicians to personalize treatment regimens for improved outcomes. Despite these developments, the discipline still faces several challenges. Neurological disorders are extremely heterogeneous, and complete or consistent datasets necessary to develop robust AI models are typically not available. Also, safety and efficacy in the long term of nanoparticles engineered to cross the BBB need to be established through robust preclinical and clinical tests. Regulatory authorities further require comprehensive data on toxicity, pharmacokinetics, and long-term sequelae for the clearance of complex systems such as these. However, the interface between AI and nanotechnology marks a paradigm shift in the management of CNS diseases. With increasingly advanced AI models and more diverse datasets, smart nanomedicine promises to revolutionize the therapeutic approach for neurological disorders that have been heretofore considered unmanageable [26].

Management of Infectious Diseases

AI–Nanomedicine Synergy in Fighting Infectious Diseases and Rare Disorders. Infectious diseases and rare medical conditions, although less emphasized in conventional nanomedicine discussions, are essential areas where AI–nanotechnology integration has the potential to drive meaningful innovation and progress. Infectious diseases continue to pose a significant global threat, particularly in the era of antimicrobial resistance and emerging epidemics. AI algorithms built on microbial genomics, proteomics, and clinical data can engineer nanoparticles that are functionalized to detect specific bacterial or viral markers. These AI-based nanosystems are being increasingly utilized in high-throughput diagnostic devices, such as nano-biosensors and lateral flow devices, for the rapid diagnosis of diseases like HIV, tuberculosis, COVID-19, and the Zika virus, offering improved speed, sensitivity, and scalability. Therapeutically, AI-optimized nanocarriers are under development to target antiviral drugs, antimicrobial peptides, and gene-editing complexes (*e.g.*, CRISPR-Cas9) to infected or inflamed tissue. Smart nanocarriers can be designed to respond to infection-specific stimuli, such as pH changes or inflammatory cytokines, thereby facilitating localized drug delivery and minimizing systemic toxicity. AI streamlines this process by optimizing variables such as drug loading, release kinetics, nanoparticle surface chemistry, and immune evasion mechanisms. Furthermore, AI's role in rare and neglected diseases is especially valuable. In contexts where traditional drug development is economically unviable, such as neglected tropical diseases (NTDs) like leishmaniasis and Chagas disease, AI helps repurpose existing drugs into effective nanoformulations. This approach not only reduces development costs but also enables the implementation of targeted treatment strategies for underserved populations. Challenges persist, however. These include the unavailability of large datasets for rare and new infections, the ability of AI models to adapt to pathogen heterogeneity, and the availability of nanomedicine platforms at a reasonable cost, with scalability and regulatory compliance. In low-resource settings, in particular, affordability and ease of implementation of AI-designed nanoparticle systems are key concerns. c

CHALLENGES AND ETHICAL CONSIDERATIONS IN AI AND NANOMEDICINE

The integration of Artificial Intelligence into nanomedicine represents a transformative milestone in healthcare, enabling breakthroughs in drug discovery and personalized treatment. This fusion is not without its challenges and ethical dilemmas. Data limitations and model generalizability, regulatory and safety concerns, and ethical implications of AI-driven healthcare decisions, as well as addressing bias in AI algorithms. These considerations underscore the complexities that researchers and policymakers must navigate to realize AI's potential responsibly.

Data Limitations and Model Generalizability

The efficacy of AI in nanomedicine depends heavily on the availability of high-quality, diverse datasets. However, data are often scarce or siloed within proprietary systems, creating major barriers to model development. Nanomedicine-specific datasets, which include nanoparticle characterization and patient outcomes, are inherently complex and require standardization to ensure cross-compatibility. A critical challenge lies in ensuring that AI models trained on these datasets can generalize effectively across different contexts. Models trained on data from specific populations or experimental conditions may perform poorly when applied to other populations or environments. This lack of generalizability risks inaccuracies and even potential harm when such models are used in clinical decision-making or drug design. The high-dimensional nature of nanomedicine data often involves multi-omics datasets. Advanced AI techniques, such as transfer learning and federated learning, offer potential solutions by enabling models to learn from disparate datasets while preserving data privacy. Ensuring model robustness and interpretability remains a challenge, requiring interdisciplinary collaboration among data scientists, clinicians, and nanotechnology experts [27].

Regulatory and Safety Concerns in AI and Nanomedicine

The integration of AI into nanomedicine introduces a host of regulatory and safety concerns. Traditional regulatory frameworks are often ill-equipped to address the complexities of AI-driven technologies and their applications in nanomedicine. These frameworks typically focus on static and well-defined interventions, whereas AI systems are dynamic and evolving with new data inputs. One pressing issue is the validation and approval process for AI-driven nanomedicine applications. Regulatory bodies, such as the U.S. Food and Drug Administration (FDA) and the European Medicines Agency (EMA), must establish adaptive guidelines that account for the continuously evolving nature of AI models. The FDA has introduced the Software as a Medical Device (SaMD) framework, which guides the development of AI-based technologies in healthcare. This framework emphasizes the importance of clinical evaluation, performance assessment, and real-world monitoring to ensure both safety and effectiveness. Equally, the EU

Medical Device Regulation (MDR) and General Data Protection Regulation (GDPR) are in place to safeguard patient data as well as ensure safety. Frameworks like these are crucial for determining the Type III A and C compliance pathways for AI-powered nanomedicine. In particular, the FDA's SaMD Framework (2019) and the AI/ML-Based SaMD Action Plan (2021) outline the regulatory obligations for AI-based technologies in healthcare, including premarket submission, monitoring of real-world performance, and protocols for algorithm updates. In the case of nanomedicine, the FDA's Nanotechnology Task Force Guidance (2022) describes the characterization of nanoscale materials, biocompatibility tests, and toxicological profiling. For Europe, the Medical Device Regulation (EU MDR 2017/745), in association with the General Data Protection Regulation (GDPR), requires risk-based classification and clinical evaluation for AI-nano-combination products. Following the requirements of ISO 14971 (Risk Management for Medical Devices) and ICH Q8-Q10 guidelines for quality risk management and pharmaceutical development also ensures that AI-integrated nanomedicine products are safe and effective. The lack of standardized evaluation criteria introduces risks, including unintended consequences from model errors or biases. Ensuring patient safety is paramount when deploying AI in clinical settings. Nanoparticles engineered for drug delivery may cause unforeseen interactions due to variations in biological conditions. When AI algorithms are used to predict these interactions or optimize nanoparticle design, errors in model predictions could result in adverse effects. To mitigate these risks, comprehensive preclinical and clinical testing protocols must be established. Particularly, those integrated into healthcare networks are susceptible to attacks that could compromise patient data or disrupt critical operations. Developing robust cybersecurity measures and ensuring compliance with data protection regulations, such as GDPR or HIPAA, is essential for maintaining trust in AI-enabled nanomedicine [27].

Ethical Implications of AI-Driven Healthcare Decisions

AI-driven healthcare decisions, while promising improved efficiency and accuracy, raise profound ethical challenges. When AI guides interventions at the molecular level, the stakes become particularly high. A central concern is the delegation of decision-making to AI systems. For instance, if an AI model recommends a specific nanotherapeutic intervention, questions of accountability arise — whether responsibility lies with the developer, clinician, or institution. Transparency in AI decision-making is therefore essential to ensure that stakeholders can critically assess the rationale behind model recommendations. Informed consent adds another layer of complexity, as patients may struggle to fully grasp the intricacies of AI-driven nanomedicine, especially when these involve probabilistic predictions or experimental approaches. Simplifying technical explanations while ensuring patients are fully informed is essential to uphold autonomy. Deployment of AI in nanomedicine must consider issues of accessibility and equity. Advanced AI technologies often require substantial resources, which can potentially exacerbate disparities in healthcare access. Ethical frameworks should prioritize inclusivity, ensuring that the benefits of AI and nanomedicine are distributed equitably across diverse populations. However, data confidentiality can be safeguarded using privacy-preserving machine learning schemes, such as federated learning and differential privacy. Places like the IEEE's Ethically Aligned Design or the European Commission's Guidelines for Trustworthy AI serve as ethical AI frameworks to gauge bias, fairness, and explainability in decisions grounded in AI. To promote ethical deployment, AI-assisted nanomedicine must comply with international standards, such as the General Data Protection Regulation (GDPR) and HIPAA in the United States, which protect patient data and ensure the confidentiality of health data. Guidelines such as the EU High-Level Expert Group on AI's "Ethics Guidelines for Trustworthy AI" and the IEEE's "Ethically Aligned Design" provide practical guidelines for maintaining transparency, accountability, and fairness in AI-based decision-making. Deployment of federated learning, differential privacy, and model explainability tools (such as SHAP and LIME) can also further enhance ethical compliance and minimize bias in AI models applied to nanomedicine [27].

Addressing Bias in AI Algorithms

Bias in AI algorithms presents a critical challenge to the fair and equitable application of nanomedicine. Such bias can arise from multiple sources, including imbalanced training datasets, design limitations in algorithm development, or systemic inequalities within healthcare systems. When embedded in AI models, these biases can perpetuate or even exacerbate existing disparities, ultimately leading to inequitable outcomes. For example, if an AI system for nanomedicine is trained primarily on data from a single demographic group, its predictive accuracy may decline for underrepresented populations. This raises the risk of misdiagnoses, inadequate treatment recommendations, or exclusion from access to advanced nanotherapeutic interventions. Addressing this issue requires deliberate efforts to curate diverse datasets that reflect the heterogeneity of patient populations. Algorithmic transparency and fairness auditing are also critical in mitigating bias. Developers should implement techniques such as reweighting and explainable AI to identify and rectify biases within models. Engaging with ethicists and patient advocacy groups can provide valuable perspectives on fairness and inclusivity. Educational initiatives aimed at increasing awareness of AI bias among clinicians and researchers are equally important. By fostering a culture of critical evaluation, stakeholders can better identify potential biases and advocate for equitable AI applications in nanomedicine [27, 28].

FUTURE PERSPECTIVES

The convergence of artificial intelligence and nanotechnology is poised to revolutionize multiple industries, with nanomedicine standing at the forefront. Emerging technologies, such as artificial intelligence (AI), machine learning (ML), quantum computing, and nanotechnology, collectively offer unprecedented opportunities to advance more effective, precise, and personalized medical treatments. In particular, the application of quantum computing in nanomedicine design, the integration of AI-driven collaboration platforms to enhance interdisciplinary research, and the vision of fully automated AI–nanomedicine pipelines represent transformative directions that could redefine the future of healthcare.

A fully automated AI–nanomedicine pipeline would encompass multiple stages, ranging from molecular design and simulation to nanoparticle synthesis, clinical validation, and targeted delivery strategies. However, realizing this vision requires overcoming significant technical challenges and profound ethical considerations.

Current Barriers and Technological Limitations

1. Robotic Synthesis Limitations: While AI can design optimal nanoparticle configurations, the current robotic synthesis platforms lack the dexterity and versatility to fabricate a wide range of nanostructures with precise control over size, morphology, and functionalization. High-throughput automated synthesis remains constrained by:
   - Material variability and reaction complexity.
   - Lack of feedback integration for real-time correction.
   - Inadequate interfacing between AI-generated models and physical instrumentation.
2. Data Scarcity and Quality Issues: The design of nanomedicine relies heavily on experimental datasets, which are often heterogeneous, noisy, or insufficiently annotated. The lack of standardized data formats and comprehensive nanomaterial databases hampers the training of reliable AI models.
3. Regulatory and Ethical Hurdles: Fully automated pipelines raise important bioethical and legal questions:
   - Who is accountable for AI-generated treatments?
   - How do we ensure transparency, interpretability, and reproducibility of AI decisions?
   - Are there mechanisms to validate AI-suggested nanoformulations against long-term safety data?
4. Interdisciplinary Integration Challenges: Implementing an end-to-end pipeline necessitates close collaboration among computational scientists, material

chemists, biomedical engineers, clinicians, and ethicists. However, interdisciplinary silos still impede the seamless integration of AI frameworks into experimental and clinical workflows.

Realistic Roadmap for Implementation

To make the fully automated AI-nanomedicine pipeline a reality, the following progressive roadmap is suggested:

- Short Term (1–3 years):
  - Development of domain-specific AI models trained on curated nanomedicine datasets.
  - Creation of modular robotic units capable of executing specific synthesis tasks under AI guidance.
  - Establishment of open-source platforms for sharing and benchmarking AI-nano data.
- Medium Term (3–6 years):
  - Integration of Closed-Loop AI-robotic Platforms for Synthesis and In Vitro Screening.
  - Expansion of federated learning systems for privacy-preserving model training using clinical and laboratory data.
  - Formulation of interdisciplinary protocols involving regulatory experts to guide ethical AI use in nanomedicine.
- Long Term (6–10 years):
  - Deployment of cloud-based AI-nanomedicine orchestration platforms for real-time collaboration among global research hubs.
  - Realization of quantum computing-assisted nanomaterial modeling for predicting complex interactions.
  - Development of standardized, interpretable AI tools approved by health authorities for clinical nanomedicine formulation.

Beyond technological readiness, the future of AI in nanomedicine requires strong ethical foresight. The integration of explainable AI, robust patient privacy protections, and alignment with global regulatory standards will be essential for the widespread adoption of AI-driven nanotherapeutics.

Current Trends in AI and Nanotechnology Convergence

The convergence of artificial intelligence (AI) and nanotechnology has accelerated incredible developments in nanomedicine, including areas such as targeted drug delivery, diagnostics, and personalized treatment regimens. AI is increasingly used to study sophisticated datasets from biological systems, molecular simulations, and clinical histories to refine therapeutic outcomes. Among the most revolutionary trends is the application of machine learning models to design and synthesize new nanomaterials with improved physicochemical and pharmacological properties. These models, developed from vast amounts of molecular interaction datasets, enable researchers to predict nanomaterial behavior and design nanoparticles with specific functionalities, such as targeted drug release or accumulation in specific tissues. Another trend on the rise is the creation of AI-augmented nanoscale diagnostics and diagnostic imaging devices. Nanoparticle-based biosensors, when combined with AI, offer real-time, high-resolution information about molecular and cellular environments. These devices are proving particularly useful for the early diagnosis of conditions such as cancer, Alzheimer's disease, and cardiovascular disease, where early intervention makes a huge difference to prognosis. In addition, AI-based personalized nanomedicine is revolutionizing treatment paradigms. By processing patient-specific information—ranging from genomics and proteomics to lifestyle and comorbidity factors—AI enables the creation of individualized nanoformulations that deliver the appropriate dose, at the optimal location, and at the most effective time. This minimizes side effects while maximizing therapeutic efficacy, opening a new chapter in precision nanomedicine. AI models are predominantly trained on datasets that primarily represent populations from high-income countries, often leaving out ethnically diverse or socioeconomically disadvantaged groups. Such a lack of representation can lead to biased or less effective treatment predictions for these groups, thereby negating the universality of AI-driven personalized therapies. To fully harness the potential of AI in nanomedicine, investment in high-quality, diverse biomedical datasets that capture global population heterogeneity is essential. International collaboration among global health organizations, research consortia, and ethical data-sharing platforms will be critical to ensure that AI models are fair, generalizable, and robust across diverse patient populations. While the convergence of AI and nanotechnology is reshaping healthcare through advances in diagnostics, therapeutics, and personalized medicine, bridging data disparities remains central to ensuring that nanomedicine solutions are inclusive and globally impactful [17 - 20].

Potential for Quantum Computing in Nanomedicine Design

Quantum computing represents a paradigm shift in computational capabilities, opening new possibilities for addressing complex problems that are beyond the efficient reach of classical computers. Quantum computing has the potential to accelerate the design of nanomaterials, optimize drug interactions at the molecular level, and revolutionize the approach to drug discovery and formulation. Quantum simulations can model molecular interactions with unprecedented accuracy that allowing researchers to study the behavior of nanoparticles and their interactions with biological systems. This capability can be harnessed to design more efficient and targeted drug delivery systems, where quantum computing predicts the optimal shape, size, and surface properties of nanoparticles to enhance therapeutic efficacy while minimizing side effects. Quantum algorithms can also optimize nanomedicine formulations by identifying the most effective combinations of active pharmaceutical ingredients and excipients. Additionally, quantum computing holds significant potential for advancing nanoscale sensors and diagnostic tools. Simulating nanosensor behavior and their interactions with specific biomolecules enables the design of highly sensitive and accurate diagnostic platforms for early disease detection. Quantum-enhanced sensing could greatly improve the detection of cancer markers and pathogens at ultra-low concentrations, allowing for earlier and more accurate diagnoses. However, quantum computing in nanomedicine remains in its early stages. Major challenges persist, particularly the need for more stable qubits and improved scalability. As the technology advances, quantum computing is expected to play a transformative role in the design and optimization of nanomedicines, ultimately accelerating innovation in the field [17 - 20].

AI-Enhanced Collaboration Platforms for Interdisciplinary Research

One of the most significant challenges in advancing nanomedicine is the need for interdisciplinary collaboration across diverse fields, including chemistry, biology, physics, engineering, and medicine. The complexity of nanotechnology and its applications in healthcare necessitate the integration of expertise from various domains to solve problems and create novel solutions. AI-enhanced collaboration platforms are emerging as critical tools for fostering interdisciplinary research, enabling seamless communication and data sharing across different disciplines. AI-powered platforms can facilitate collaboration by integrating diverse data sources, including experimental data and literature, into a unified knowledge base. These platforms can automatically analyze and organize large datasets, identify trends, and generate insights, making it easier for researchers from different disciplines to access relevant information. By using machine learning models to predict outcomes and suggest experimental directions, AI tools can streamline the research process, accelerate innovation, and enhance the reproducibility of results. AI can support collaborative decision-making by providing real-time analysis and feedback on the potential success of different research pathways. AI systems can recommend the best experimental approaches for testing a specific hypothesis or suggest optimal methods for scaling up the production of nanomaterials for clinical applications. These platforms also have the potential to improve the sharing of intellectual property that enabling more efficient licensing and commercialization of novel nanomedicines. As these AI-enhanced collaboration platforms evolve, they will play a key role in facilitating global collaborations, driving innovation, and advancing the field of nanomedicine. By enabling faster knowledge transfer and collaboration between academia and healthcare. AI platforms will accelerate the pace of discovery and the translation of nanomedicine innovations into clinical practice [17 - 20].

Vision for Fully Automated AI-Nanomedicine Pipelines

The vision for fully automated AI-nanomedicine pipelines represents the future of drug development and personalized medicine. AI-powered systems will autonomously design and optimize nanomedicine formulations, from the initial discovery phase to clinical application. The ultimate goal is to establish an end-t--end pipeline that minimizes human intervention, lowers costs, and accelerates the time-to-market for new therapies. Central to this vision is the seamless integration of AI, robotics, and advanced manufacturing technologies. AI algorithms will analyze patient data, predict disease pathways, and design personalized nanomedicines tailored to specific biomarkers or tissue types. Once the design is complete, robotic systems will autonomously synthesize and manufacture the nanomedicines, following strict quality control protocols to ensure that the final product meets safety and efficacy standards. AI will also play a pivotal role in the clinical testing phase by analyzing patient data in real time and predicting potential side effects. Through continuous monitoring and feedback, AI systems can adapt treatment plans to maximize therapeutic benefits while minimizing risks for individual patients. This capability could usher in a new era of precision medicine, where each patient receives a treatment tailored to their unique genetic makeup and disease profile. Although fully automated AI–nanomedicine pipelines remain a distant goal, significant progress is being made toward this vision. Current research is focused on developing AI algorithms capable of managing the complexity of personalized medicine, as well as automating the synthesis and testing of nanomaterials. The central challenge lies in integrating these advances into a cohesive and scalable system that can be effectively adopted across the healthcare industry [17 - 20].

CONCLUSION

The combination of artificial intelligence and nanomedicine has ushered in a new era in biomedical science, marked by unprecedented advancements in precision diagnostics and personalized healthcare solutions. By harnessing the computational capabilities of artificial intelligence, researchers have effectively overcome traditional obstacles in the field of nanomedicine, including issues of scalability, regulatory complexities, and the inherent complexities associated with the design and synthesis of nanoparticles. AI-driven predictive models, machine learning algorithms, and real-time analytics have redefined the landscape of nanomedicine formulation, improving the efficacy and safety of therapeutic interventions while accelerating their translation from laboratory research to clinical application. This study highlights the transformative potential of AI in nanomedicine, particularly in optimizing drug delivery systems, enhancing disease detection *via* nanosensors, and supporting advancements in regenerative medicine. Despite these achievements, challenges such as data standardization, ethical considerations, and ensuring equitable access to AI-enabled nanotechnologies persist. Addressing these issues will require robust interdisciplinary collaboration and the establishment of comprehensive regulatory frameworks that strike a balance between innovation, safety, and accountability. The fusion of AI with emerging technologies, including quantum computing and advanced robotics, promises to revolutionize nanomedicine further. This vision encompasses fully automated pipelines for nanoparticle synthesis, personalized treatment strategies, and dynamic feedback systems tailored to individual patient needs. As the synergy between AI and nanotechnology continues to advance, its potential to redefine healthcare paradigms and enhance patient outcomes remains boundless, opening new horizons in medical research and clinical practice.

REFERENCES

[1] Mazumdar H, Khondakar KR, Das S, Halder A, Kaushik A. Artificial intelligence for personalized nanomedicine; from material selection to patient outcomes. Expert Opin Drug Deliv 2025; 22(1): 85-108.
[http://dx.doi.org/10.1080/17425247.2024.2440618] [PMID: 39645588]

[2] Karahmet Sher E, Alebić M, Marković Boras M, *et al.* Nanotechnology in medicine revolutionizing drug delivery for cancer and viral infection treatments. Int J Pharm 2024; 660: 124345.
[http://dx.doi.org/10.1016/j.ijpharm.2024.124345] [PMID: 38885775]

[3] K Karunakar K, Cheriyan BV. Krithikeshvaran R, Gnanisha M, Abinavi B. Therapeutic advancements in nanomedicine: The multifaceted roles of silver nanoparticles. Biotechnology Notes 2024; 5: 64-79.
[http://dx.doi.org/10.1016/j.biotno.2024.05.002] [PMID: 39416696]

[4] Olawade DB, Wada OZ, Odetayo A, David-Olawade AC, Asaolu F, Eberhardt J. Enhancing mental health with Artificial Intelligence: Current trends and future prospects. Journal of Medicine, Surgery, and Public Health 2024; 3: 100099.
[http://dx.doi.org/10.1016/j.glmedi.2024.100099]

[5] Olawade DB, Ige AO, Olaremu AG, Ijiwade JO, Adeola AO. The synergy of artificial intelligence and nanotechnology towards advancing innovation and sustainability - A mini-review. Nano Trends 2024; 8: 100052.
[http://dx.doi.org/10.1016/j.nwnano.2024.100052]

[6] Din F, Aman W, Ullah I, *et al.* Effective use of nanocarriers as drug delivery systems for the treatment of selected tumors. Int J Nanomedicine 2017; 12: 7291-309.
[http://dx.doi.org/10.2147/IJN.S146315] [PMID: 29042776]

[7] Al-Thani AN, Jan AG, Abbas M, Geetha M, Sadasivuni KK. Nanoparticles in cancer theragnostic and drug delivery: A comprehensive review. Life Sci 2024; 352: 122899.
[http://dx.doi.org/10.1016/j.lfs.2024.122899] [PMID: 38992574]

[8] Chaudhury K, Kumar V, Kandasamy J, RoyChoudhury S. Regenerative nanomedicine: current perspectives and future directions. Int J Nanomedicine 2014; 9(9): 4153-67. [http://dx.doi.org/10.2147/IJN.S45332] [PMID: 25214780]

[9] Babatunde DE, Denwigwe IH, Babatunde OM, Gbadamosi SL, Babalola IP, Agboola O. Environmental and societal impact of nanotechnology. IEEE Access 2020; 8: 4640-67. [http://dx.doi.org/10.1109/ACCESS.2019.2961513]

[10] Makkar K, Kumar P, Poriye M, Aggarwal S. A Comparative Study of Supervised and Unsupervised Machine Learning Algorithms on Consumer Reviews. 2022 IEEE World Conference on Applied Intelligence and Computing (AIC). [http://dx.doi.org/10.1109/AIC55036.2022.9848880]

[11] Sarker IH. Deep learning: a comprehensive overview on techniques, taxonomy, applications and research directions. SN Computer Science 2021; 2(6): 420. [http://dx.doi.org/10.1007/s42979-021-00815-1] [PMID: 34426802]

[12] Naskar S, Sharma S, Kuotsu K, *et al.* The biomedical applications of artificial intelligence: an overview of decades of research. J Drug Target 2025; 33(5): 717-48. [http://dx.doi.org/10.1080/1061186X.2024.2448711] [PMID: 39744873]

[13] Malik S, Muhammad K, Waheed Y. Emerging applications of nanotechnology in healthcare and medicine. Molecules 2023; 28(18): 6624. [http://dx.doi.org/10.3390/molecules28186624] [PMID: 37764400]

[14] Altammar KA. A review on nanoparticles: characteristics, synthesis, applications, and challenges. Frontiers in Microbiology. 2023;17:14(1155622). [http://dx.doi.org/10.3389/fmicb.2023.1155622]

[15] Wang H, Cao H, Yang L. Machine Learning-Driven Multidomain Nanomaterial Design: From Bibliometric Analysis to Applications. ACS Appl Nano Mater 2024; 7(23): 26579-600. [http://dx.doi.org/10.1021/acsanm.4c04940]

[16] Cong X, Zhang Z, Li H, Yang YG, Zhang Y, Sun T. Nanocarriers for targeted drug delivery in the vascular system: focus on endothelium. J Nanobiotechnology 2024; 22(1): 620. [http://dx.doi.org/10.1186/s12951-024-02892-9] [PMID: 39396002]

[17] Vora LK, Gholap AD, Jetha K, Thakur RRS, Solanki HK, Chavda VP. Artificial Intelligence in Pharmaceutical Technology and Drug Delivery Design. Pharmaceutics 2023; 15(7): 1916-6. [http://dx.doi.org/10.3390/pharmaceutics15071916] [PMID: 37514102]

[18] Vora LK, Gholap AD, Jetha K, Thakur RRS, Solanki HK, Chavda VP. Artificial Intelligence in Pharmaceutical Technology and Drug Delivery Design. Pharmaceutics 2023; 15(7): 1916-6. [http://dx.doi.org/10.3390/pharmaceutics15071916] [PMID: 37514102]

[19] Wasilewski T, Kamysz W, Gębicki J. AI-Assisted Detection of Biomarkers by Sensors and Biosensors for Early Diagnosis and Monitoring. Biosensors (Basel) 2024; 14(7): 356. [http://dx.doi.org/10.3390/bios14070356] [PMID: 39056632]

[20] Huanbutta K, Burapapadh K, Kraisit P, *et al.* Artificial intelligence-driven pharmaceutical industry: A paradigm shift in drug discovery, formulation development, manufacturing, quality control, and post-market surveillance. Eur J Pharm Sci 2024; 203: 106938-8. [http://dx.doi.org/10.1016/j.ejps.2024.106938] [PMID: 39419129]

[21] Vaquero JJ, Kinahan P. Positron Emission Tomography: Current Challenges and Opportunities for Technological Advances in Clinical and Preclinical Imaging Systems. Annu Rev Biomed Eng 2015; 17(1): 385-414. [http://dx.doi.org/10.1146/annurev-bioeng-071114-040723] [PMID: 26643024]

[22] Krishani M, Shin WY, Suhaimi H, Sambudi NS. Development of Scaffolds from Bio-Based Natural Materials for Tissue Regeneration Applications: A Review. Gels 2023; 9(2): 100. [http://dx.doi.org/10.3390/gels9020100] [PMID: 36826270]

[23] Bikash Medhi . Artificial Intelligence: A Catalyst for Breakthroughs in Nanotechnology and Pharmaceutical Research. International Journal of Pharmaceutical Sciences and Nanotechnology(IJPSN) 2024; 17(4): 7439-45.
[http://dx.doi.org/10.37285/ijpsn.2024.17.4.1]

[24] Omidian H, Babanejad N, Cubeddu LX. Nanosystems in Cardiovascular Medicine: Advancements, Applications, and Future Perspectives. Pharmaceutics 2023; 15(7): 1935-5.
[http://dx.doi.org/10.3390/pharmaceutics15071935] [PMID: 37514121]

[25] Farhoudi L, Fobian SF, Oei AL, Amin M, Jaafari MR, ten Hagen TLM. Applications of biomimetic nanoparticles in breast cancer as a blueprint for improved next-generation cervical cancer therapy. Nano Today 2023; 53: 102032-2.
[http://dx.doi.org/10.1016/j.nantod.2023.102032]

[26] Schmidt TJN, Berarducci B, Konstantinidou S, Raffa V. CRISPR/Cas9 in the era of nanomedicine and synthetic biology. Drug Discov Today 2023; 28(1): 103375.
[http://dx.doi.org/10.1016/j.drudis.2022.103375] [PMID: 36174966]

[27] Mahadik SS, Pawar PM, Muthalagu R, *et al.* Digital Privacy in Healthcare: State-of-the-Art and Future Vision. IEEE Access 2024; 12: 84273-91.
[http://dx.doi.org/10.1109/ACCESS.2024.3410035]

[28] Seh AH, Zarour M, Alenezi M, *et al.* Healthcare data breaches: Insights and implications. Healthcare (Basel) 2020; 8(2): 133.
[http://dx.doi.org/10.3390/healthcare8020133] [PMID: 32414183]

SUBJECT INDEX

E

F

G

H

I

K

L

M

N

O

P

Q

R

S

T

U

V

W

Z

www.ingramcontent.com/pod-product-compliance
Lightning Source LLC
LaVergne TN
LVHW070951210926
848482LV00002B/171

9798898813147